The Cardiovascular System at a Glance

The Cardiovascular System at a Glance

Philip I. Aaronson

Reader in Pharmacology
Division of Asthma, Allergy and Lung Biology
King's College, London

Jeremy P. T. Ward

Head of Department of Physiology
& Professor of Respiratory Cell Physiology
King's College, London

Third edition

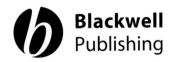
Blackwell
Publishing

First published 1999
Second edition 2004
Third edition 2007

1   2007

Library of Congress Cataloging-in-Publication Data

Aaronson, Philip Irving, 1953–
    The cardiovascular system at a glance / Philip I. Aaronson, Jeremy P. T. Ward. — 3rd ed.
        p.   ;   cm.
    Includes bibliographical references and index.
    ISBN 978-1-4051-5044-6 (alk. paper)
    1. Cardiovascular system—Physiology.   2. Cardiovascular system—Pathophysiology.
I. Ward, Jeremy P. T.   II. Title.
    [DNLM: 1. Cardiovascular System—anatomy & histology.   2. Cardiovascular Diseases.
3. Cardiovascular Physiology. WG 100 A113c 2007

    QP101.c293 2007
    616.1—dc22

                                                            2007017560

A catalogue record for this title is available from the British Library

Set in 9/11.5pt Times by Graphicraft Limited, Hong Kong
Printed and bound in Singapore by Fabulous Printers Pte Ltd

Commissioning Editor: Martin Sugden/Vicki Donald
Editorial Assistant: Robin Harries
Development Editor: Hayley Salter
Production Controller: Debbie Wyer

For further information on Blackwell Publishing, visit our website:
http://www.blackwellpublishing.com

The publisher's policy is to use permanent paper from mills that operate a sustainable forestry policy,
and which has been manufactured from pulp processed using acid-free and elementary chlorine-free
practices. Furthermore, the publisher ensures that the text paper and cover board used have met acceptable
environmental accreditation standards.

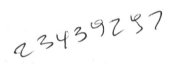

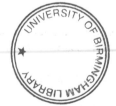

Contents

Preface 6
Acknowledgements 6
Sources of illustrations 7
List of abbreviations 8

Introduction
1   Overview of the cardiovascular system 10

Anatomy and histology
2   Gross anatomy and histology of the heart 12
3   Vascular anatomy 14
4   Vascular histology and smooth muscle cell ultrastructure 16

Blood and body fluids
5   Constituents of blood 18
6   Erythropoiesis, haemoglobin and anaemia 20
7   Haemostasis and thrombosis 22
8   Blood groups and transfusions 24

Cellular physiology
9   Membrane potential, ion channels and pumps 26
10   Electrophysiology of cardiac muscle and the origin of
     the heart beat 28
11   Excitation–contraction coupling in cardiac muscle cells 30
12   Electrical conduction system in the heart 32
13   Vascular smooth muscle excitation–contraction coupling 34

Form and function
14   Cardiac cycle 36
15   Control of cardiac output and Starling's law of the heart 38
16   Haemodynamics 40
17   Blood pressure and flow in the arteries and arterioles 42
18   The microcirculation and lymphatic system 44
19   Fluid filtration in the microcirculation 46
20   The venous system 48
21   Local control of blood flow 50
22   Regulation of the vasculature by the endothelium 52
23   The coronary, skeletal muscle, cutaneous and cerebral
     circulations 54
24   The pulmonary and fetal circulations 56

Integration and regulation
25   Cardiovascular reflexes 58
26   Autonomic control of the cardiovascular system 60

27   The control of blood volume 62
28   Cardiovascular effects of exercise 64
29   Shock and haemorrhage 66

History, examination and investigations
30   History and examination of the cardiovascular system 68
31   Cardiovascular investigations 70
32   The electrocardiogram 72

Pathology and therapeutics
33   Risk factors for cardiovascular disease 74
34   Beta-blockers, angiotensin-converting
     enzyme inhibitors, angiotensin receptor
     blockers, and Ca^{2+}-channel blockers 76
35   Hyperlipidaemias 78
36   Atherosclerosis 80
37   Treatment of hypertension 82
38   Mechanisms of primary hypertension 84
39   Stable and variant angina 86
40   Pharmacological management of stable and
     variant angina 88
41   Unstable angina and non-ST segment elevation
     myocardial infarction 90
42   Revascularization 92
43   Pathophysiology of acute myocardial infarction 94
44   Clinical aspects of acute myocardial infarction
     (STEMI) 96
45   Thrombosis, anticoagulants and thrombolytics 98
46   Chronic heart failure 100
47   Treatment of chronic heart failure 102
48   Mechanisms of arrhythmia 104
49   Supraventricular tachyarrhythmias 106
50   Ventricular tachyarrhythmias and non-pharmacological
     treatment of arrhythmias 108
51   Pharmacological treatment of arrhythmias 110
52   Diseases of the aortic valve 112
53   Diseases of the mitral valve 114
54   Congenital heart disease 116

Self-assessment case studies
Case studies and questions 118
Answers 123

Index 129

Preface

This book aims to provide a comprehensive yet concise description of the cardiovascular system which integrates normal structure, function and regulation with pathophysiology, pharmacology and therapeutics. It is directed mainly at preclinical medical students taking systems-based courses. It should, however, serve equally well as an introduction to this subject suitable for other biomedical students and scientists, as well as a focused 'refresher course' for clinicians, nurses and other healthcare professionals. Each chapter is based around one or more diagrams, and is designed to contain an amount of information roughly equivalent to that presented in an hour-long lecture.

For this third edition we have substantially updated and revised many of the topics. However, the most striking change that our previous readers will notice is that all figures are now presented in full colour, a change that we hope will make some of our complex diagrams more user-friendly. In addition, we have also added new chapters on examination of the cardiovascular system, key cardiovascular drugs and arrhythmias. Sample ECGs demonstrating abnormalities associated with many common arrhythmias have also been included, and the number of case studies has been expanded from four to eight.

Recommended Reading

Braunwald, 7th edition, 2004
Braunwald's Heart Disease: A Textbook of Cardiovascular Medicine
Saunders

Levick 4th RevEd edition, 2003
An Introduction to Cardiovascular Physiology
JR Levick
Hodder Arnold

Lilly, 4th edition, 2006
Braunwald's Heart Disease Review and Assessment
Leonard Lilly
Saunders

Acknowledgements

The case study on pulmonary embolism was written by Dr Richard Leach, and that on hypertension by Michelle Connolly. We are enormously grateful to Richard, author of *Critical Care Medicine at a Glance* and director of the High-Dependency Unit at St Thomas's Hospital in London, and to Michelle, who somehow manages to combine studying for her medical degree with acting as editor and co-editor, respectively, of the UK magazines *Trauma* and *Junior Dr*, for finding the time to contribute. We also greatly appreciate the assistance of Dr Albert Ferro, Senior Lecturer and Honorary Consultant in Clinical Pharmacology at King's College London, who read and revised several of the case studies.

We would also like to thank our editors Martin Sugden and Hayley Salter, who continued the tradition of earlier editors by gracefully ignoring our missed deadlines and lack of enthusiasm for sorting those last few boring but crucial details associated with publication. Finally, we would like to express our appreciation to our readers, and especially our students at King's College London, whose comments and criticisms over the years have encouraged and enabled us to carry on trying to improve this book.

Sources of illustrations

Fig. 2(d) Reproduced from *J Cell Biol*, 1969; **42**: 1–45 by copyright permission of The Rockefeller University Press.

Fig. 3 (top) Reproduced with permission from Gosling JA *et al. Human Anatomy—color atlas and text*, 3rd edn. Mosby Wolfe, London, 1996.

Fig. 4(a) Reproduced with permission from Berne RM. *Handbook of Physiology*. Oxford University Press, New York, 1980.

Fig. 16 Reproduced with permission from Berne RM & Levy MN. *Cardiovascular Physiology*, 7th edn. Mosby, St Louis, 1997.

Fig. 17 (inset). Reproduced with permission from Nichols WW, O'Rourke MF. *McDonald's Blood Flow in Arteries: Theoretical, Experimental and Clinical Principles*, 5th edn, Hodder Arnold, London, 2005.

Fig. 23(b) Reproduced with permission from Levick JR. *An Introduction to Cardiovascular Physiology*, 4th edn. Hodder Arnold, London, 2003.

Fig. 28(a) Reproduced with permission from Berne RM, Levy MN. *Cardiovascular Physiology*, 8th edn. Mosby, St Louis, 2001.

Table 28.1 Reproduced with permission from Mitchell JH, Blomqvist G. Maximal oxygen uptake. *N Engl J Med* 1971; **284**: 1018. © Massachusetts Medical Society. All rights reserved.

Figs 31(b) and (d) Reproduced with permission from Patel, Lecture Notes: Radiology 2e. Blackwell Publishing, 2005.

Fig. 39 Reproduced in part with permission from Opie LH, ed. *Drugs for the Heart*, 3rd edn. WB Saunders, Philadelphia, 1991.

Fig. 41 Reproduced in part with permission from Opie LH, *Drugs for the Heart*, 5th edn. WB Saunders, Philadelphia, 2001.

Fig. 42 Reproduced with permission from Lilly LS. *Pathophysiology of Heart Disease*, 3rd edn. Lippincott Williams & Wilkins, Philadelphia, 2003.

List of abbreviations

5-HT	5-hydroxytryptamine (serotonin)		DM2	type 2 diabetes mellitus
ABP	arterial blood pressure		DVT	deep venous/vein thrombosis
ACE	angiotensin-converting enzyme		EAD	early afterdepolarization
ACEI	angiotensin-converting enzyme inhibitor/s		ECF	extracellular fluid
ACS	acute coronary syndromes		ECG	electrocardiogram/electrocardiograph (EKG)
ADH	antidiuretic hormone		ECM	extracellular matrix
ADMA	asymmetrical dimethyl arginine		EDHF	endothelium-derived hyperpolarizing factor
ADP	adenosine diphosphate		EDP	end-diastolic pressure
AF	atrial fibrillation		EDRF	endothelium-derived relaxing factor
ANP	atrial natriuretic peptide		EDV	end-diastolic volume
ANS	autonomic nervous system		eNOS	endothelial NOS
AP	action potential		ERP	effective refractory period
APC	active protein C		ESR	erythrocyte sedimentation rate
APD	action potential duration		FDP	fibrin degradation product
APSAC	anistreplase		HDL	high-density lipoprotein
aPTT	activated partial thromboplastin time		HPV	hypoxic pulmonary vasoconstriction
AR	aortic regurgitation		HR	heart rate
ARB	angiotensin II receptor blocker		IDL	intermediate-density lipoprotein
ARDS	acute respiratory distress syndrome		IML	intermediolateral
AS	aortic stenosis		iNOS	inducible NOS
ASD	atrial septal defect		INR	international normalized ratio
AV	atrioventricular		ISH	isolated systolic hypertension
AVA	arteriovenous anastomosis		JVP	jugular venous pressure
AVM	arteriovenous malformation		LA	left atrium
AVN	atrioventricular node		LAD	left anterior descending
AVNRT	atrioventricular nodal re-entrant tachycardia		LDL	low-density lipoprotein
AVRT	atrioventricular re-entrant tachycardia		LITA	left internal thoracic artery
BBB	blood–brain barrier		LMWH	low molecular weight heparin
BMI	body mass index		L-NAME	L-nitro arginine methyl ester
BP	blood pressure		LPL	lipoprotein lipase
CABG	coronary artery bypass grafting		LQT	long QT
CAD	coronary artery disease		LV	left ventricle/left ventricular
CaM	calmodulin		LVH	left ventricular hypertrophy
CCB	calcium-channel blocker		MABP	mean arterial blood pressure
CHD	congenital heart disease		MAP	mean arterial pressure
CHD	coronary heart disease		MCH	mean cell haemoglobin
CHF	chronic heart failure		MCHC	mean cell haemoglobin concentration
CICR	calcium-induced calcium release		MCV	mean cell volume
CK-MB	creatine kinase MB		MI	myocardial infarction
CNS	central nervous system		MLCK	myosin light-chain kinase
CO	cardiac output		MOF	multiorgan failure
COPD	chronic obstructive pulmonary disease		MR	mitral regurgitation
COX	cyclooxygenase		MRI	magnetic resonance imaging
CRP	C-reactive protein		MS	mitral stenosis
CSF	cerebrospinal fluid		MW	molecular weight
CT	computed tomography		NCX	Na/Ca exchanger
CVD	cardiovascular disease		NO	nitric oxide
CVP	central venous pressure		NOS	nitric oxide synthase
CXR	chest X-ray		NSAIDs	non-steroidal anti-inflammatory drugs
DAD	delayed afterdepolarization		NSCC	non-selective cation channel
DAG	diacylglycerol		NSTEMI	non-ST segment elevation myocardial infarction
DBP	diastolic blood pressure		NTS	nucleus tractus solitarius
DC	direct current		OS	opening snap
DHP	dihydropyridine		PA	postero-anterior
DIC	disseminated intravascular coagulation		PAI-1	plasminogen activator inhibitor-1

PCI	percutaneous coronary intervention	**SK**	streptokinase
PCV	packed cell volume	**SOC**	store-operated Ca^{2+} channel
PDA	patent ductus arteriosus	**SPECT**	single photon emission computed tomography
PGI₂	prostacyclin	**SR**	sarcoplasmic reticulum
PI3K	phosphatidylinositol 3-kinase	**STEMI**	ST elevation myocardial infarction
PKC	protein kinase C	**SV**	stroke volume
PKG	cyclic GMP-dependent protein kinase	**SVR**	systemic vascular resistance
PLD	phospholipid	**SVT**	supraventricular tachycardia
PMCA	plasma membrane Ca^{2+}-ATPase	**TF**	tissue factor thromboplastin
PND	paroxysmal nocturnal dyspnoea	**TFPI**	tissue factor pathway inhibitor
PRU	peripheral resistance unit	**TOE**	transoesophageal echocardiography
PT	prothrombin time	**tPA**	tissue plasminogen activator
PTCA	percutaneous transcoronary angioplasty	**TPR**	total peripheral resistance
PVC	premature ventricular contraction	**TRP**	transient receptor potential
PVR	pulmonary vascular resistance	**TXA₂**	thromboxane A_2
RAA	renin–angiotensin–aldosterone	**UA**	unstable angina
RAP	right atrial pressure	**UH**	unfractionated heparin
RCC	red cell count	**uPA**	urokinase
RGC	receptor-gated channel	**VF**	ventricular fibrillation
RMP	resting membrane potential	**VGC**	voltage-gated channel
RVLM	rostral ventrolateral medulla	**VLDL**	very low density lipoprotein
PVR	pulmonary vascular resistance	**VSD**	ventricular septal defect
RAP	right atrial pressure	**VSM**	vascular smooth muscle
RVOT	right ventricular outflow tract tachycardia	**VT**	ventricular tachycardia
RyR	ryanodine receptor	**VTE**	venous thromboembolism
SAN	sinoatrial node	**V/Q**	ventilation/perfusion
SERCA	smooth endoplasmic reticulum Ca^{2+}-ATPase	**vWF**	von Willebrand factor
SHO	senior house officer	**WPW**	Wolff–Parkinson–White

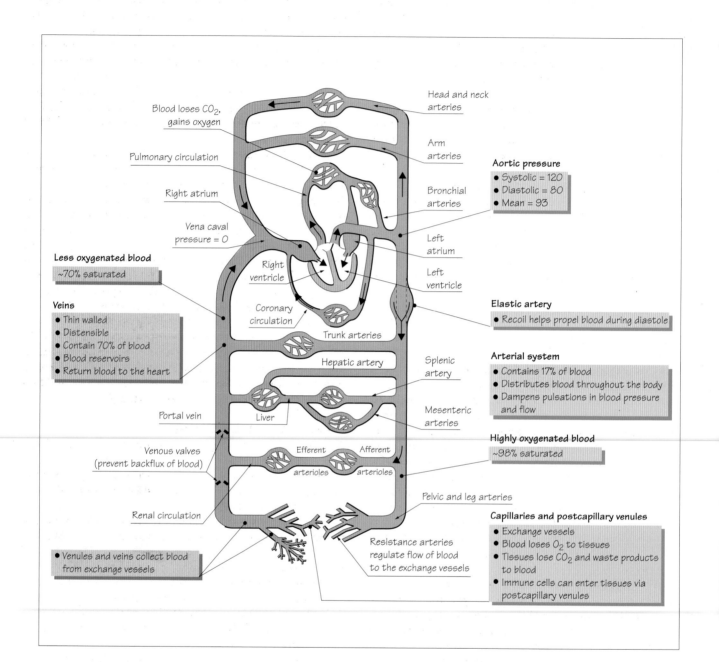

Blood loses CO_2, gains oxygen

Pulmonary circulation

Right atrium

Vena caval pressure = 0

Head and neck arteries

Arm arteries

Bronchial arteries

Left atrium

Left ventricle

Aortic pressure
- Systolic = 120
- Diastolic = 80
- Mean = 93

Less oxygenated blood

~70% saturated

Right ventricle

Coronary circulation

Trunk arteries

Veins
- Thin walled
- Distensible
- Contain 70% of blood
- Blood reservoirs
- Return blood to the heart

Hepatic artery

Splenic artery

Portal vein

Liver

Mesenteric arteries

Venous valves (prevent backflux of blood)

Efferent arterioles

Afferent arterioles

Renal circulation

Pelvic and leg arteries

Venules and veins collect blood from exchange vessels

Resistance arteries regulate flow of blood to the exchange vessels

Elastic artery
- Recoil helps propel blood during diastole

Arterial system
- Contains 17% of blood
- Distributes blood throughout the body
- Dampens pulsations in blood pressure and flow

Highly oxygenated blood

~98% saturated

Capillaries and postcapillary venules
- Exchange vessels
- Blood loses O_2 to tissues
- Tissues lose CO_2 and waste products to blood
- Immune cells can enter tissues via postcapillary venules

The cardiovascular system is composed of the heart, blood vessels and blood. In simple terms, its main functions are:

1 distribution of O_2 and nutrients (e.g. glucose, amino acids) to all body tissues

2 transportation of CO_2 and metabolic waste products (e.g. urea) from the tissues to the lungs and excretory organs

3 distribution of water, electrolytes and hormones throughout the body

4 contributing to the infrastructure of the immune system

5 thermoregulation.

Blood is composed of **plasma**, an aqueous solution containing electrolytes, proteins and other molecules, in which **cells** are suspended. The cells comprise 40–45% of blood volume and are mainly **erythrocytes**, but also **white blood cells** and **platelets**. Blood volume is about 5.5 L in an 'average' 70-kg man.

The figure illustrates the 'plumbing' of the cardiovascular system.

Blood is driven through the cardiovascular system by the **heart**, a muscular pump divided into left and right sides. Each side contains two chambers, an **atrium** and a **ventricle**, composed mainly of cardiac muscle cells. The thin-walled atria serve to fill or 'prime' the thick-walled ventricles, which when full constrict forcefully, creating a pressure head that drives the blood out into the body. Blood enters and leaves each chamber of the heart through separate one-way valves, which open and close reciprocally (i.e. one closes before the other opens) to ensure that flow is unidirectional.

Consider the flow of blood, starting with its exit from the left ventricle.

When the ventricles contract, the left ventricular internal pressure rises from 0 to 120 mmHg (atmospheric pressure = 0). As the pressure rises, the aortic valve opens and blood is expelled into the **aorta**, the first and largest artery of the **systemic circulation**. This period of ventricular contraction is termed **systole**. The maximal pressure during systole is called the **systolic pressure**, and it serves both to drive blood through the aorta and to distend the aorta, which is quite elastic. The aortic valve then closes, and the left ventricle relaxes so that it can be refilled with blood from the left atrium via the mitral valve. The period of relaxation is called **diastole**. During diastole aortic blood flow and pressure diminish but do not fall to zero, because *elastic recoil* of the aorta continues to exert a **diastolic pressure** on the blood, which gradually falls to a minimum level of about 80 mmHg. The difference between systolic and diastolic pressures is termed the **pulse pressure**. **Mean arterial blood pressure** (MABP) is pressure averaged over the entire cardiac cycle. Because the heart spends approximately 60% of the cardiac cycle in diastole, the MABP is approximately equal to the diastolic pressure + one-third of the pulse pressure, rather than to the arithmetic average of the systolic and diastolic pressures.

The blood flows from the aorta into the **major arteries**, each of which supplies blood to an organ or body region. These arteries divide and subdivide into smaller **muscular arteries**, which eventually give rise to the **arterioles** – arteries with diameters of < 100 μm. Blood enters the arterioles at a mean pressure of about 60–70 mmHg.

The walls of the arteries and arterioles have circumferentially arranged layers of **smooth muscle cells**. The lumen of the entire vascular system is lined by a monolayer of **endothelial cells**. These cells secrete vasoactive substances and serve as a barrier, restricting and controlling the movement of fluid, molecules and cells into and out of the vasculature.

The arterioles lead to the smallest vessels, the **capillaries**, which form a dense network within all body tissues. The capillary wall is a layer of overlapping endothelial cells, with no smooth muscle cells. The pressure in the capillaries ranges from about 25 mmHg on the arterial side to 15 mmHg at the venous end. The capillaries converge into small **venules**, which also have thin walls of mainly endothelial cells. The venules merge into larger venules, with an increasing content of smooth muscle cells as they widen. These then converge to become **veins**, which progressively join to give rise to the **superior** and **inferior venae cavae**, through which blood returns to the right side of the heart. Veins have a larger diameter than arteries, and thus offer relatively little resistance to flow. The small pressure gradient between venules (15 mmHg) and the venae cavae (0 mmHg) is therefore sufficient to drive blood back to the heart.

Blood from the venae cavae enters the **right atrium**, and then the **right ventricle** through the **tricuspid valve**. Contraction of the right ventricle, simultaneous with that of the left ventricle, forces blood through the pulmonary valve into the pulmonary artery, which progressively subdivides to form the arteries, arterioles and capillaries of the **pulmonary circulation**. The pulmonary circulation is shorter and has a much lower pressure than the systemic circulation, with systolic and diastolic pressures of about 25 and 10 mmHg, respectively. The pulmonary capillary network within the lungs surrounds the alveoli of the lungs, allowing exchange of CO_2 for O_2. Oxygenated blood enters pulmonary venules and veins, and then the **left atrium**, which pumps it into the left ventricle for the next systemic cycle.

The output of the right ventricle is slightly lower than that of the left ventricle. This is because 1–2% of the systemic blood flow never reaches the right atrium, but is shunted to the left side of the heart via the bronchial circulation (see figure) and a small fraction of coronary blood flow drains into the thebesian veins (see Chapter 23).

Blood vessel functions

Each vessel type has important functions in addition to being a conduit for blood.

The branching system of elastic and muscular arteries progressively reduces the pulsations in blood pressure and flow imposed by the intermittent ventricular contractions.

The smallest arteries and arterioles have a crucial role in regulating the amount of blood flowing to the tissues by dilating or constricting. This function is regulated by the sympathetic nervous system, and factors generated locally in tissues. These vessels are referred to as **resistance arteries**, because their constriction resists the flow of blood.

Capillaries and small venules are the **exchange vessels**. Through their walls, gases, fluids and molecules are transferred between blood and tissues. White blood cells can also pass through the venule walls to fight infection in the tissues.

Venules can constrict to offer resistance to the blood flow, and the ratio of arteriolar and venular resistance exerts an important influence on the movement of fluid between capillaries and tissues, thereby affecting blood volume.

The veins are thin walled and very *distensible*, and therefore contain about 70% of all blood in the cardiovascular system. The arteries contain just 17% of total blood volume. Veins and venules thus serve as volume reservoirs, which can shift blood from the peripheral circulation into the heart and arteries by constricting. In doing so, they can help to increase the **cardiac output** (volume of blood pumped by the heart per unit time), and they are also able to maintain the blood pressure and tissue perfusion in essential organs if **haemorrhage** (blood loss) occurs.

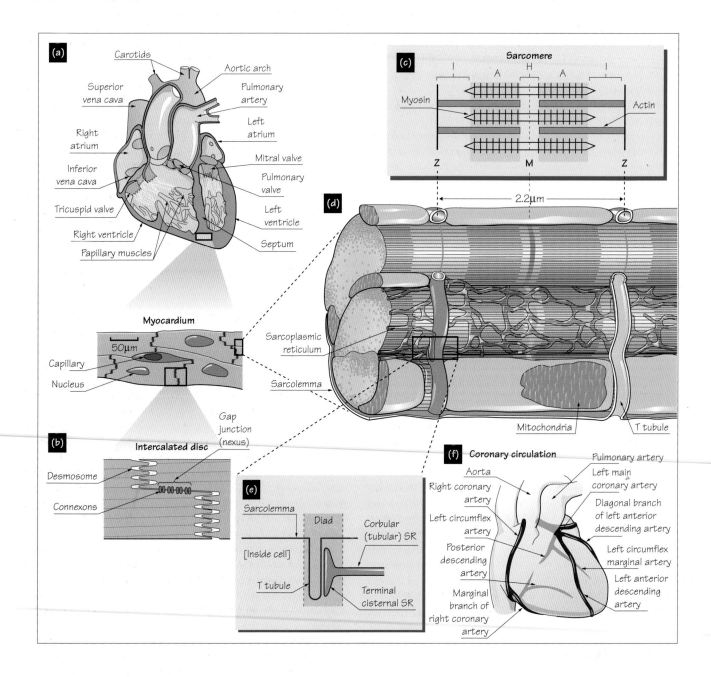

(a)
Carotids
Aortic arch
Superior vena cava
Pulmonary artery
Left atrium
Right atrium
Mitral valve
Inferior vena cava
Pulmonary valve
Tricuspid valve
Left ventricle
Right ventricle
Septum
Papillary muscles

(c) Sarcomere
Myosin
Actin
I A H A I
Z M Z
2.2μm

(d)
Sarcoplasmic reticulum
Sarcolemma
Mitochondria
T tubule

Myocardium
50μm
Capillary
Nucleus

(b) Intercalated disc
Gap junction (nexus)
Desmosome
Connexons

(e)
Sarcolemma
Diad
Corbular (tubular) SR
[Inside cell]
T tubule
Terminal cisternal SR

(f) Coronary circulation
Aorta
Pulmonary artery
Right coronary artery
Left main coronary artery
Left circumflex artery
Diagonal branch of left anterior descending artery
Posterior descending artery
Left circumflex marginal artery
Marginal branch of right coronary artery
Left anterior descending artery

Gross anatomy of the heart (Figure 2a)

The heart consists of four chambers. Blood flows into the right atrium via the superior and inferior venae cavae. The left and right atria connect to the ventricles via the mitral (two cusps) and tricuspid (three cusps) atrioventricular (AV) valves, respectively. The AV valves are passive and close when the ventricular pressure exceeds that in the atrium. They are prevented from being everted into the atria during systole by fine cords (**chordae tendineae**) attached between the free margins of the cusps and the papillary muscles, which contract during systole. The outflow from the right ventricle passes through the pulmonary semilunar valve to the pulmonary artery, and that from the left ventricle enters the aorta via the aortic semilunar valve. These valves close passively at the end of systole, when ventricular pressure falls below that of the arteries. Both semilunar valves have three cusps.

The cusps or leaflets of the cardiac valves are formed of fibrous connective tissue, covered in a thin layer of cells similar to and contiguous with the **endocardium** (AV valves and ventricular surface of semilunar valves) and **endothelium** (vascular side of semilunar valves). When closed, the cusps form a tight seal (come to apposition) at the **commissures** (line at which the edges of the leaflets meet).

The atria and ventricles are separated by a band of fibrous connective tissue called the **annulus fibrosus**, which provides a skeleton for attachment of the muscle and insertion of the valves. It also prevents electrical conduction between the atria and ventricles except at the **atrioventricular node** (AVN). This is situated near the interatrial septum and the mouth of the coronary sinus and is an important element of the cardiac electrical conduction system (see Chapter 12).

The ventricles fill during diastole; at the initiation of the heart beat the atria contract and complete ventricular filling. As the ventricles contract the pressure rises sharply, closing the AV valves. When ventricular pressure exceeds the pulmonary artery or aortic pressure, the semilunar valves open and ejection occurs (see Chapter 14). As systole ends and ventricular pressure falls, the semilunar valves are closed by backflow of blood from the arteries.

The force of contraction is generated by the muscle of the heart, the **myocardium**. The atrial walls are thin. The greater pressure generated by the left ventricle compared with the right is reflected by its greater wall thickness. The inside of the heart is covered in a thin layer of cells called the **endocardium**, which is similar to the endothelium of blood vessels. The outer surface of the myocardium is covered by the **epicardium**, a layer of mesothelial cells. The whole heart is enclosed in the **pericardium**, a thin fibrous sheath or sac, which prevents excessive enlargement. The **pericardial space** contains interstitial fluid as a lubricant.

Structure of the myocardium

The myocardium consists of **cardiac myocytes** (*muscle cells*) that show a striated subcellular structure, although they are less organized than skeletal muscle. The cells are relatively small (100×20 µm) and branched, with a single nucleus, and are rich in mitochondria. They are connected together as a network by **intercalated discs** (Figure 2b), where the cell membranes are closely opposed. The intercalated discs provide both a structural attachment by 'glueing' the cells together at **desmosomes**, and an electrical connection through **gap junctions** formed of pores made up of proteins called **connexons**. As a result, the myocardium acts as a **functional syncytium**, in other words as a single functional unit, even though the individual cells are still separate. The gap junctions play a vital part in conduction of the electrical impulse through the myocardium (see Chapter 12).

The myocytes contain **actin** and **myosin** filaments which form the contractile apparatus, and exhibit the classical M and Z lines and A, H and I bands (Figure 2c). The intercalated discs always coincide with a Z line, as it is here that the actin filaments are anchored to the cytoskeleton. At the Z lines the **sarcolemma** (cell membrane) forms tubular invaginations into the cells known as the **transverse** (T) **tubular system**. The **sarcoplasmic reticulum** (SR) is less extensive than in skeletal muscle, and runs generally in parallel with the length of the cell (Figure 2d). Close to the T tubules the SR forms **terminal cisternae** that with the T tubule make up **diads** (Figure 2e), an important component of excitation–contraction coupling (see Chapter 11). The typical *triad* seen in skeletal muscle is less often present. The T tubules and SR never physically join, but are separated by a narrow gap. The myocardium has an extensive system of capillaries.

Coronary circulation (Figure 2f)

The heart has a rich blood supply, derived from the **left and right coronary arteries**. These arise separately from the aortic sinus at the base of the aorta, behind the cusps of the aortic valve. They are not blocked by the cusps during systole because of eddy currents, and remain patent throughout the cardiac cycle. The **right coronary artery** runs forward between the pulmonary trunk and right atrium, to the AV sulcus. As it descends to the lower margin of the heart, it divides to **posterior descending** and **right marginal** branches. The **left coronary artery** runs behind the pulmonary trunk and forward between it and the left atrium. It divides into the **circumflex**, **left marginal** and **anterior descending** branches. There are anastomoses between the left and right marginal branches, and the anterior and posterior descending arteries, although these are not sufficient to maintain perfusion if one side of the coronary circulation is occluded.

Most of the blood returns to the right atrium via the **coronary sinus**, and **anterior cardiac veins**. The **large** and **small** coronary veins run parallel to the left and right coronary arteries, respectively, and empty into the sinus. Numerous other small vessels empty into the cardiac chambers directly, including **thebesian veins** and **arteriosinusoidal vessels**.

The coronary circulation is capable of developing a good collateral system in ischaemic heart disease, when a branch or branches are occluded by, for example, atheromatous plaques. Most of the left ventricle is supplied by the left coronary artery, and occlusion can therefore be very dangerous. The AVN and **sinus node** are supplied by the right coronary artery in the majority of people; disease in this artery can cause a slow heart rate and AV block (see Chapters 10, 12).

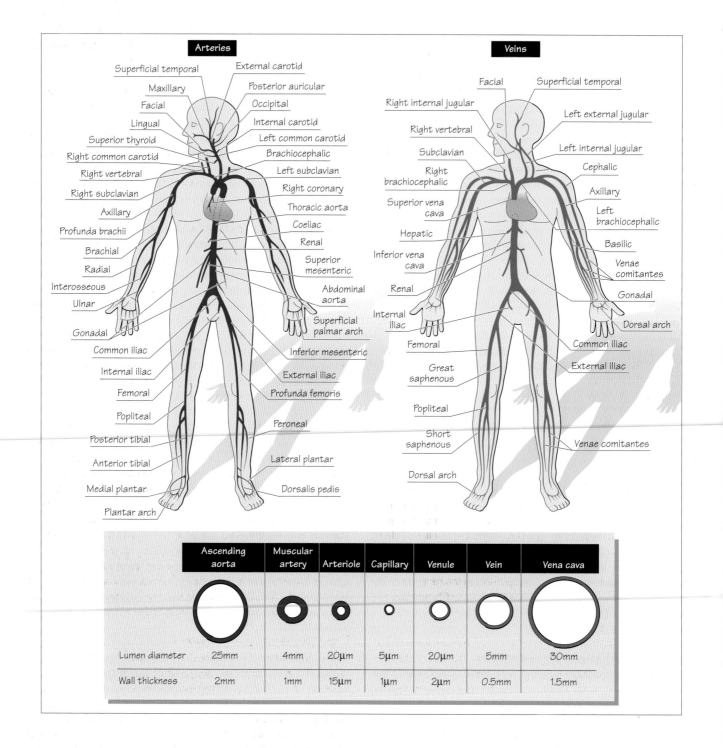

Arteries

Superficial temporal
Maxillary
Facial
Lingual
Superior thyroid
Right common carotid
Right vertebral
Right subclavian
Axillary
Profunda brachii
Brachial
Radial
Interosseous
Ulnar
Gonadal
Common iliac
Internal iliac
Femoral
Popliteal
Posterior tibial
Anterior tibial
Medial plantar
Plantar arch

External carotid
Posterior auricular
Occipital
Internal carotid
Left common carotid
Brachiocephalic
Left subclavian
Right coronary
Thoracic aorta
Coeliac
Renal
Superior mesenteric
Abdominal aorta
Superficial palmar arch
Inferior mesenteric
External iliac
Profunda femoris
Peroneal
Lateral plantar
Dorsalis pedis

Veins

Facial
Superficial temporal
Right internal jugular
Left external jugular
Right vertebral
Left internal jugular
Subclavian
Cephalic
Right brachiocephalic
Axillary
Superior vena cava
Left brachiocephalic
Hepatic
Basilic
Inferior vena cava
Venae comitantes
Renal
Gonadal
Internal iliac
Dorsal arch
Femoral
Common iliac
Great saphenous
External iliac
Popliteal
Short saphenous
Venae comitantes
Dorsal arch

	Ascending aorta	Muscular artery	Arteriole	Capillary	Venule	Vein	Vena cava
Lumen diameter	25mm	4mm	20μm	5μm	20μm	5mm	30mm
Wall thickness	2mm	1mm	15μm	1μm	2μm	0.5mm	1.5mm

The blood vessels of the cardiovascular system are for convenience of description classified into **arteries** (elastic and muscular), **resistance vessels** (small arteries and arterioles), **capillaries, venules** and **veins**. Typical dimensions for the different types of vessel are illustrated.

The systemic circulation

Arteries

The **systemic (or greater) circulation** begins with the pumping of blood by the left ventricle into the largest artery, the **aorta**. This ascends from the top of the heart, bends downward at the **aortic arch** and descends just anterior to the spinal column. The aorta bifurcates into the left and right **iliac arteries**, which supply the pelvis and legs. The major arteries supplying the head, the arms and the heart arise from the aortic arch, and the main arteries supplying the visceral organs branch from the descending aorta. All of the major organs except the liver (see below) are therefore supplied with blood by arteries which arise from the aorta. The fundamentally *parallel* organization of the systemic vasculature has a number of advantages over the alternative *series* arrangement, in which blood would flow sequentially through one organ after another. The parallel arrangement of the vascular system ensures that the supply of blood to each organ is relatively independent, is driven by a large pressure head, and also that each organ receives highly oxygenated blood.

The aorta and its major branches (**brachiocephalic, common carotid, subclavian** and **common iliac** arteries) are termed **elastic arteries**. In addition to conducting blood away from the heart, these arteries distend during systole and recoil during diastole, damping the pulse wave and evening out the discontinuous flow of blood created by the heart's intermittent pumping action.

Elastic arteries branch to give rise to **muscular arteries** with relatively thicker walls; this prevents their collapse when joints bend. The muscular arteries give rise to **resistance vessels**, so named because they present the greatest part of the resistance of the vasculature to the flow of blood. These are sometimes subclassified into *small arteries*, which have multiple layers of smooth muscle cells in their walls, and *arterioles*, which have one or two layers of smooth muscle cells. Resistance vessels have the highest wall to lumen ratio in the vasculature. The degree of constriction or **tone** of these vessels regulates the amount of blood flowing to each small area of tissue. All but the smallest resistance vessels tend to be heavily innervated (especially in the *splanchnic, renal* and *cutaneous* vasculatures) by the **sympathetic nervous system**, the activity of which usually causes them to constrict (see Chapter 26).

Arterial anastomoses

In addition to branching to give rise to smaller vessels, arteries and arterioles may also merge to form **anastomoses**. These are found in many circulations (e.g. the brain, mesentery, uterus, around joints) and provide an alternative supply of blood if one artery is blocked. If this occurs, the anastamosing artery gradually enlarges, providing a **collateral circulation**.

The smallest arterioles, capillaries and postcapillary venules comprise the **microcirculation**, the structure and function of which is described in Chapters 18 and 19.

Veins

The venous system can be divided into the **venules**, which contain one or two layers of smooth muscle cells, and the **veins**. The veins of the limbs, particularly the legs, contain paired semilunar **valves** which ensure that the blood cannot move backwards. These are orientated so that they are pressed against the venous wall when the blood is flowing forward, but are forced out to occlude the lumen when the blood flow reverses.

The veins from the head, neck and arms come together to form the **superior vena cava**, and those from the lower part of the body merge into the **inferior vena cava**. These deliver blood to the right atrium, which pumps it into the right ventricle.

The one or two veins draining a body region typically run next to the artery supplying that region. This promotes heat conservation, because at low temperatures the warmer arterial blood gives up its heat to the cooler venous blood, rather than to the external environment. The pulsations of the artery caused by the heart beat also aid the venous flow of blood.

The pulmonary circulation

The **pulmonary (or lesser) circulation** begins when blood is pumped by the right ventricle into the **main pulmonary artery**, which immediately bifurcates into the **right** and **left pulmonary arteries** supplying each lung. This 'venous' blood is oxygenated during its passage through the pulmonary capillaries. It then returns to the heart via the **pulmonary veins** to the left atrium, which pumps it into the left ventricle. The metabolic demands of the lungs are not met by the pulmonary circulation, but by the **bronchial circulation**. This arises from the **intercostal arteries**, which branch from the aorta. Most of the veins of the bronchial circulation terminate in the right atrium, but some drain into the pulmonary veins (see Chapter 24).

The splanchnic circulation

The arrangement of the **splanchnic circulation** (liver and digestive organs) is a partial exception to the parallel organization of the systemic vasculature (see figure in Chapter 1). Although a fraction of the blood supply to the liver is provided by the hepatic artery, the liver receives most (~70%) of its blood via the **portal vein**. This vessel carries venous blood that has passed through the capillary beds of the stomach, spleen, pancreas and intestine. Most of the liver's circulation is therefore *in series* with that of the digestive organs. This arrangement facilitates hepatic uptake of nutrients and detoxification of foreign substances which have been absorbed during digestion. This type of sequential perfusion of two capillary beds is referred to as a **portal circulation**. A somewhat different type of portal circulation is also found within the kidney.

The lymphatic system

The body contains a parallel circulatory system of **lymphatic vessels** and **nodes** (see Chapter 18). The lymphatic system functions to return to the cardiovascular system the approximately 8 L/day of interstitial fluid that leaves the exchange vessels to enter body tissues. The larger lymphatic vessels pass through nodes containing lymphocytes, which act to mount an immune response to microbes, bacterial toxins and other foreign material carried into the lymphatic system with the interstitial fluid.

Vascular histology and smooth muscle cell ultrastructure

4

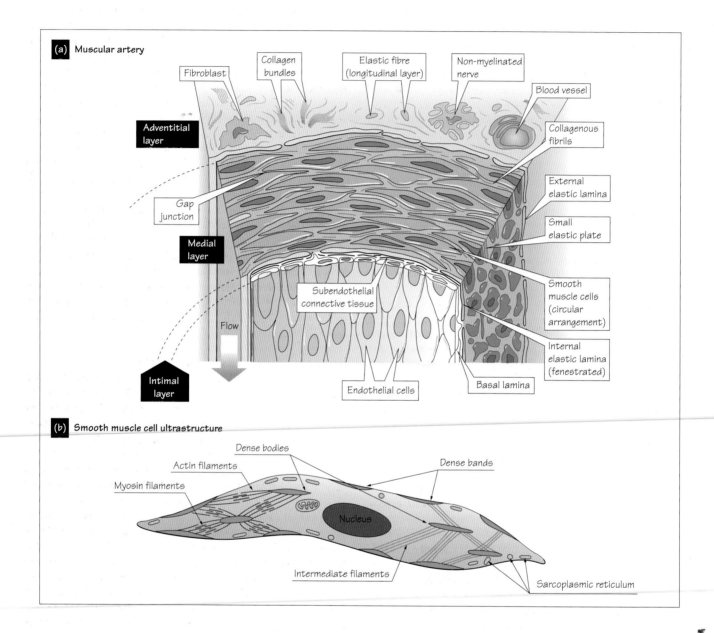

(a) Muscular artery

Fibroblast

Collagen bundles

Elastic fibre (longitudinal layer)

Non-myelinated nerve

Blood vessel

Adventitial layer

Collagenous fibrils

Gap junction

External elastic lamina

Medial layer

Small elastic plate

Subendothelial connective tissue

Smooth muscle cells (circular arrangement)

Flow

Internal elastic lamina (fenestrated)

Intimal layer

Endothelial cells

Basal lamina

(b) Smooth muscle cell ultrastructure

Dense bodies

Actin filaments

Dense bands

Myosin filaments

Nucleus

Intermediate filaments

Sarcoplasmic reticulum

Larger blood vessels share a common three-layered structure. Figure (a) illustrates the arrangement of these layers, or *tunics*, in a muscular artery.

A thin inner layer, the **tunica intima**, comprises an *endothelial cell monolayer* (*endothelium*) supported by connective tissue. The endothelial cells lining the vascular lumen are sealed to each other by *tight junctions*, which restrict the diffusion of large molecules across the endothelium. The endothelial cells have a crucial role in controlling vascular permeability, vasoconstriction, angiogenesis (growth of new blood vessels) and regulation of haemostasis. The intima is relatively thicker in larger arteries, and contains some smooth muscle cells in large and medium-sized arteries and veins.

The thick middle layer, the **tunica media**, is separated from the intima by a fenestrated (perforated) sheath, the *internal elastic lamina*, mostly composed of elastin. The media contains *smooth muscle cells* embedded in an extracellular matrix composed mainly of collagen, elastin and proteoglycans. The cells are shaped like elongated and irregular spindles or cylinders with tapering ends, and are 15–100 μm long. In the arterial system, they are orientated circularly or in a low-pitch spiral, so that the vascular lumen narrows when they contract. Individual cells are long enough to wrap around small arterioles several times.

Adjacent smooth muscle cells form **gap junctions**. These are areas of close cellular contact in which arrays of large channels called **connexons** span both cell membranes, allowing ions to flow from one cell to the other. The smooth muscle cells therefore form a **syncytium**, in which depolarization spreads from each cell to its neighbours.

An *external elastic lamina* separates the tunica media from the outer layer, the **tunica adventitia**. This contains collagenous tissue supporting *fibroblasts* and *nerves*. In large arteries and veins, the adventitia contains **vasa vasorum**, small blood vessels which also penetrate into the outer portion of the media and supply the vascular wall with oxygen and nutrients.

These three layers are also present in the venous system, but are less distinct. Compared to arteries, veins have a thinner tunica media containing a smaller amount of smooth muscle cells, which also tend to have a more random orientation.

The protein **elastin** is found mainly in the arteries. Molecules of elastin are arranged into a network of randomly coiled fibres. These molecular 'springs' allow arteries to expand during systole and then rebound during diastole to keep the blood flowing forward. This is particularly important in the aorta and other large elastic arteries, in which the media contains fenestrated sheets of elastin separating the smooth muscle cells into multiple concentric layers (**lamellae**).

The fibrous protein **collagen** is present in all three layers of the vascular wall, and functions as a framework that anchors the smooth muscle cells in place. At high internal pressures, the collagen network becomes very rigid, limiting vascular distensibility. This is particularly important in veins, which have a higher collagen content than arteries.

Exchange vessel structure

Capillaries and postcapillary venules are tubes formed of a single layer of overlapping endothelial cells. This is supported and surrounded on the external side by the *basal lamina*, a 50–100-nm-thick layer of fibrous proteins including collagen, and glycoproteins. *Pericytes*, isolated cells which can give rise to smooth muscle cells during angiogenesis, adhere to the outside of the basal lamina, especially in postcapillary venules. The luminal side of the endothelium is coated by *glycocalyx*, a dense glycoprotein network attached to the cell membrane.

There are three types of capillaries, and these differ in their locations and permeabilities. Their structures are illustrated in Chapter 18.

Continuous capillaries occur in skin, muscles, lungs and the central nervous system. They have a low permeability to molecules that cannot pass readily through cell membranes, owing to the presence of tight junctions which bring the overlapping membranes of adjacent endothelial cells into close contact. The tight junctions run around the perimeter of each cell, forming a seal restricting the paracellular flow of molecules of molecular weight (MW) > 10 000. These junctions are especially tight in most capillaries of the central nervous system, and form an integral part of the **blood–brain barrier** (see Chapter 18).

Fenestrated capillaries are much more permeable than continuous capillaries. These are found in endocrine glands, renal glomeruli, intestinal villi and other tissues in which large amounts of fluid or metabolites enter or leave capillaries. In addition to having leakier intercellular junctions, the endothelial cells of these capillaries contain *fenestrae*, circular pores of diameter 50–100 nm spanning areas of the cells where the cytoplasm is thinned. Except in the renal glomeruli, fenestrae are usually covered by a thin perforated diaphragm.

Discontinuous capillaries or **sinusoids** are found in liver, spleen and bone marrow. These are large irregularly shaped capillaries with gaps between the endothelial cells wide enough to allow large proteins and even erythrocytes to cross the capillary wall.

Smooth muscle cell ultrastructure

The cytoplasm of vascular smooth muscle cells contains thin **actin** and thick **myosin** filaments (Figure 4b). Instead of being aligned into sarcomeres as in cardiac myocytes, groups of actin filaments running roughly parallel to the long axis of the cell are anchored at one end into elongated **dense bodies** in the cytoplasm and **dense bands** along the inner face of the cell membrane. Dense bodies and bands are linked by bundles of **intermediate filaments** composed mainly of the proteins **desmin** and **vimentin** to form the **cytoskeleton**, an internal scaffold giving the cell its shape. The free ends of the actin filaments interdigitate with myosin filaments. The myosin crossbridges are structured so that the actin filaments on either side of a myosin filament are pulled in opposite directions during crossbridge cycling. This draws the dense bodies towards each other, causing the cytoskeleton, and therefore the cell, to shorten. The dense bands are attached to the extracellular matrix (ECM) by membrane-spanning proteins called **integrins**, allowing force development to be distributed throughout the vascular wall. The interaction between the ECM and integrins is a dynamic process which is affected by forces exerted on the matrix by the pressure inside the vessel. This allows the integrins, which are signalling molecules capable of influencing both cytoskeletal structure and signal transduction, to orchestrate cellular responses to changes in pressure.

The **sarcoplasmic reticulum** (SR, also termed smooth endoplasmic reticulum) occupies 2–6% of cell volume. This network of tubes and flattened sacs permeates the cell and contains a high concentration (~50 mmol/L) of Ca^{2+}. Elements of the SR closely approach the cell membrane. Several types of Ca^{2+}-regulated ion channels and transporters are concentrated in these areas of the plasmalemma, which may have an important role in cellular excitation.

The nucleus is located in the central part of the cell. Organelles including rough endoplasmic reticulum, Golgi complex and mitochondria are mainly found in the perinuclear region.

5 Constituents of blood

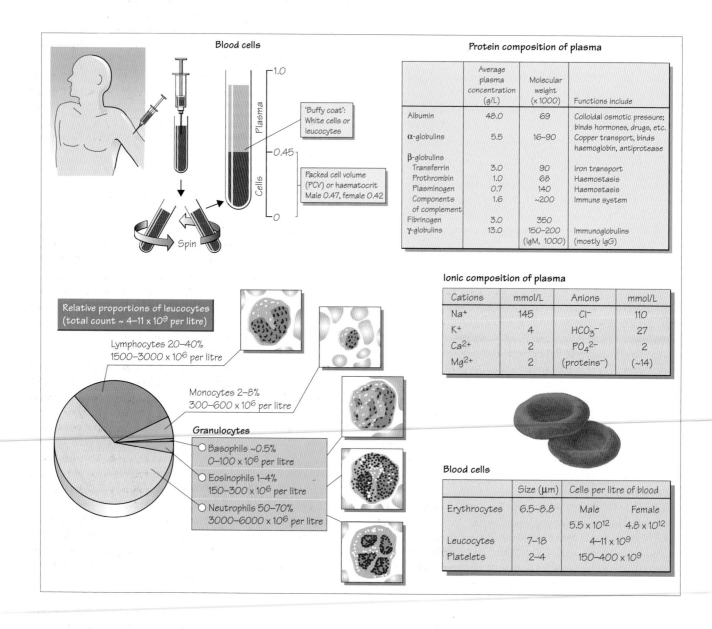

Blood cells

'Buffy coat': White cells or leucocytes

Packed cell volume (PCV) or haematocrit Male 0.47, female 0.42

Spin

Protein composition of plasma

	Average plasma concentration (g/L)	Molecular weight (×1000)	Functions include
Albumin	48.0	69	Colloidal osmotic pressure; binds hormones, drugs, etc.
α-globulins	5.5	16–90	Copper transport, binds haemoglobin, antiprotease
β-globulins			
Transferrin	3.0	90	Iron transport
Prothrombin	1.0	68	Haemostasis
Plasminogen	0.7	140	Haemostasis
Components of complement	1.6	~200	Immune system
Fibrinogen	3.0	350	
γ-globulins	13.0	150–200 (IgM, 1000)	Immunoglobulins (mostly IgG)

Ionic composition of plasma

Cations	mmol/L	Anions	mmol/L
Na^+	145	Cl^-	110
K^+	4	HCO_3^-	27
Ca^{2+}	2	PO_4^{2-}	2
Mg^{2+}	2	(proteins⁻)	(~14)

Relative proportions of leucocytes (total count ~ 4–11 × 10⁹ per litre)

Lymphocytes 20–40%
1500–3000 × 10⁶ per litre

Monocytes 2–8%
300–600 × 10⁶ per litre

Granulocytes

Basophils ~0.5%
0–100 × 10⁶ per litre

Eosinophils 1–4%
150–300 × 10⁶ per litre

Neutrophils 50–70%
3000–6000 × 10⁶ per litre

Blood cells

	Size (μm)	Cells per litre of blood	
		Male	Female
Erythrocytes	6.5–8.8	5.5×10^{12}	4.8×10^{12}
Leucocytes	7–18	$4–11 \times 10^9$	
Platelets	2–4	$150–400 \times 10^9$	

The primary function of blood is to deliver O_2 and energy sources to the tissues, and to remove CO_2 and waste products. It contains important elements of the defence and immune systems, is important for regulation of temperature, and transports hormones and other signalling molecules between tissues. In a 70-kg man blood volume is ~5500 mL, or 8% of body weight. Blood consists of **plasma** and **blood cells**. If 100 mL of blood is spun in a centrifuge, the cells sediment and this **packed cell volume** (PCV, haematocrit) is normally ~45 mL (0.45) in men, less (~0.42) in women.

Plasma

The plasma volume is ~5% of the body weight. It consists of ions in solution and a wide range of plasma proteins. After clotting, a straw-coloured fluid called **serum** remains, which differs from plasma only in that fibrinogen and other clotting factors have been removed. The

relative osmotic pressures of plasma, interstitial and intracellular fluid are critical for maintenance of tissue cell volume, and are related to the amount of osmotically active particles (molecules) per litre, or **osmolarity** (mosmol/L); as plasma is not an ideal fluid (e.g. it contains slow diffusing proteins), in physiology and medicine **osmolality** (mosmol/kg H_2O) is often used instead. Plasma **osmolality** is ~300 mosmol/kg H_2O, mostly due to dissolved ions and small diffusible molecules (glucose and urea). These diffuse easily across capillaries, and the pressure they exert (**crystalloid osmotic pressure**) is therefore the same either side of the capillary wall. Proteins do not pass through capillary walls easily, and are responsible for the **colloidal osmotic pressure** (or **oncotic** pressure) of the plasma. This is much smaller than crystalloid osmotic pressure, but is critical for fluid transfer across the capillary wall because it differs between plasma and interstitial fluid (see Chapter 19). It is thus more meaningfully expressed in terms of pressure, and in plasma the colloidal osmotic pressure is normally ~25 mmHg. Maintenance of plasma osmolality is vital for regulation of both cell and blood volume (see Chapter 27).

Ionic composition

Na^+ is the most prevalent ion in plasma, and the main determinant of plasma osmolality and thus blood volume. The concentration of the major ions is shown in the figure; others are present in smaller amounts. Changes in ionic concentration can have major consequences for excitable tissues (e.g. K^+, Ca^{2+}). Na^+, K^+ and Cl^- are completely dissociated in the plasma, but Ca^{2+} and Mg^{2+} are partly bound to plasma proteins, so that free concentration is ~50% of the total.

Proteins

Normal total plasma protein concentration is 65–83 g/L; as proteins vary widely in molecular weight the molar concentration is an approximation. Most plasma proteins other than γ-globulins (see below) are synthesized in the liver. Proteins can ionize as either acids or bases because of the presence of both NH_2 and COOH groups. At pH 7.4 they are mostly in the anionic (acidic) form. Their ability to accept or donate H^+ means they can act as buffers, although they account for only ~15% of the buffering capacity of blood. Plasma proteins have an important transport function. They bind with many hormones (e.g. cortisol and thyroxine) and metals (e.g. iron), and are important for blood transport of many drugs. They may therefore modulate the free concentration of such agents, and thus their biological activity.

Plasma proteins are classified into **albumin** (~48 g/L), **globulin** (~25 g/L) and **fibrinogen** (~2–4 g/L) fractions. Globulins are further classified as α-, β- and γ-globulins, each of which may include many different proteins. β-Globulins include transferrin (iron transport), components of complement (immune system), and prothrombin and plasminogen, which with fibrinogen are involved in blood clotting (see Chapter 7). The most important γ-globulins are the immunoglobulins.

Blood cells

In the adult, all blood cells are produced in the **red bone marrow**, although in the fetus, and following bone marrow damage in the adult, they are also produced in the liver and spleen. The marrow contains a small number of **uncommitted stem cells**, which differentiate into specific **committed stem cells** for each blood cell type. The average number of the main cell types is shown in the figure.

Erythrocytes

Erythrocytes (red cells) are by far the most numerous cells in the blood, with ~5.5×10^{12}/L in males (red cell count, RCC). The haemoglobin they contain is responsible for carriage of O_2, and plays an important part in acid–base buffering. Erythrocytes are biconcave discs and have no nucleus. Their shape and flexibility allows them to deform easily and pass through the capillaries. The **erythrocyte sedimentation rate (ESR)** is the rate at which cells sediment from blood when allowed to stand in the presence of an anticoagulant. This is increased when cells stack together (form *rouleaux*), and in pregnancy and inflammatory disease. It is decreased by low plasma fibrinogen. Erythrocytes have a normal volume of 85 fL (85×10^{-15}/L; mean cell volume, **MCV**), and ~30 pg of haemoglobin (30×10^{-12}/g; mean cell haemoglobin, **MCH**). The mean cell haemoglobin concentration (**MCHC**) is thus ~350 g/L. Blood contains ~160 g/L (male) and ~140 g/L (female) haemoglobin. Erythrocytes have an average lifespan of 120 days. Their formation (erythropoiesis) and related diseases are discussed in Chapter 6.

$$MCV = \frac{PCV}{RCC}; \; MCH = \frac{Hb}{RCC}; \; MCHC = \frac{MCH}{MCV} \text{ or } \frac{Hb}{PCV}$$

Leucocytes (white cells)

Leucocytes defend the body against infection by foreign material. The normal total count in adults is $4–11 \times 10^9$/L, although considerable variations occur. In the newborn the count is ~20×10^9/L. Three main types are present in blood: **granulocytes**, **lymphocytes** and **monocytes**. Granulocytes are further classified as **neutrophils** (containing neutral-staining granules), **eosinophils** (acid-staining granules) and **basophils** (basic-staining granules). All are involved in inflammation and release inflammatory mediators.

Neutrophils migrate to areas of infection (**chemotaxis**) and destroy bacteria by **phagocytosis**. They have a short half-life of ~6 h. Eosinophils are less motile and are effective against larger parasites. They are increased in allergic diseases and release proinflammatory mediators. Basophils contain histamine and heparin and are similar to tissue **mast** cells.

Lymphocytes originate in the marrow but mature in the lymph nodes, thymus and spleen before returning to the circulation. Most remain in the lymphatic system. They are critical components of the **immune** system and produce immunoglobulins (antibodies).

Monocytes have a clear cytoplasm and are larger than granulocytes. After formation in the marrow they circulate in the blood for ~72 h before entering the tissues and becoming **macrophages**, to form the **reticuloendothelial system** in the liver, spleen and lymph nodes.

Platelets

Platelets have a critical role in haemostasis (Chapter 7). They are small (~3-μm) vesicle-like structures formed from **megakaryocytes** in the bone marrow, and have a lifespan in the blood of ~4 days. Clearly visible **dense granules** contain mediators such as serotonin (5-HT) and adenosine diphosphate (ADP), which are released on platelet activation.

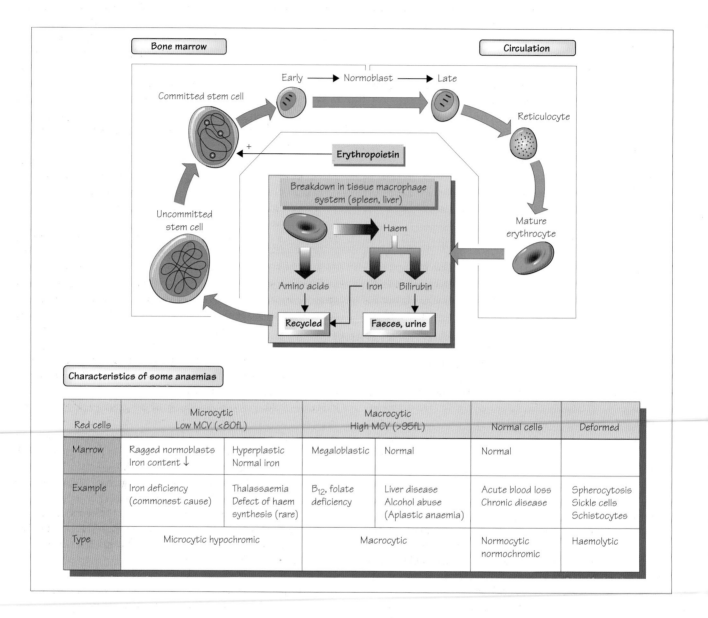

Red cells	Microcytic Low MCV (<80fL)		Macrocytic High MCV (>95fL)		Normal cells	Deformed
Marrow	Ragged normoblasts Iron content ↓	Hyperplastic Normal iron	Megaloblastic	Normal	Normal	
Example	Iron deficiency (commonest cause)	Thalassaemia Defect of haem synthesis (rare)	B_{12}, folate deficiency	Liver disease Alcohol abuse (Aplastic anaemia)	Acute blood loss Chronic disease	Spherocytosis Sickle cells Schistocytes
Type	Microcytic hypochromic		Macrocytic		Normocytic normochromic	Haemolytic

Erythropoiesis leads to the formation of new red blood cells (**erythrocytes**). **Anaemia** is any condition in which there is a reduced blood haemoglobin, resulting in impaired ability of the blood to transport O_2. Some anaemias are associated with abnormal haemoglobins.

Erythropoiesis

Erythrocytes originate from **committed stem cells** in the bone marrow of the adult, and liver and spleen of the fetus. Damage to the marrow can result in erythropoiesis from the liver and spleen of adults. Committed stem cells differentiate into **erythroblasts (early normoblasts)**, which are relatively large (~15 μm) and nucleated. As differentiation proceeds the cells shrink, haemoglobin is synthesized, and in the **late normoblast** the nucleus breaks up and disappears. The young erythrocyte shows a reticulum on staining, and is called a **reticulocyte**. As it ages, the reticulum disappears and the characteristic biconcave shape develops.

Normally 1–2% of circulating red cells are reticulocytes. This increases when erythropoiesis is enhanced, for example by increased **erythropoietin**. About 2×10^{11} erythrocytes are produced from the marrow each day.

Erythropoietin is a glycoprotein hormone produced mainly by the kidneys in adults. In the fetus the main source is the liver. Erythropoietin increases the number of committed stem cells and promotes the production of erythrocytes. The key stimulus for increased erythropoietin is hypoxia. Altitude and chronic respiratory diseases cause the Po_2 of the blood to fall, and there is a greatly increased number of erythrocytes (**polycythaemia**) and haematocrit. In kidney disease, chronic inflammation and cirrhosis of the liver erythropoietin levels can fall, resulting in anaemia.

Erythrocytes are destroyed by **macrophages** in the liver and spleen after ~120 days. The spleen also sequesters and eradicates defective erythrocytes. The haem group is split from haemoglobin and converted to **biliverdin** and then **bilirubin**. The iron is conserved and recycled via **transferrin**, an iron transport protein, or stored in **ferritin**. Bilirubin is a brown-yellow compound which is excreted in the bile. An increased rate of haemoglobin breakdown results in excess bilirubin, which stains the tissues (**jaundice**).

Haemoglobin

Haemoglobin has four subunits, each containing a polypeptide **globin** chain and an iron-containing porphyrin, **haem**. Haem is synthesized from succinic acid and glycine, and contains one atom of iron in the **ferrous** state (Fe^{2+}). One molecule of haemoglobin has therefore four atoms of iron, and binds four molecules of O_2. There are several types of haemoglobin, relating to the globin chains. The haem moiety is unchanged. Adult haemoglobin (Hb A) has two α and two β chains. Fetal haemoglobin (Hb F) has two γ chains in place of the β chains, and a high affinity for O_2. There are several **haemoglobinopathies** due to abnormal haemoglobins.

Sickle cell anaemia is the most important and occurs in 10% of the Black population. It is caused by substitution of one glutamic acid by valine in the β chain; this haemoglobin is called Hb S. At a low Po_2 Hb S gels, causing deformation (*sickling*) of the erythrocyte. The cell is less flexible and prone to fragmentation, and there is an increased rate of erythrocyte breakdown by macrophages. The Hb S variant is inherited in a Mendelian fashion. Heterozygous offspring with less than 40% Hb S normally have no symptoms (**sickle cell trait**). Homozygous offspring with more than 70% Hb S develop full **sickle cell anaemia**. There are acute episodes of pain relating to blockage of blood vessels, congestion of the liver and spleen with red cells, and commonly leg ulcers.

Thalassaemia is caused by a defect in synthesis of either the α- or β-globin chains. Several genes are involved. In β thalassaemia there are either fewer or no β chains available. The α chains therefore bind to γ (Hb F) or δ chains (Hb A_2). Thalassaemia major (severe β thalassaemia) has high levels of Hb A_2 and Hb F, and severe anaemia. The liver and spleen are enlarged and bone expansion causes typical features. Regular transfusions are required, leading to iron overload. In heterozygous β thalassaemia minor there are no symptoms, although Hb A_2 is elevated and erythrocytes are **microcytic** and **hypochromic**, i.e. **mean cell volume** (MCV), **mean cell haemoglobin content** (MCH) and **mean cell haemoglobin concentration** (MCHC) are reduced. In α thalassaemia there are fewer or no α chains. In the latter case the haem binds four γ chains (Hb Barts), and does not bind O_2. Infants have huge spleens and livers and oedema (**hydrops fetalis**), and do not survive. When some α chains are present, patients surviving as adults may produce some Hb H (four β chains); this precipitates in the red cells which are then destroyed in the spleen, and this is therefore enlarged.

Anaemia

Some anaemias result from simple blood loss (e.g. haemorrhage, heavy menstruation) or chronic disease (e.g. infection, tumours, renal failure). When the cells have an otherwise normal MCV and MCH (see Chapter 5), the condition is termed **normocytic normochromic** anaemia.

Aplastic anaemia results from an aplastic (non-functional) bone marrow and causes **pancytopenia** (reduced red, white and platelet cell count). It is dangerous but uncommon. It can be caused by certain chemicals and drugs (particularly anticancer drugs), radiation, infections (e.g. viral hepatitis, TB) and pregnancy, where it has a 90% mortality. There is a rare inherited condition, **Fanconi's anaemia**, which gives rise to a defect in stem cell production and differentiation. Clinical signs include anaemia, bleeding and infections. The condition is variable, and can show either spontaneous remission or gradual and persistent deterioration. Transfusions can be used for maintenance, but long-term treatment may require a bone marrow transplant.

Haemolytic anaemia results from an excessive rate of erythrocyte destruction, and thus causes jaundice. It is associated with blood transfusion mismatch, **haemolytic anaemia of the newborn** (see Chapter 8), abnormal erythrocyte fragility and haemoglobins, and several other disorders including autoimmune, liver and hereditary diseases.

In **hereditary haemolytic anaemia** (familial spherocytosis) erythrocytes have a more spheroid appearance, are more fragile, and are more rapidly destroyed in the spleen. It is relatively common, affecting 1 in 5000 Caucasians. Jaundice is common but not invariable at birth, and may appear after several years. Patients may develop aplastic anaemia after infections, and **megaloblastic anaemia** from folate deficiency as a result of high bone marrow activity. Removal of the spleen is normally recommended.

Megaloblastic anaemia. Maturation of the normoblast requires **vitamin B_{12}** (cyanocobalamin) and **folate**, which is commonly given in pregnancy with iron. A reduction in vitamin B_{12} or folate leads to the formation of unusually large normoblasts (**megaloblasts**), which mature as **macrocytes**. These have a large MCV and MCH, although MCHC is normal. The number of red cells is greatly reduced, and the rate of destruction increased. **Folate deficiency** is mostly related to poor diet, in particular in the old or poor. Alcoholism also impairs utilization. Certain anticonvulsant drugs (e.g. phenytoin) have an antifolate action. **Pernicious anaemia** is caused by vitamin B_{12} deficiency as there is defective absorption from the gut. B_{12} is transported across the ileum as a complex with **intrinsic factor**, which is produced by the gastric mucosa. Damage to the gastric mucosa results in pernicious anaemia. B_{12} deficiency can also occur in strict vegans.

Iron deficiency. The daily requirement for **iron** in the diet is small, as the body has an efficient recycling system. It is increased when there is significant blood loss. As a result of menstrual blood loss women have a higher requirement for dietary iron than men. This is also increased during pregnancy. **Iron deficiency** causes defective haemoglobin formation and a **microcytic hypochromic** anaemia.

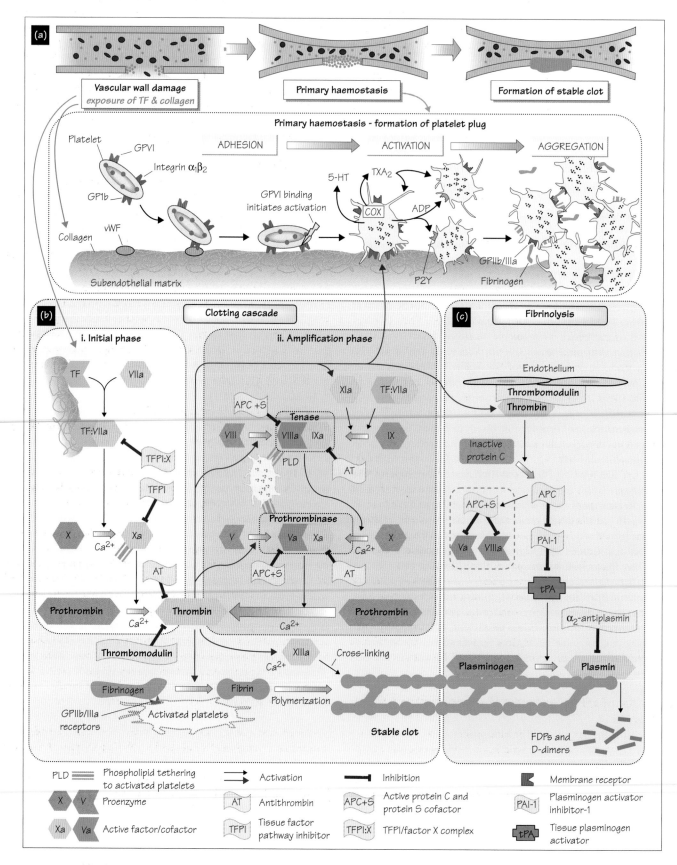

Primary haemostasis (Figure 7a)

Initially, damage to the blood vessel wall causes transient vasoconstriction, reducing blood flow. **Platelet adhesion** is initiated when **GPIb** (glycoprotein) receptors on platelet membranes bind to **von Willebrand factor (vWF)** attached to collagen in the exposed subendothelial matrix. This initial tethering promotes binding of platelet **integrin** $\alpha_2\beta_1$ and **GPVI** receptors directly to collagen. GPVI receptor binding initiates **activation** – platelets change shape, put out pseudopodia and make thromboxane A$_2$ (**TXA$_2$**) via cyclooxygenase (**COX**), fibrinogen (GPIIb/IIIa) receptors are activated and **phospholipid** (PLD) is exposed on their surface. TXA$_2$ releases mediators from platelet **dense granules**, including **serotonin** (5-HT) and adenosine diphosphate (**ADP**). TXA$_2$ and 5-HT cause further vasoconstriction, and ADP activates more platelets via **P2Y** purinergic receptors; **thrombin** (see below) binds to PAR1 receptors and is a potent platelet activator. Plasma fibrinogen sticks to activated platelets (via GPIIb/IIIa) so they **aggregate**, forming a soft **platelet plug** (Figure 7a). This is fragile, and is stabilized with **fibrin** during clotting.

Formation of the blood clot (Figure 7b)

Fibrin monomers are cleaved from fibrinogen by the protease **thrombin**, a key component in clotting. Activation of thrombin involves sequential conversion of proenzymes to active enzymes (e.g. factor X → Xa) in a **cascade**. This is initiated by exposure of **tissue factor** (TF; thromboplastin) in the subendothelial matrix, which binds to factor VIIa in plasma. The **TF:VIIa** complex activates **factors X** and IX (see below). When tethered to activated platelets via PLD, **factor Xa** converts **prothrombin** to thrombin. This **initial phase** of coagulation (Figure 7bi; previously *extrinsic pathway*) produces comparatively little thrombin, but initiates an **amplification phase** (Figure 7bii; previously *intrinsic pathway*) because thrombin activates factors **XI, VIII** and **V**, and more platelets.

Factor XIa activates IX (tethered to platelet PLD), which complexes with VIIIa to form **tenase (X-ase)**, a more powerful activator of factor X than TF:VIIa. Similarly, factors Va and Xa combine to form **prothrombinase**, a much more efficient prothrombin activator than Xa alone. The amplification phase accounts for > 90% of thrombin produced. As key clotting factors (e.g. IXa, Xa) only work when tethered to activated platelets via PLD, clotting is confined to the platelet plug. Factor XII (not shown) is probably of limited significance; it activates XI and may be involved in pathological clotting in the brain.

Once formed, fibrin **polymerizes**, and is **cross-linked** by factor **XIIIa** (activated by thrombin), creating a tough network of fibrin fibres and a **stable clot**. Retraction of platelet pseudopodia contracts the clot by ~60%, making it tougher and assisting repair by drawing the edges of the wound together. Ca^{2+} is required for activation of factors X, XIII and prothrombin; Ca^{2+} chelators (e.g. citrate, EDTA) can therefore be used to prevent clotting in stored blood.

Inhibitors of haemostasis and dissolution of the clot

Haemostasis involves positive feedback, so inhibitory mechanisms are vital. **Prostacyclin** (PGI$_2$) and nitric oxide from endothelium impede platelet adhesion and activation. Tissue factor pathway inhibitor (**TFPI**) forms a complex with and inhibits factor Xa, and this complex inhibits TF:VIIa (Figure 7bi). **Antithrombin** inhibits thrombin, factor Xa and IXa/tenase; its activity is strongly potentiated by **heparin**, a polysaccharide. *Heparan* on endothelial cells is similar. **Thrombomodulin** on endothelial cells binds thrombin and prevents it cleaving fibrinogen; instead, it activates **protein C (APC)** which with its cofactor **protein S** inactivates factors Va and VIIIa, and hence tenase and prothrombinase (Figure 7bii).

Plasmin breaks down fibrin (**fibrinolysis**; Figure 7c) into soluble fibrin degradation products (**FDPs**) including small **D-dimers**. Plasmin is formed from fibrin-bound **plasminogen** by tPA (**tissue plasminogen activator**); **urokinase** (uPA) is similar. APC inactivates an inhibitor of tPA (plasminogen activator inhibitor-1; **PAI-1**), and so promotes fibrinolysis (Figure 7c). Plasmin can also inactivate factors Va and VIIIa, and is itself inactivated by α_2-antiplasmin.

Defects in haemostasis

The most common hereditary disorder is **haemophilia A**, a deficiency of factor VIII sex linked to males. Others are **Christmas disease**, a deficiency of factor IX, and **von Willebrand disease**, a deficiency of vWF. The latter leads to defective platelet adhesion and reduced availability of factor VIII, which is stabilized by vWF. The liver requires **vitamin K** for correct synthesis of prothrombin and factors VII, IX and X. As vitamin K is obtained from intestinal bacteria and food, disorders of fat absorption or liver disease can result in deficiency and defective clotting. **Purpura** refers to easy bruising and spontaneous haemorrhages in skin and mucous membranes, and is caused by defective primary haemostasis, e.g. low platelet numbers (**thrombocytopenia**). **Antiphospholipid syndrome** is due to phospholipid-binding antibodies and associated with recurrent thromboses. It is linked to 20% of strokes in people over 50 years.

Laboratory investigations

Platelet count: normally $150–400 \times 10^9$ per litre. Low: **thrombocytopenia**; high: **thrombocytosis**.

Bleeding time: time to cessation of bleeding when clot formation is prevented by wiping every 30 s. A measure of primary haemostasis, normally 3–10 min. Prolonged by e.g. thrombocytopenia.

Prothrombin time (PT): time to clot formation following addition of thromboplastin (TF) (fibrinogen and Ca^{2+} in excess); normally ~14 s. A measure of activity of vitamin K-dependent clotting factors, and thus important for titrating dose of **warfarin** (see Chapter 45). It is expressed as **international normalized ratio (INR)**, the ratio of the patient's PT to that of a standardized reference sample. INR is normally 1.

Activated partial thromboplastin time (aPTT): time to clot formation following addition of a surface activator (kaolin; activates factor XII), PLD and Ca^{2+} to plasma. Measures activity of factors in the amplification phase (i.e. not factor VIIa) (Figure 7bii). Normally 35–45 s. Prolonged by relevant deficiencies or inhibitors.

D-dimers and FDPs: indicative of fibrinolysis; therefore raised in disseminated intravascular coagulation (**DIC**) and other thrombotic conditions.

Thrombosis and embolism are major causes of death, and are discussed with associated therapies in Chapter 45.

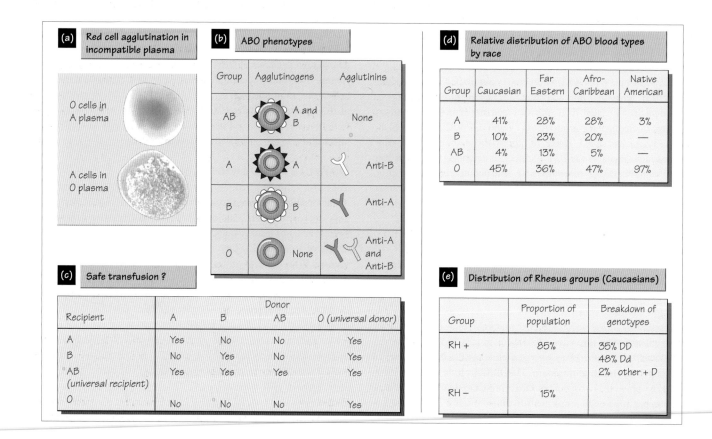

(a) Red cell agglutination in incompatible plasma

O cells in A plasma

A cells in O plasma

(b) ABO phenotypes

Group	Agglutinogens	Agglutinins
AB	A and B	None
A	A	Anti-B
B	B	Anti-A
O	None	Anti-A and Anti-B

(c) Safe transfusion ?

Recipient	Donor A	B	AB	O (universal donor)
A	Yes	No	No	Yes
B	No	Yes	No	Yes
AB (universal recipient)	Yes	Yes	Yes	Yes
O	No	No	No	Yes

(d) Relative distribution of ABO blood types by race

Group	Caucasian	Far Eastern	Afro-Caribbean	Native American
A	41%	28%	28%	3%
B	10%	23%	20%	—
AB	4%	13%	5%	—
O	45%	36%	47%	97%

(e) Distribution of Rhesus groups (Caucasians)

Group	Proportion of population	Breakdown of genotypes
RH +	85%	35% DD 48% Dd 2% other + D
RH −	15%	

Blood groups

If samples of blood from different individuals are mixed together, some combinations result in red cells sticking together as clumps (Figure 8a). This is called **agglutination**, and occurs when the **blood groups** are incompatible. It is caused when antigens (or **agglutinogens**) on the red cell membrane react with specific antibodies (or **agglutinins**) in the plasma. If the quantity (or **titre**) of antibodies is sufficiently high, they bind to their antigens on several red cells and glue the cells together, which then rupture (**haemolyse**). If this occurs following a blood transfusion it can lead to anaemia and other serious complications. The most important blood groups are the **ABO system** and **Rh** (**Rhesus**) groups.

The ABO system

The ABO system consists of four blood groups: A, B, AB and O. The precise group depends on the presence or absence of two antigens, A and B, on the red cells, and their respective antibodies, α and β, in the plasma (Figure 8b). The A and B antigens on red cells are mostly glycolipids that differ in respect of their terminal sugar. The antigens are also found as glycoproteins in other tissues, including salivary glands, pancreas, lungs and testes, and in saliva and semen.

Group A blood contains the A antigen and β antibody, and group B the B antigen and α antibody. Group AB has both A and B antigens, but neither antibody. Group O blood contains neither antigen, but both α and β antibodies. Group A blood cannot therefore be transfused into people of group B, or vice versa, because antibodies in the recipient

react with their respective antigens on the donor red cells and cause agglutination (Figure 8c). As people of group AB have neither α nor β antibodies in the plasma, they can be transfused with blood from any group, and are called **universal recipients**. Group O red cells have neither antigen, and can therefore be transfused into any patient. People of group O are therefore called **universal donors**. Although group O blood contains both antibodies, this can normally be disregarded as they are diluted during transfusion and are bound and neutralized by free A or B antigens in the recipient's plasma. If large or repeated transfusions are required, blood of the same group is used.

Inheritance of ABO blood groups

The expression of A and B antigens is determined genetically. A and B allelomorphs (alternative gene types) are dominant, and O recessive. Therefore AO (**heterozygous**) and AA (**homozygous**) genotypes both have group A phenotypes. An AB genotype produces both antigens, and is thus group AB. The proportion of each blood group varies according to race (Figure 8d), although group O is most common (35–50%). Native Americans are almost exclusively group O.

Rh groups

In ~85% of the population the red cells have a D antigen on the membrane (Figure 8e). Such people are called Rh+ (Rhesus positive), while those who lack the antigen are Rh− (Rhesus negative). Unlike ABO antigens, the D antigen is not found in other tissues. The antibody to D antigen (**anti-D agglutinin**) is not normally found in the plasma of Rh– individuals, but sensitization and subsequent antibody production occurs if a relatively small amount of Rh+ blood is introduced. This can result from transfusion, or when an Rh– mother has an Rh+ child, and fetal red blood cells enter the maternal circulation during birth. Occasionally, fetal cells may cross the placenta earlier in the pregnancy.

Inheritance of Rh groups

The gene corresponding to the D antigen is also called D, and is dominant. When D is absent from the chromosome, its place is taken by the allelomorph of D called d, which is recessive. Individuals who are homozygous and heterozygous for D will be Rh+. About 50% of the population are heterozygous for D, and ~35% homozygous. Blood typing for Rh groups is routinely performed for prospective parents to determine the likelihood of **haemolytic disease** in the offspring.

Haemolytic disease of the newborn

Most pregnancies with Rh– mothers and Rh+ fetuses are normal, but in some cases a severe reaction may occur. Anti-D antibody in the mother's blood can cross the placenta and agglutinate fetal red cells expressing D antigen. The titre of antibody is generally too low to be of consequence during a first pregnancy with a Rh+ fetus, but it can be dangerously increased during subsequent pregnancies, or if the mother was previously sensitized with Rh+ blood. Agglutination of the fetal red cells and consequent haemolysis can result in anaemia and other complications. This is known as **haemolytic disease of the newborn** or **erythroblastosis fetalis**. The haemoglobin released is broken down to bilirubin, which in excess results in **jaundice** (yellow staining of the tissues). If the degree of agglutination and anaemia is severe, the fetus develops severe jaundice and is grossly oedematous (**hydrops fetalis**), and often dies *in utero* or shortly after birth.

Prevention and treatment In previously unsensitized mothers, sensitization can be prevented by treatment with anti-D immunoglobulin after birth. This destroys any fetal Rh+ red cells in the maternal circulation before sensitization of the mother can occur. If haemolytic disease is evident in the fetus or newborn, the Rh+ blood can be replaced by Rh– blood immediately after birth. By the time the newborn has regenerated its own Rh+ red cells, the anti-D antibody from the mother will have been reduced to safe levels. Phototherapy is commonly used for jaundice, as light converts bilirubin to a more rapidly eliminated compound.

Other blood groups

Although there are other blood groups, these are of little clinical importance, as humans rarely develop antibodies to the respective antigens. They may, however, be of importance in medicolegal situations, such as determination of paternity. An example is the MN group, which is a product of two genes (M and N). A person can therefore be MM, MN or NN, each genome coming from one parent. As with the other groups, analysis of the respective parties' genomes can only determine that the man is *not* the father. This method has been largely superceded by DNA profiling.

Complications of blood transfusions

Blood type incompatibility When the recipient of a blood transfusion has a significant plasma titre of α, β or anti-D antibodies, donor red cells expressing the respective antigen will rapidly agglutinate and haemolyse (**haemolytic transfusion reaction**). If the subsequent accumulation of bilirubin is sufficiently large, **haemolytic jaundice** develops. In severe cases renal failure may develop. Antibodies in the donor blood are rarely problematical, as they are diluted and removed in the recipient.

Transmission of infection due to bacteria, viruses and parasites. Most important are hepatitis, HIV, prions and in endemic areas parasites such as malaria.

Iron overload due to frequent transfusions and breakdown of red cells (*transfusion haemosiderosis*), for example in **thalassaemia** (see Chapter 6). Can cause damage to heart, liver, pancreas and glands. Treatment: iron chelators and vitamin C.

Fever due to an immune response to transfused leucocytes which release pyrogens. Relatively common but mild in patients who have previously been transfused, and in pregnancy.

Electrolyte changes and **suppression of haemostasis** following massive transfusions (e.g. major surgery) with stored blood (see below).

Blood storage

Blood is stored for transfusions at 4°C in the presence of an agent that chelates free Ca^{2+} to prevent clotting, for example citrate, oxalate and EDTA (see Chapter 7). Even under these conditions the red cells deteriorate, although they last much longer in the presence of glucose, which provides a metabolic substrate. The cell membrane Na^+ pump works more slowly in the cold, with the result that Na^+ enters the cell, and K^+ leaves. This causes water to move into the cell so that it swells, and becomes more spherocytic. On prolonged storage the cells become fragile, and **haemolyse** (fragment) easily. Neither leucocytes nor platelets survive storage well, and disappear within a day of transfusion. Blood banks normally remove all the donor agglutinins (antibodies), although for small transfusions these would be sufficiently diluted to be of no threat. Great care is taken to screen potential donors for blood-borne diseases (e.g. hepatitis, HIV).

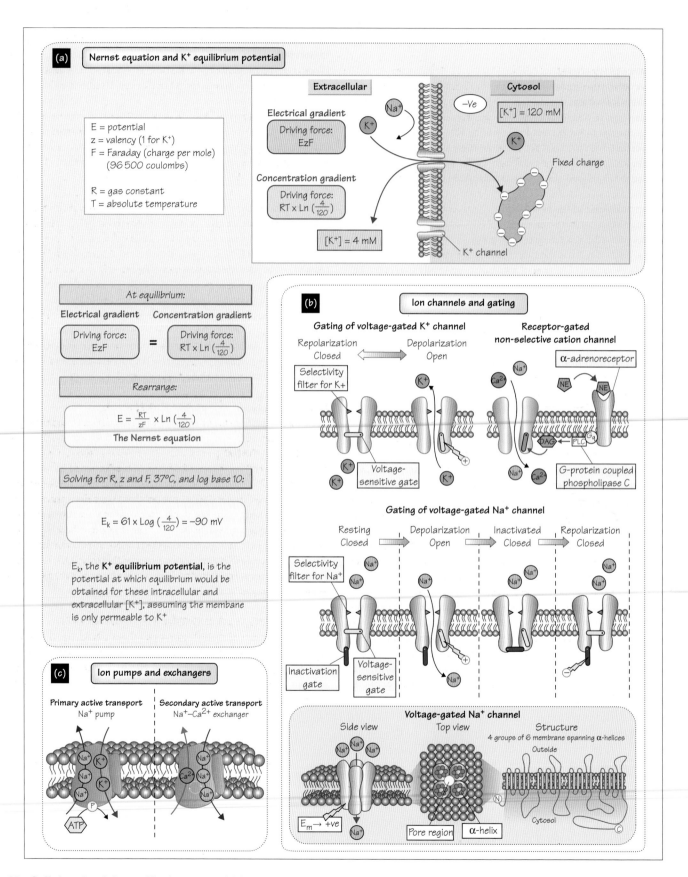

(a) Nernst equation and K⁺ equilibrium potential

E = potential
z = valency (1 for K⁺)
F = Faraday (charge per mole)
    (96 500 coulombs)

R = gas constant
T = absolute temperature

Extracellular

Electrical gradient

Driving force:
EzF

Concentration gradient

Driving force:
$RT \times Ln \left(\frac{4}{120}\right)$

$[K^+] = 4$ mM

K⁺ channel

Cytosol

$[K^+] = 120$ mM

Fixed charge

At equilibrium:

Electrical gradient   Concentration gradient

Driving force: =   Driving force:
EzF $RT \times Ln \left(\frac{4}{120}\right)$

Rearrange:

$$E = \frac{RT}{zF} \times Ln \left(\frac{4}{120}\right)$$

The Nernst equation

Solving for R, z and F, 37°C, and log base 10:

$$E_k = 61 \times Log \left(\frac{4}{120}\right) = -90 \text{ mV}$$

E_k, the **K⁺ equilibrium potential**, is the potential at which equilibrium would be obtained for these intracellular and extracellular [K⁺], assuming the membane is only permeable to K⁺

(b) Ion channels and gating

Gating of voltage-gated K⁺ channel

Repolarization   Depolarization
Closed   Open

Selectivity filter for K+

Voltage-sensitive gate

Receptor-gated non-selective cation channel

α-adrenoreceptor

NE

DAG   PLC

Gₐ

G-protein coupled phospholipase C

Gating of voltage-gated Na⁺ channel

Resting   Depolarization   Inactivated   Repolarization
Closed   Open   Closed   Closed

Selectivity filter for Na⁺

Inactivation gate

Voltage-sensitive gate

Voltage-gated Na⁺ channel

Side view   Top view   Structure
4 groups of 6 membrane spanning α-helices

Outside

$E_m \to +ve$

Pore region   α-helix

Cytosol

N   C

(c) Ion pumps and exchangers

Primary active transport
Na⁺ pump

Secondary active transport
Na⁺–Ca²⁺ exchanger

ATP

The cell membrane is a lipid bilayer with an intrinsically low permeability to charged ions. However, a variety of structures span the membrane through which ions can enter or leave the cell. These include **ion channels** through which ions passively diffuse and **ion pumps** that actively transport ions across the membrane. Pumps regulate ionic gradients, and channels determine membrane potential and underlie action potentials.

The resting membrane potential (Figure 9a)

The resting membrane is more permeable to K^+ and Cl^- than other ions, and is therefore **semipermeable**. The cell contains negatively charged molecules (e.g. proteins) that cannot cross the membrane. This fixed negative charge attracts K^+ but repels Cl^-, leading to accumulation of K^+ within the cell and loss of Cl^-. However, the consequent increase in K^+ concentration gradient drives K^+ back out of the cell. An equilibrium is reached where the *electrical* forces exactly balance those due to *concentration* differences (**Gibbs–Donnan equilibrium**); the net force or **electrochemical gradient** for K^+ is then zero. The opposing effect of the concentration gradient means fewer K^+ ions move into the cell than are required by the fixed negative charges. The inside of the cell is therefore negatively charged compared to the outside (*charge separation*), and a potential develops across the membrane. Only a small charge separation (e.g. 1 in ~100 000 K^+ ions) is required to cause a potential of ~−100 mV. If the membrane was only permeable to K^+ and no other cations, the potential at equilibrium (**K^+ equilibrium potential**, E_K) would be defined by the K^+ concentration gradient, and calculated from the **Nernst equation**. As cardiac muscle intracellular $[K^+]$ is ~120 mM and extracellular $[K^+]$ ~4 mM, $E_K = ~−90$ mV (Figure 9a).

In real membranes K^+ permeability (P_K) at rest is indeed greater than for other ions, so the **resting membrane potential** (RMP) is close to E_K (~−85 mV). RMP does not equal E_K because there *is* some permeability to other ions; most notably Na^+ permeability (P_{Na}) is ~1% of P_K. The Na^+ concentration gradient is also opposite to that for K^+ (intracellular $[Na^+]$ ~10 mM, extracellular ~140 mM), because the **Na^+ pump** (see below) actively removes Na^+ from the cell. As a result, the theoretical equilibrium potential for Na^+ (E_{Na}) is ~+65 mV, far from the actual RMP. Both concentration and electrical gradients are therefore in the same direction, and this inward electrochemical gradient drives Na^+ into the cell. As P_{Na} at rest is relatively low, the amount of Na^+ leaking into the cell is small, but is still sufficient to cause an inward current that slightly depolarizes the membrane. RMP is thus less negative than E_K. RMP can be calculated using the **Goldman equation**, a derivation of the Nernst equation taking into account other ions and their permeabilities.

A consequence of the above is that if P_{Na} was increased to more than P_K, then the membrane potential would shift towards E_{Na}. This is exactly what happens during an action potential, when Na^+ channels open so that P_{Na} becomes 10-fold greater than P_K, and the membrane depolarizes (see Chapter 10). An equivalent situation arises for Ca^{2+}, as intracellular $[Ca^{2+}]$ is ~100 nM at rest, much smaller than the extracellular $[Ca^{2+}]$ of ~1 mM.

Ion channels and gating (Figure 9b)

Channels differ in ion selectivity and activation mechanisms. They are either **open** or **closed**; transition between these states is called **gating**. When channels open ions move passively down their electrochemical gradient. As ions are charged, this causes an electrical current (*ionic current*); positive ions entering the cell cause **inward currents** and depolarization. Phosphorylation of channel proteins by e.g. cyclic AMP can modify function, for example of Ca^{2+} channels (see Chapter 11). There are several types of gating; two are described.

Voltage-gated channels (VGCs) are regulated by membrane potential. Some (e.g. certain K^+ channels) simply switch between **open** and **shut** states according to the potential across them (Figure 9b). Others, such as the **fast inward Na^+ channel** responsible for the upstroke of the action potential in nerves, skeletal and cardiac muscle (Figure 9b; see Chapter 10), have three states: open, shut and **inactive**. When a cell depolarizes sufficiently to activate these Na^+ channels (i.e. reaches their **threshold** potential), they open and the cell depolarizes towards E_{Na}. After a short period (< ms) the channels spontaneously **inactivate**, as though another gate had closed. Inactivated channels can only be reactivated once the membrane potential becomes negative again. This is essential for generation of action potentials (see Chapter 11).

Receptor-gated channels (RGCs; important in smooth muscle, see Chapter 13) are commonly **non-selective cation channels** (NSCCs; permeable to Na^+ and Ca^{2+}). They open when a hormone or neurotransmitter (e.g. norepinephrine) binds to a receptor and initiates production of a second messenger, such as **diacylglycerol** (Figure 9b).

Ion pumps and exchangers (Figure 9c)

Ion pumps use energy to transfer ions against their electrochemical gradient. **Primary active transport** consumes ATP for energy, the prime example being the **Na^+ pump** (Na^+-K^+-ATPase), which pumps three Na^+ out of the cell in exchange for two K^+. Another is the Ca^{2+}-ATPase that pumps Ca^{2+} into intracellular stores (see Chapters 11, 13). **Secondary active transport** uses the Na^+ electrochemical gradient generated by the Na^+ pump to drive the transfer of other ions or molecules across the membrane. An example is the **Na^+–Ca^{2+} exchanger**, which exchanges three Na^+ ions for a Ca^{2+} ion (see Chapter 11). Na^+ pump inhibitors (e.g. **digoxin**) reduce the Na^+ gradient, and thus indirectly inhibit secondary transport. Pumps are regulated by ion concentrations, and modulated by second messengers.

Ion pumps and membrane potential

The Na^+ pump and Na^+–Ca^{2+} exchanger are **electrogenic** as unequal amounts of charge are transported, and thus a small ionic current is generated. They can therefore both affect, and be affected by, membrane potential. An example is Na^+–Ca^{2+} exchange during the cardiac muscle action potential (see Chapters 10, 11).

Electrophysiology of cardiac muscle and origin of the heart beat

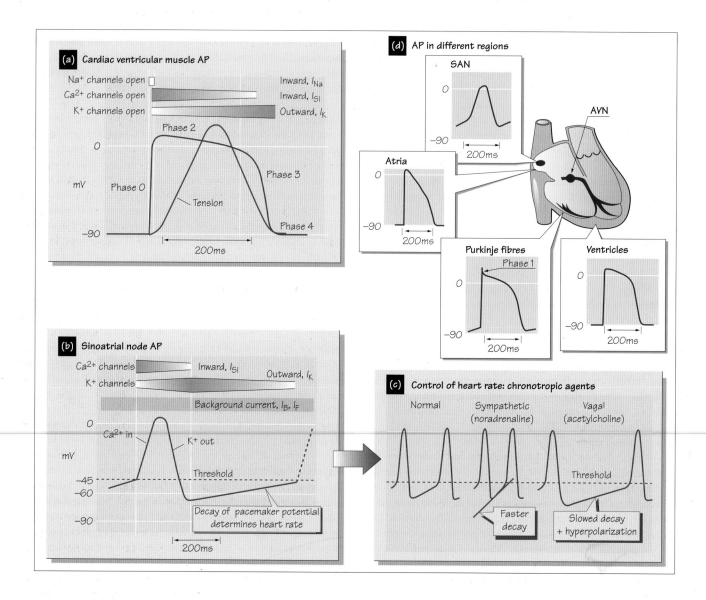

An action potential (AP) is the transient depolarization of a cell as a result of activity of ion channels. The cardiac AP is considerably longer than those occurring in nerve or skeletal muscle (~300 ms vs ~1–3 ms). This is due to the presence of a **plateau phase** in cardiac muscle, lasting for 200–300 ms.

Ventricular muscle action potential (Figure 10a)
Initiation of the action potential

At rest, the membrane is most permeable to K^+ and the **resting membrane potential** (RMP) is primarily dependent on the K^+ concentration gradient (see Chapter 9). An AP is initiated when the membrane is depolarized to a **threshold potential** (~ -65 mV) by transmission from adjacent cells through **gap junctions** (see Chapter 2). At threshold, sufficient **voltage-gated Na$^+$ channels** open for the inward current caused by entry of Na^+ (I_{Na}) to overcome the outward current through K^+ channels, causing further depolarization. More Na^+ channels there-

fore open, and depolarization becomes self-generating (*positive feedback*); this results in a very rapid upstroke (phase 0; ~500 V/s). The membrane is now more permeable to Na^+ than K^+ and so the membrane potential moves towards the Na^+ equilibrium potential ($\sim +65$ mV) (see Chapter 9). It does not reach it because of the remaining K^+ permeability, and also because the Na^+ channels start to **inactivate** (see Chapter 9). As these channels cannot be reactivated until the potential returns to < -60 mV, another AP cannot be initiated until the cell repolarizes *to at least* this potential (**absolute refractory period**). At more negative potentials increasing numbers of Na^+ channels reactivate, allowing an AP to be initiated by a sufficiently large stimulus (**relative refractory period**). When the cell is completely repolarized all Na^+ channels are in their resting state. As the AP and thus refractory period are similar in length to the twitch (Figure 10a), cardiac muscle cannot be tetanized.

The plateau phase

By the end of the upstroke all Na^+ channels are inactivated and Na^+ permeability returns to resting values. In skeletal muscle the cell therefore repolarizes within ~3 ms. In cardiac muscle, however, the membrane potential remains close to 0 mV for ~250 ms. This **plateau phase** (phase 2) is due to Ca^{2+} entering the cell via **voltage-sensitive (L-type) Ca^{2+} channels**, which activate relatively slowly when the membrane potential becomes more positive than ~ −35 mV. The resultant Ca^{2+} current (**slow inward current** or I_{SI}), coupled with a reduced K^+ outward current, is sufficient to slow repolarization until the potential falls to ~ −20 mV. The length of the plateau is related to slow **inactivation** of Ca^{2+} channels. Ca^{2+} entry during the plateau is vital for cardiac muscle contraction (see Chapter 11).

Repolarization (phase 3)

At the end of the plateau the K^+ permeability and outward current increase, and membrane potential returns to resting levels (phase 4). Several types of K^+ channel contribute to repolarization. Factors that influence these channels will affect the rate of repolarization, and hence the length of AP (see Chapter 51).

Role of Na^+–Ca^{2+} exchange during the action potential

In the early stages of the plateau, when it is most positive and the Na^+ electrochemical gradient is therefore smallest, the Na^+–Ca^{2+} exchanger (see Chapter 9) may reverse, and contribute to inward movement of Ca^{2+}. As the plateau decays and becomes more negative the Na^+ gradient increases, and the Na^+–Ca^{2+} exchanger returns to its usual function of expelling Ca^{2+}. The resulting influx of Na^+ ions causes an inward current that may slow repolarization and reduce the rate of decay of the plateau, thus lengthening the AP.

Sinoatrial node and the origin of the heart beat

The AP of the **sinoatrial node** (SAN, Figure 10b) differs in several important aspects from that of the ventricle. The upstroke in the SAN is much slower than in the ventricle. This is because there are no functional Na^+ channels, and depolarization is caused by Ca^{2+} entry via slowly activating L-type Ca^{2+} channels. The slower upstroke leads to slower conduction from cell to cell (see Chapter 12). This is of particular importance in the **atrioventricular node** (AVN), which has a similar AP to the SAN.

In contrast to the ventricle, the SAN has an unstable resting potential which decays from ~ −60 mV to a threshold potential of ~ −40 mV, at which point an AP is initiated. The threshold potential is more positive than in the ventricle, because voltage-gated Ca^{2+} channels, responsible for the upstroke in the SAN, have a more positive threshold than voltage-gated Na^+ channels, responsible for the upstroke in the ventricle. The rate of decay of the SAN resting potential determines the rate at which APs are generated, and hence heart rate. The resting potential is therefore commonly called the **pacemaker potential**. It primarily relies on a K^+ outward current that slowly decays with time (I_K), and two relatively stable inward currents, mostly due to the inward movement of Na^+. These are I_b, which is also present in other cardiac cells, and I_f ('*funny*'), which appears to be specific to the SAN. As the outward I_K decays, this allows the contribution from the inward I_f and I_b to become more dominant, and the membrane depolarizes.

Factors influencing these currents alter the slope of the pacemaker and thus heart rate, and are called **chronotropic agents**. The sympathetic neurotransmitter norepinephrine increases heart rate by increasing the slope of the pacemaker, caused by an increase in the size of I_f. It also reduces the length of the AP by increasing the rate of Ca^{2+} entry and hence the slope of the upstroke. The parasympathetic transmitter acetylcholine reduces the slope of the pacemaker, and causes a small hyperpolarization, both of which increase the time required to reach threshold, and reduce heart rate (Figure 10c).

Action potentials in other regions of the heart (Figure 10d)

AVN APs are similar to those of the SAN. Atrial muscle has a similar AP to ventricular muscle, although the shape is more triangular. **Purkinje fibres** in the conduction system have a spike at the peak of upstroke (phase 1). This relates to a greater inward Na^+ current and more rapid upstroke, and contributes to faster conduction. The AVN, bundle of His and Purkinje system may also have decaying resting potentials that can act as pacemakers. However, the SAN is normally fastest and predominates. This is called **dominance** or **overdrive suppression**.

Effects of plasma [K^+]

Several conditions increase plasma [K^+] (e.g. renal failure, tissue damage). If it rises above ~5.5 mM (**hyperkalaemia**) there can be serious consequences, as the membrane depolarizes and becomes closer to threshold potential. This can cause dangerous arrhythmias (e.g. ventricular fibrillation), especially where the myocardium is diseased (see Chapter 48). Hyperkalaemia also slows and weakens the AP upstroke due to partial inactivation of Na^+ channels, and slows conduction. Above 8 mM this leads to complete cessation of conduction (**heart block**). Conversely **hypokalaemia** (<~3 mM [K^+]) hyperpolarizes the membrane, making it more difficult to reach threshold and also affecting conduction. Hypokalaemia is commonly associated with diuretic therapy in heart disease (e.g. Chapter 47).

11 Excitation–contraction coupling in cardiac muscle cells

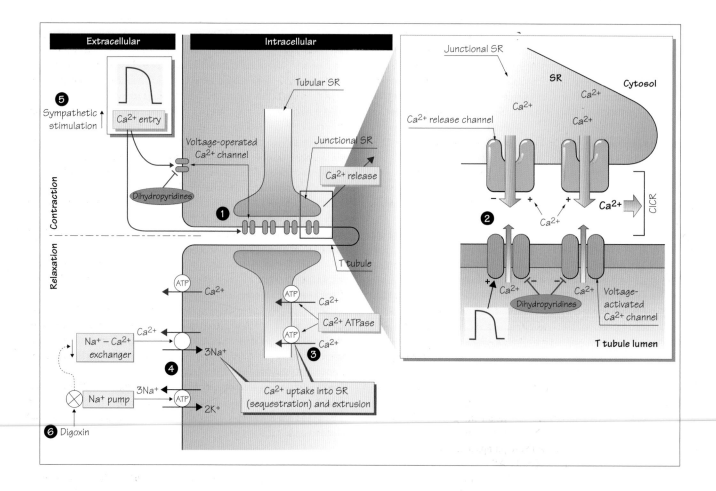

Cardiac muscle contracts when cytosolic [Ca^{2+}] rises above about 100 nM. This rise in [Ca^{2+}] couples the action potential (AP) to contraction, and the mechanisms involved are referred to as **excitation–contraction coupling**. The relationship between cardiac muscle force and stretch is discussed in Chapter 15. The ability of cardiac muscle to generate force *for any given fibre length* is described as its **contractility**. This depends on cytosolic [Ca^{2+}], and to a lesser extent on factors that affect Ca^{2+} sensitivity of the contractile apparatus. The contractility of cardiac muscle is primarily dependent on the way that the cell handles Ca^{2+}.

Initiation of contraction

During the **plateau phase** of the AP, Ca^{2+} enters the cell through L-**type voltage-gated Ca^{2+} channels** in the **sarcolemma** (figure). L-type channels are specifically blocked by **dihydropyridines** (e.g. **nifedipine**) and *verapamil*. However, the amount of Ca^{2+} that enters the cell is less than 20% of that required for the observed rise in cytosolic [Ca^{2+}] ([Ca^{2+}]$_i$). The rest is released from the **sarcoplasmic reticulum** (SR), where Ca^{2+} is stored in high concentrations associated with **calsequestrin**. The action potential travels down the **T tubules** which are close to, but do not touch, the **terminal cisternae** of the SR ❶. During the first 1–2 ms of the plateau Ca^{2+} enters and causes a rise in [Ca^{2+}] in the gap between the sarcolemma and the SR. This rise in [Ca^{2+}]

activates Ca^{2+}-sensitive **Ca^{2+} release channels** in the SR ❷, through which stored Ca^{2+} floods into the cytoplasm down its concentration gradient. This process is called **calcium-induced calcium release (CICR)**. The combination of Ca^{2+} release and Ca^{2+} entry across the membrane causes a rapid increase in [Ca^{2+}]$_i$ over the next 10 ms, and initiates contraction. Note that cardiac muscle differs from skeletal muscle, in that CICR is entirely responsible for Ca^{2+} release from the SR. The action potential itself in the absence of Ca^{2+} entry cannot cause Ca^{2+} release, and in the *absence of external Ca^{2+} there is no contraction of cardiac muscle*.

The amount of Ca^{2+} released depends both on how much is stored in the SR and on the amount of Ca^{2+} entering across the sarcolemma. Modulation of the latter is a key way in which cardiac function is regulated (see 'Inotropic agents' below). Peak [Ca^{2+}]$_i$ normally rises to ~2 μM, although maximum contraction occurs when [Ca^{2+}]$_i$ rises above 10 μM.

Generation of tension

The physical arrangement of **actin** and **myosin** filaments is discussed in Chapter 2. Force is generated when the myosin heads protruding from the thick filament bind to sites on actin to form **crossbridges**, and drag the actin past in a ratchet fashion, using ATP bound to myosin as an energy source. This is the **sliding filament** or **crossbridge mechanism** of muscle contraction.

Regulation of crossbridge formation

In cardiac muscle as in skeletal muscle, $[Ca^{2+}]_i$ controls crossbridge formation via the regulatory proteins **tropomyosin** and **troponin**. Tropomyosin is a coiled strand which, at rest, lies in the cleft between the two actin chains that form the thin filament helix, and covers the myosin binding sites on the actin. The myosin heads therefore cannot bind, and there is no tension. Troponin is formed from a complex of three smaller globular proteins (**troponin C, I and T**), which is bound to tropomyosin by **troponin T** at intervals of 40 nm. When $[Ca^{2+}]_i$ rises above 100 nM, Ca^{2+} binds to **troponin C** and there is a conformational change involving dissociation of **troponin I** from actin, which allows tropomyosin to shift out of the actin cleft. The binding sites are uncovered, myosin crossbridges form, and tension develops. Tension is related to the number of active crossbridges, and will increase until all troponin C is bound to Ca^{2+} ($[Ca^{2+}]_i > 10$ μM).

Relaxation mechanisms

When $[Ca^{2+}]_i$ rises above the resting level (~100 nM), ATP-dependent Ca^{2+} pumps (**Ca^{2+}-ATPase**) in the tubular part of the SR are activated, and start to pump (**sequester**) Ca^{2+} from the cytosol back into the SR ❸. As the AP repolarizes and voltage-dependent Ca^{2+} channels inactivate, this mechanism reduces $[Ca^{2+}]_i$ towards resting levels, Ca^{2+} ions dissociate from troponin C, and the muscle relaxes.

If there were no other mechanisms to remove Ca^{2+} from the cell, the size of the SR Ca^{2+} store would gradually increase as more Ca^{2+} enters during each AP. Excess Ca^{2+} is transported out of the cell by the **Na^+–Ca^{2+} exchanger** in the sarcolemma ❹ (see Chapter 9). This uses the inward Na^+ electrochemical gradient as an energy source to pump Ca^{2+} out, and in the process three Na^+ ions enter the cell for each Ca^{2+} ion removed. There are also Ca^{2+}-ATPase pumps in the sarcolemma, but their importance is minor. At the end of the AP about 80% of the Ca^{2+} will have been resequestered into the SR, and most of the rest ejected from the cell. The remainder is slowly pumped out during the diastolic interval.

Regulation of contractility

Inotropic agents

Factors that alter the contractility of cardiac muscle are called **inotropic agents**. A positive inotropic agent increases contractility, whereas a negative one decreases it. Most act via mechanisms that regulate $[Ca^{2+}]_i$, although some may alter Ca^{2+} binding to troponin C. For example, a high plasma $[Ca^{2+}]$ increases contractility by increasing Ca^{2+} entry during the AP.

Norepinephrine from sympathetic nerve endings, and to a lesser extent circulating **epinephrine**, are the most important physiological inotropic agents. They also increase heart rate (positive **chronotropes**; see Chapter 10). Norepinephrine binds to β_1-adrenoceptors on the sarcolemma, and thus increases cAMP. cAMP-mediated phosphorylation of Ca^{2+} channels increases Ca^{2+} entry during the AP ❺ (see Chapter 9), and thus elevates $[Ca^{2+}]_i$, largely by increasing Ca^{2+} release from the SR (❷; see above). Norepinephrine may also activate Ca^{2+} channels directly via G-proteins (see Chapter 9). The rate of Ca^{2+} reuptake into the SR, and hence the rate of relaxation, is also increased by norepinephrine, via cAMP-mediated phosphorylation of **phospholamban**, a regulatory protein associated with the Ca^{2+}-ATPase ❸.

Cardiac glycosides such as **digoxin** inhibit the **Na^+ pump** which removes $[Na^+]$ from the cell ❻. Intracellular $[Na^+]$ therefore increases, so reducing the Na^+ gradient across the sarcolemma that drives Na^+–Ca^{2+} exchange ❹ (see Chapter 9). Consequently, less Ca^{2+} is pumped out of the cell, so more is left in the SR. There is therefore more available for release, and peak $[Ca^{2+}]_i$ and tension increases. The clinical use of digoxin is discussed in Chapter 47.

Overstimulation by positive inotropes can lead to **Ca^{2+} overload**, and damage due to excessive uptake of Ca^{2+} by the SR and mitochondria. This is important for the progressive decline in myocardial function seen in **chronic heart failure** (see Chapter 46), when sympathetic stimulation is high.

Acidosis is *negatively* inotropic, largely by interfering with the actions of Ca^{2+}. This is important in **myocardial ischaemia** and **heart failure** (see Chapter 46), where poor perfusion can lead to **lactic acidosis** and so depress cardiac function.

The influence of heart rate

When heart rate increases there is a proportional rise in cardiac muscle force. This phenomenon is known as the **staircase**, **Treppe** or **Bowditch** effect. It can be attributed both to an increase in cytosolic $[Na^+]$ due to the greater frequency of APs, with a consequent inhibition of the Na^+–Ca^{2+} exchanger (see above), and to a decreased diastolic interval over which Ca^{2+} can be extruded from the cell, resulting in more Ca^{2+} in the SR.

12 Electrical conduction system in the heart

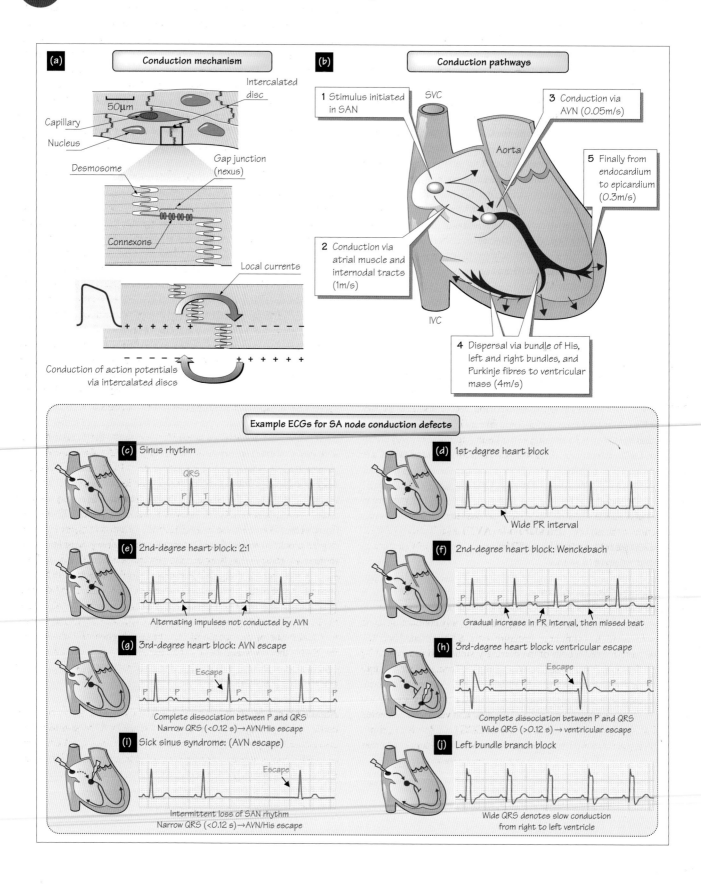

(a) Conduction mechanism

Intercalated disc

50 μm

Capillary

Nucleus

Desmosome

Gap junction (nexus)

Connexons

Local currents

Conduction of action potentials via intercalated discs

(b) Conduction pathways

1 Stimulus initiated in SAN

SVC

3 Conduction via AVN (0.05m/s)

Aorta

5 Finally from endocardium to epicardium (0.3m/s)

2 Conduction via atrial muscle and internodal tracts (1m/s)

IVC

4 Dispersal via bundle of His, left and right bundles, and Purkinje fibres to ventricular mass (4m/s)

Example ECGs for SA node conduction defects

(c) Sinus rhythm

QRS

P   T

(d) 1st-degree heart block

Wide PR interval

(e) 2nd-degree heart block: 2:1

P   P   P   P

Alternating impulses not conducted by AVN

(f) 2nd-degree heart block: Wenckebach

P   P   P   P   P   P

Gradual increase in PR interval, then missed beat

(g) 3rd-degree heart block: AVN escape

Escape

P   P   P   P   P   P

Complete dissociation between P and QRS
Narrow QRS (<0.12 s)→AVN/His escape

(h) 3rd-degree heart block: ventricular escape

Escape

P   P   P   P   P   P

Complete dissociation between P and QRS
Wide QRS (>0.12 s) → ventricular escape

(i) Sick sinus syndrome: (AVN escape)

Escape

Intermittent loss of SAN rhythm
Narrow QRS (<0.12 s)→AVN/His escape

(j) Left bundle branch block

Wide QRS denotes slow conduction from right to left ventricle

Electrical conduction in cardiac muscle
(Figure 12b)

Cardiac muscle cells are connected via **intercalated discs** (see Chapter 2). These incorporate regions where the membranes of adjacent cells are very close, called **gap junctions.** Gap junctions consist of proteins known as **connexons**, which form low-resistance junctions between cells. They allow the transfer of small ions and thus electrical current. As all cells are therefore electrically connected, cardiac muscle is said to be a **functional** (or electrical) **syncytium.** If an action potential (AP) is initiated in one cell, local currents via gap junctions will cause adjacent cells to depolarize, initiating their own AP. A wave of depolarization will therefore be conducted from cell to cell throughout the myocardium. The rate of conduction is partly dependent on gap junction resistance and the *size of the depolarizing current.* This is related to the **upstroke velocity of the AP** (phase 0). Drugs that slow phase 0 slow conduction (e.g. lidocaine, class I antiarrhythmics). Pathological conditions such as ischaemia may increase gap junction resistance, and slow or abolish conduction. Retrograde conduction does not normally occur because the original cell is refractory (see Chapter 10). Transfer of the pacemaker signal from the sinoatrial node (SAN) and synchronous contraction of the ventricles is facilitated by **conduction pathways** formed from modified muscle cells.

Conduction pathways in the heart (Figure 12a)
Sinoatrial node

The heart beat is normally initiated in the **sinoatrial node** (SAN), located at the junction of the superior vena cava and right atrium. The SAN is a ~2-mm-wide group of small elongated muscle cells that extends for ~2 cm down the sulcus terminalis. It has a rich capillary supply and sympathetic and parasympathetic (right vagal) nerve endings. The SAN generates an AP about once a second (sinus rhythm, see Figure 12c; see Chapter 10).

Atrial conduction

The impulse spreads from the SAN across the atria at ~1 m/s. Conduction to the **atrioventricular node** (AVN) is facilitated by larger cells in the three **internodal tracts** of Bachmann (anterior), Wenckebach (middle) and Thorel (posterior).

The atrioventricular node

The atria and ventricles are separated by the non-conducting **annulus fibrosus.** The AVN marks the upper region of the only conducting route through this band. It is similar in structure to the SAN, situated near the interatrial septum and mouth of the coronary sinus, and innervated by sympathetic and left vagal nerves. The complex arrangement of small cells and slow AP upstroke (see Chapter 10) result in a very slow conduction velocity (~0.05 m/s). This provides a functionally significant delay of ~0.1 s between contraction of the atria and ventricles, reflected by the **PR interval** of the electrocardigram (**ECG**). Sympathetic stimulation increases conduction velocity and reduces the delay, whereas vagal stimulation slows conduction and increases the delay.

Bundle of His and Purkinje system

The **bundle of His** transfers the impulse from the AVN to the top of the interventricular septum. Close to the attachment of the tricuspid septal cusp it branches to form the **left** and **right bundle branches**. The left bundle divides into the posterior and anterior fascicles. The bundles travel under the endocardium down the walls of the septum, and at the base divide into the multiple fibres of the **Purkinje system**. This distributes the impulse over the inner walls of the ventricles. Cells in the bundle of His and Purkinje system have large diameters (~40 µm) and rapid AP upstroke, and consequently fast conduction (~4 m/s). The impulse spreads from the Purkinje cells through the ventricular wall to the epicardium at 0.3–1 m/s, thereby initiating contraction.

Abnormalities of impulse generation or conduction (see also Chapters 48–50)

Sinus tachycardia (100–200 beats/min;) is normal in exercise or excitement, but also occurs when pathological stimuli (e.g. phaeochromocytoma, heart failure, thyrotoxicosis) elevate sympathetic tone and accelerate SAN firing. Sinus tachycardia generally starts and stops gradually. Treatment, if required, involves removing the underlying cause. The ECG is otherwise normal. Conversely **sick sinus syndrome**, generally caused by SAN fibrosis, causes slowed impulse generation and **bradycardia** (slow heart rate), or a sustained or intermittent failure of the impulse to reach the AVN, termed **sinoatrial block** (Figure 12i). Since other parts of the conduction system also exhibit pacemaking activity (see Chapter 10), sick sinus syndrome can result in the emergence of **escape** beats or rhythms in which impulses arising elsewhere (usually the AVN) can activate ventricular depolarization. Sick sinus syndrome can be treated by implantation of a pacemaker.

Heart block Abnormally slow conduction in the AVN can result in incomplete (**first-degree**) heart block (Figure 12d), where the delay is greater than normal, resulting in an extended PR interval. **Second-degree** heart block occurs when only a fraction of impulses from the atria are conducted; for example, ventricular contraction is only initiated every second or third atrial contraction (**2:1 or 3:1 block**; Mobitz II; Figure 12e). **Wenckebach block** (Mobitz I) is another type of second-degree block, in which the PR interval progressively lengthens until there is no transmission from atria to ventricles and a QRS complex is missed; the cycle then begins again (Figure 12f). Patients with first- or second-degree block are often asymptomatic. Complete (**third-degree**) heart block occurs when conduction between atria and ventricles is abolished (Figures 12g and 12h). This can result from ischaemic damage to nodal tissue or the bundle of His. In the absence of a signal from the SAN, the AVN and bundle of His can generate a heart rate of ~40 beats/min. Some ventricular cells spontaneously generate APs, but at a rate less than 20/min.

Bundle branch block When one branch of the bundle of His does not conduct, the part of the ventricle that it serves will be stimulated by conduction through the myocardium from unaffected areas. As this form of conduction is slower, activation is delayed and the QRS complex broadened (Figure 12j). This is left or right bundle branch block.

13 Vascular smooth muscle excitation–contraction coupling

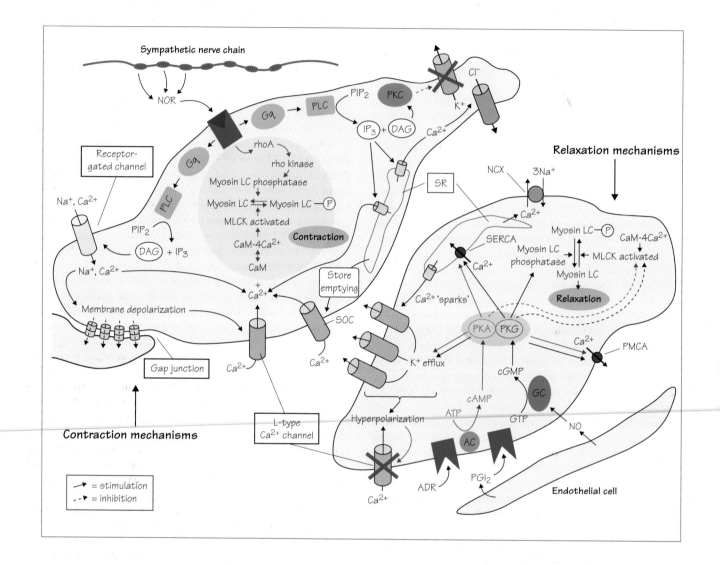

Vascular smooth muscle (VSM) contraction is, like that of cardiac muscle, controlled by the *intracellular Ca^{2+} concentration* $[Ca^{2+}]_i$. Unlike cardiac muscle cells, however, VSM cells lack troponin and utilize a *myosin-based system* to regulate contraction.

Regulation of contraction by Ca^{2+} and myosin phosphorylation (see shaded area in left cell of figure)

Vasoconstricting stimuli initiate VSM cell contraction by increasing $[Ca^{2+}]_i$ from its basal level of ~100 nM. Force development is proportional to the increase in $[Ca^{2+}]_i$, with maximal contraction occurring at ~1 µM $[Ca^{2+}]_i$. The rise in $[Ca^{2+}]_i$ promotes its binding to the cytoplasmic regulatory protein **calmodulin (CaM)**. Once a calmodulin molecule has bound four Ca^{2+} ions, it can activate the enzyme **myosin light-chain kinase** (MLCK). MLCK in turn phosphorylates two 20-kDa subunits ('**light chains**') contained within the 'head' of each myosin molecule. Phosphorylated myosin then forms crossbridges with actin, using ATP hydrolysis as an energy source to produce contraction.

Actin–myosin interactions during crossbridge cycling are similar to those in cardiac myocytes (see Chapter 11).

The degree of myosin light-chain phosphorylation, which determines crossbridge turnover, is a balance between the activity of MLCK and a **myosin light-chain phosphatase** which dephosphorylates the light chains. Once $[Ca^{2+}]_i$ falls, MLCK activity diminishes and relaxation occurs as light-chain phosphorylation is returned to basal levels by the phosphatase.

VSM cells *in vivo* maintain a tonic level of partial contraction that varies with fluctuations in the vasoconstricting and vasodilating influences to which they are exposed. VSM cells avoid fatigue during prolonged contractions because their rate of ATP consumption is 300-fold lower than that of skeletal muscle fibres. This is possible because the crossbridge cycle is much slower than in striated muscles. The maximum crossbridge cycling rate of smooth muscle during shortening is only about 1/10 of that in striated muscles, as a result of differences in the types of myosin present. In addition, once they have shortened, vascular cells can maintain contraction with an even lower expenditure of ATP because the myosin crossbridges remain attached to actin for a longer time, thus 'locking in' shortening.

Vasoconstricting mechanisms

The binding to receptors of **norepinephrine** and other important vasoconstrictors such as **endothelin, thromboxane A_2, angiotensin II** and **vasopressin** stimulates VSM contraction via common **G-protein-mediated** pathways (see left cell).

Effects of IP_3 and diacylglycerol

Binding of vasoconstrictors to receptors activates the G-protein **Gq**, which stimulates the enzyme **phospholipase C**. Phospholipase C splits the membrane phospholipid phosphatidylinositol 1,4-bisphosphate (PIP_2), generating the second messengers inositol 1,4,5-triphosphate (IP_3), and diacylglycerol (**DAG**). IP_3 binds to and opens Ca^{2+} channels on the membrane of the **sarcoplasmic reticulum** (SR). This allows Ca^{2+}, which is stored in high concentrations within the SR, to flood out into the cytoplasm and rapidly increase $[Ca^{2+}]_i$. DAG activates **protein kinase C** (PKC). This activates the protein CPI-17, which phosphorylates and inhibits myosin phosphatase, promoting contraction.

Ca^{2+} influx mechanisms

Vasoconstrictors also cause **membrane depolarization** via several mechanisms. First, the release of SR Ca^{2+}, which they initiate, opens **Ca^{2+}-activated chloride channels** in the plasma membrane. Second, vasoconstrictors may act via DAG and PKC to cause depolarization by *inhibiting* the activity of **K^+ channels**. Third, vasoconstrictors induce both membrane depolarization and Ca^{2+} entry into VSM cells by opening **receptor-gated cation channels**, which allow the influx of both Na^+ and Ca^{2+} ions.

The membrane depolarization elicited by vasoconstrictors opens L-type voltage-gated Ca^{2+} channels similar to those found in cardiac myocytes. With sufficient depolarization, some blood vessels may fire brief Ca^{2+} channel-mediated APs that cause transient contractions. More often, however, vasoconstrictors cause graded depolarizations, during which sufficient Ca^{2+} influx occurs to cause more sustained contractions. Vasoconstrictors further enhance Ca^{2+} influx through L-type channels by evoking channel phosphorylation. Furthermore, depletion of Ca^{2+} from the SR due to the action of IP_3 opens a **store-operated Ca^{2+} channel** (SOC) in the cell membrane which admits Ca^{2+} to the cell.

As well as raising $[Ca^{2+}]_i$, vasoconstrictors also promote contraction by a process termed **Ca^{2+} sensitization**. Ca^{2+} sensitization is caused by the inhibition of myosin phosphatase. This increases myosin light-chain phosphorylation, and therefore force development, even with minimal increases in $[Ca^{2+}]_i$ and MLCK activity. Although PKC has this effect (see above), phosphatase inhibition is primarily caused by **rhoA kinase**, an enzyme stimulated by the *ras* type G-protein rhoA, which is activated by vasoconstrictors by an as yet unknown mechanism.

The relative importance of the excitatory mechanisms listed above varies between different vasoconstrictors and vascular beds. In resistance arteries depolarization and Ca^{2+} influx through voltage-gated channels are probably most important.

Ca^{2+} removal and vasodilator mechanisms
(see right cell of figure)

Several mechanisms serve to remove Ca^{2+} from the cytoplasm. These are continually active, allowing cells both to recover from stimulation and to maintain a low basal $[Ca^{2+}]_i$ in the face of the enormous electrochemical gradient tending to drive Ca^{2+} into cells even when they are not stimulated. The **smooth endoplasmic reticulum Ca^{2+}-ATPase** (**SERCA**) pumps Ca^{2+} from the cytoplasm into the SR. This process is referred to as **Ca^{2+} sequestration**. An analogous **plasma membrane Ca^{2+}-ATPase** (**PMCA**) pumps Ca^{2+} from the cytoplasm into the extracellular space (**Ca^{2+} extrusion**). Cells also extrude Ca^{2+} via a **Na^+-Ca^{2+} exchanger** (**NCX**) located in the cell membrane, which is similar to that found in cardiac cells (see Chapter 11). The NCX may be localized to areas of the plasma membrane which are approached closely by the sarcoplasmic reticulum, allowing any Ca^{2+} leaking from the SR to be quickly ejected from the cell without causing tension development.

Most vasodilators acting on smooth muscle cells cause relaxation by activating either the cyclic **GMP** (e.g. nitric oxide, atrial natriuretic peptide) or cyclic **AMP** (e.g. adenosine, prostacyclin, β-receptor agonists) second messenger systems. Both second messengers activate kinases, which act by phosphorylating overlapping sets of cellular proteins. cGMP activates **cyclic GMP-dependent protein kinase (protein kinase G or PKG)**. PKG has multiple vasodilating effects. It activates K^+ channels by phosphorylating them, leading to a membrane hyperpolarization which inhibits Ca^{2+} influx by switching off voltage-gated Ca^{2+} channels, a fraction of which are open even at the resting membrane potential. PKG also stimulates the sequestration and extrusion of Ca^{2+} sequestration by activating the Ca^{2+} pumps, and it stimulates myosin phophatase by inhibiting rho kinase.

Cyclic AMP exerts its effects via **cyclic AMP-dependent protein kinase (protein kinase A or PKA)**, although high levels of cAMP have also been shown to stimulate PKG. PKA lowers $[Ca^{2+}]_i$ by stimulating Ca^{2+} pumps, and also by opening K^+ channels (again via phosphorylation). The stimulation of SERCA and consequent loading of SR $[Ca^{2+}]$ by PKA may also indirectly activate **Ca^{2+}-activated K^+ (BK_{Ca}) channels** by increasing the frequency of 'Ca^{2+} sparks'. These are transient elevations of $[Ca^{2+}]_i$ near the cell membrane caused by the opening of ryanodine receptors (RyRs). PKA can also phosphorylate MLCK, thereby inhibiting its activity. The contribution of this mechanism to relaxation under physiological conditions is, however, controversial.

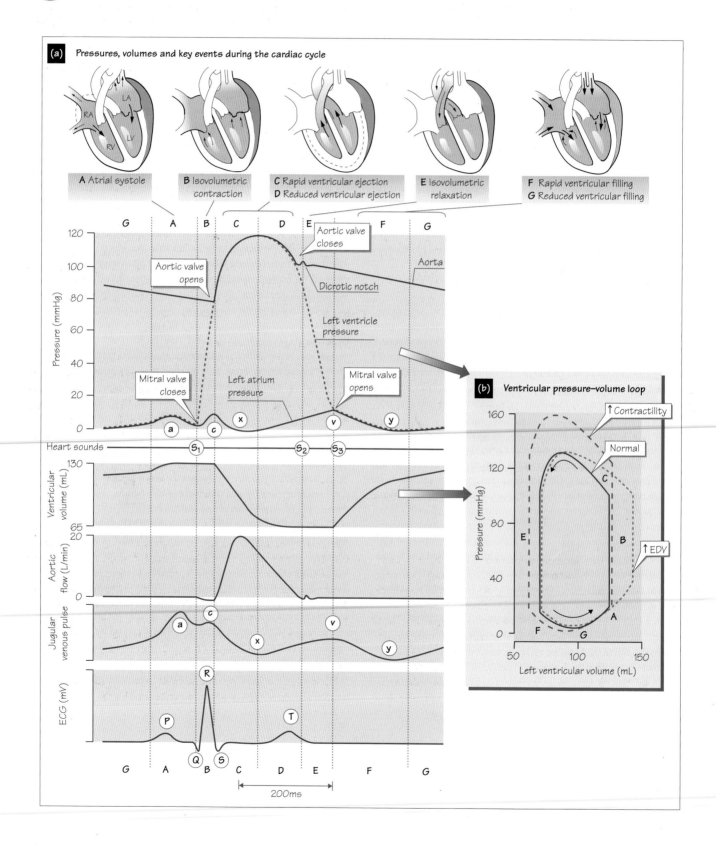

The **cardiac cycle** is the sequence of mechanical events that occurs during a single heart beat (Figure 14a).

Towards the end of **diastole** (G) all chambers of the heart are relaxed. The valves between the atria and ventricles are open (**AV valves**: right, **tricuspid**; left, **mitral**), because atrial pressure remains slightly greater than ventricular pressure until the ventricles are fully distended. The **pulmonary** and **aortic** (semilunar) **outflow valves** are closed, as pulmonary artery and aortic pressure is greater than ventricular pressure. The cycle begins when the **sinoatrial node** initiates the heart beat.

Atrial systole (A)

Contraction of the atria completes ventricular filling. At rest, the atria contribute less than 20% of ventricular volume, but this proportion increases with heart rate, as diastole shortens and there is less time for ventricular filling. There are no valves between the veins and atria, and some blood regurgitates into the veins. The **a wave** of atrial and venous pressure traces reflects atrial systole. Ventricular volume after filling is known as **end-diastolic volume** (EDV), and is ~120–140 mL. The equivalent pressure (**end-diastolic pressure**, EDP) is less than 10 mmHg, and is higher in the left ventricle than in the right due to the more muscular and therefore stiffer left ventricular wall. EDV is an important determinant of the strength of the subsequent contraction (Starling's law; see Chapter 15). Atrial depolarization causes the **P wave** of the ECG.

Ventricular systole

Ventricular contraction causes a sharp rise in ventricular pressure, and the atrioventricular (AV) valves close once this exceeds atrial pressure. Closure of the AV valves causes the **first heart sound** (S_1). Ventricular depolarization is associated with the **QRS complex** of the ECG. During the initial phase of ventricular contraction pressure is less than that in the pulmonary artery and aorta, so the outflow valves remain closed. This is **isovolumetric contraction** (B), as ventricular volume does not change. The increasing pressure causes the AV valves to bulge into the atria, resulting in the small atrial pressure wave (**c wave**), followed by a fall (**x descent**).

Ejection

The outflow valves open when pressure in the ventricle exceeds that in its respective artery. Note that pulmonary artery pressure (~15 mmHg) is considerably less than that in the aorta (~80 mmHg). Flow into the arteries is initially very rapid (**rapid ejection phase**, C), but as contraction wanes ejection is reduced (**reduced ejection phase**, D). Rapid ejection can sometimes be heard as a **murmur**. Active contraction ceases during the second half of ejection, and the muscle repolarizes. This is associated with the **T wave** of the ECG. Ventricular pressure during the reduced ejection phase is slightly less than that in the artery, but blood continues to flow out of the ventricle because of momentum.

Eventually the flow briefly reverses, causing closure of the outflow valve and a small increase in aortic pressure, the **dicrotic notch**. Closure of the semilunar valves is associated with the second heart sound (S_2).

The amount of blood ejected by the ventricle in one beat is the **stroke volume**, ~70 mL. About 50 mL of blood is therefore left in the ventricle at the end of systole (**end-systolic volume**). The proportion of EDV that is ejected (stroke volume/EDV) is the **ejection fraction**. During the last two-thirds of systole atrial pressure rises as a result of filling from the veins (**v wave**).

Diastole – relaxation and refilling

Following closure of the outflow valves the ventricles are rapidly relaxing. Ventricular pressure is still greater than atrial pressure however, and the AV valves remain closed. This is **isovolumetric relaxation** (E). When ventricular pressure falls below atrial pressure, the AV valves open, and atrial pressure falls (**y descent**) as the ventricles refill (**rapid ventricular refilling**, F). This is assisted by elastic recoil of the ventricular walls, essentially sucking in the blood. A **third heart sound** (S_3) may be heard in young people, or when EDP is high. As the ventricles relax completely refilling slows (**reduced refilling**, G). This continues during the last two-thirds of diastole due to venous flow. At rest, diastole is twice the length of systole, but decreases proportionately during exercise and as heart rate increases.

The pressure–volume loop

Ventricular pressure plotted against volume generates a loop (Figure 14b). The shape of the loop is affected by **contractility** (see Chapters 11, 15) and **compliance** (*'stretchiness'*) of the ventricle, and factors that alter **refilling** or **ejection** (e.g. CVP, afterload). The bottom dotted line shows the passive elastic properties of the ventricle (compliance). If compliance was decreased as a result of fibrotic damage following an infarct, the curve would be steeper. The area of the loop (Δ pressure $\times \Delta$ volume) is a measure of work done during a beat, and is an indicator of cardiac function. A clinical estimate of **stroke work** is calculated from mean arterial pressure $\times$ stroke volume.

The pulse

The pulse is caused by pressure waves travelling down the vascular tree. The shape of the arterial pulse is modified by the compliance and size of the artery. A stiff artery, as in advancing age or atherosclerosis, results in a sharper pulse. The pulse also becomes sharper as artery size decreases (see Chapter 17). Reflections back up the artery from points where resistance to flow increases, e.g. where the artery divides, can give rise to further peaks. The **jugular venous pulse** reflects the right atrial pressure, and has corresponding **a, c** and **v waves**, and **x** and **y descents** (see above).

Basic examination of the cardiac cycle, including cardiac auscultation, pulses and blood pressure, is described in Chapter 30.

Control of cardiac output and Starling's law of the heart

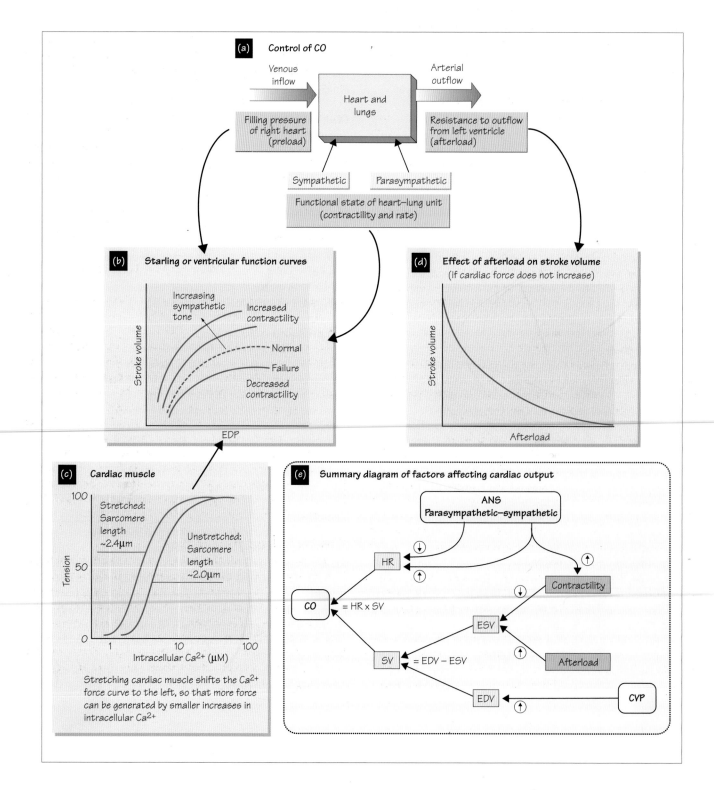

(a) Control of CO

Venous inflow

Arterial outflow

Heart and lungs

Filling pressure of right heart (preload)

Resistance to outflow from left ventricle (afterload)

Sympathetic

Parasympathetic

Functional state of heart–lung unit (contractility and rate)

(b) Starling or ventricular function curves

Increasing sympathetic tone

Increased contractility

Normal

Failure

Decreased contractility

Stroke volume

EDP

(d) Effect of afterload on stroke volume
(if cardiac force does not increase)

Stroke volume

Afterload

(c) Cardiac muscle

Stretched: Sarcomere length ~2.4μm

Unstretched: Sarcomere length ~2.0μm

Tension

Intracellular Ca^{2+} (μM)

Stretching cardiac muscle shifts the Ca^{2+} force curve to the left, so that more force can be generated by smaller increases in intracellular Ca^{2+}

(e) Summary diagram of factors affecting cardiac output

ANS Parasympathetic–sympathetic

HR

Contractility

CO = HR × SV

ESV

SV = EDV − ESV

Afterload

EDV

CVP

Cardiac output (CO) is the volume of blood pumped through the heart per minute, i.e. stroke volume (SV) × heart rate (HR). In a normal 70-kg man, cardiac output at rest is about 5 L/min, but during strenuous exercise this can rise to 25 L/min or more. Stroke volume is influenced by the filling pressure (**preload**), the force developed by the cardiac muscle, and the pressure against which the heart has to pump (**afterload**). Both heart rate and force development are modulated by the **autonomic nervous system** (Figure 15a).

Filling pressure and stroke volume

The volume of blood in the ventricle at the start of systole (**end-diastolic volume**, EDV) depends on the **end-diastolic pressure** (EDP) and **compliance** of the ventricular wall (how easy it is to inflate). Right ventricular EDP is primarily dependent on **central venous pressure** (CVP). If EDP (and thus EDV) is increased, the force of the next contraction and stroke volume also increases (Figure 15b). This is known as the **Frank–Starling** relationship. The graph relating stroke volume to EDP is called a **Starling** or **ventricular function** curve. The force of contraction is related to the degree of stretch of the muscle, and **Starling's law of the heart** can be quoted as '*The energy released during contraction depends on the initial fibre length*'.

In skeletal muscle the relationship between muscle length and force generation can be explained by the **sliding filament theory** of muscle function; as muscle is stretched, more crossbridges can form between myosin and actin, and thus force increases. Cardiac muscle, however, has a much steeper relationship between stretch and force, because Ca^{2+} sensitivity is increased so that more force is generated for any given rise in intracellular $[Ca^{2+}]$ (Figure 15c). This mechanism involves troponin C (see Chapter 11), and provides a greater sensitivity to small degrees of stretch than the sliding filament mechanism.

The importance of Starling's law

The most important consequence of Starling's law is that the stroke volumes of the left and right ventricles are matched. Small transient differences in output occur all the time, e.g. during breathing or rising from a supine position. However, if right ventricular output was greater than that from the left for any significant period, pulmonary blood volume and pressure would rise dramatically, and fluid would be forced into the lung (**pulmonary oedema**). This does not normally happen because any increase in pulmonary blood pressure increases the filling pressure, and hence EDV, of the left ventricle. Left ventricular stroke volume then increases according to Starling's law, until it matches right ventricular output and so preventing any further rise in pulmonary venous pressure.

This also explains how an increase in CVP, which only directly affects the output of the right ventricle, causes an increase in cardiac output. Starling's law will therefore also contribute to the rise in cardiac output during exercise when CVP may increase, and to the initial fall in cardiac output seen on standing, when CVP falls due to blood pooling in the legs. Starling's law is an important compensatory mechanism in heart failure (see Chapter 46).

Afterload

Afterload is the load against which the heart has to work, and it should be intuitive that an increase in afterload will reduce output if cardiac force is not increased (Figure 15d). Afterload is normally related to the aortic pressure for the left ventricle, and pulmonary artery pressure for the right ventricle. It increases if blood pressure rises, or there is stenosis (narrowing) of the outflow valves. If the increase is not severe, cardiac output can be maintained as a consequence of Starling's law. When afterload increases, there is initially a decline in **ejection fraction** (proportion of EDV ejected per beat) and stroke volume. However, more blood is therefore left in the ventricle after systole, and also the output of two sides of the heart no longer match. As a result, blood accumulates on the venous side and filling pressure rises. Contractile force therefore increases according to Starling's law until it can overcome the increased afterload, and after a few beats cardiac output is restored.

Influence of the autonomic nervous system

Starling's law is intrinsic to cardiac muscle. The autonomic nervous system provides an important extrinsic influence on cardiac output, and is central to control of blood pressure (see Chapters 25, 26). Sympathetic stimulation and circulating epinephrine cause an increase in heart rate and contractile force, whereas **parasympathetic** stimulation decreases heart rate; agents that alter heart rate are called **chronotropes** (see Chapter 10). Sympathetic stimulation causes the ventricular function curve to shift upwards, so that more force is generated for any given EDV (Figure 15b), that is, any given degree of stretch. This increase in force *without a change in length* is called an increase in **contractility**, and agents that do this are called positive **inotropic** agents, or inotropes. By definition, Starling's law does *not* cause an increase in contractility. Parasympathetic stimulation does not decrease contractility, as ventricular parasympathetic innervation is sparse. The mechanisms underlying the actions of inotropic agents are discussed in Chapter 11.

Control of cardiac output

The compensation provided by Starling's law means that cardiac output is only really affected by the filling pressure of the right heart, i.e. CVP, and the effects of the autonomic nervous system on heart rate and contractility (Figure 15e). Cardiac output can thus be maintained in moderate heart disease, though at the expense of increased filling pressures. However, even if stroke volume is normal, the ejection fraction is reduced because EDV has to be large to maintain this output. Thus, a **reduced ejection fraction** (< 50%) and an **enlarged heart** are diagnostic for underlying heart disease.

16 Haemodynamics

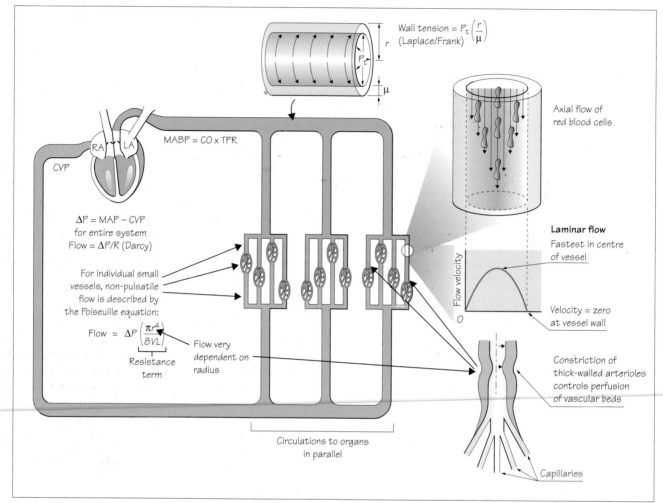

Fig. 16.1

Relationships between pressure, resistance and flow

Haemodynamics is the study of the relationships between **pressure**, **resistance** and the **flow of blood** in the cardiovascular system. Although the properties of this flow are enormously complex, they can largely be derived from simpler physical laws governing the flow of liquids through single tubes.

When a fluid is pumped through a closed system, its flow (Q) is determined by the pressure head developed by the pump (P_1-P_2 or ΔP), and by the resistance (R) to that flow, according to **Darcy's law** (analogous to Ohm's law):

$$Q = \Delta P/R$$

or for the cardiovascular system as a whole:

$$CO = (MABP - CVP)/TPR$$

where CO is cardiac output, $MABP$ is mean arterial blood pressure, TPR is total peripheral resistance and CVP is central venous pressure. Since CVP is ordinarily close to zero, $MABP$ is equal to $CO \times TPR$.

Resistance to flow is caused by frictional forces within the fluid, and depends on the viscosity of the fluid and the dimensions of the tube, as described by **Poiseuille's law**:

$$\text{resistance} = 8VL/\pi r^4$$

so that:

$$\text{flow} = \Delta P (\pi r^4/8VL)$$

Here, V is the viscosity of the fluid, L is the tube length, and r is the inner radius ($= 1/2$ the diameter) of the tube. Because flow depends on the 4th power of the tube radius in this equation, *small changes in radius have a powerful effect on flow*. For example, a 20% decrease in radius reduces flow by about 60%.

Considering the cardiovascular system as a whole, the different types or sizes of blood vessels (e.g. arteries, arterioles, capillaries) are arranged sequentially, or in *series*. In this case, the resistance of the entire system is equal to the *sum of all the resistances* offered by each type of vessel: +

$$R_{total} = R_{arteries} + R_{arterioles} + R_{capillaries} + R_{venules} + R_{veins}$$

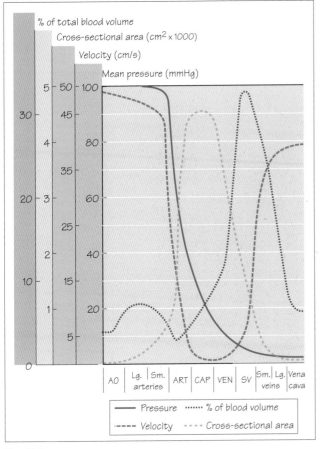

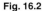

Fig. 16.2

Calculations taking into account the estimated lengths, radii and numbers of the various sizes of blood vessels show that the arterioles, and to a lesser extent the capillaries and venules, are primarily responsible for the resistance of the cardiovascular system to the flow of blood. In other words, $R_{\text{arteriole}}$ makes the largest contribution to R_{total}. Because according to Darcy's law the pressure drop in any section of the system is proportional to the resistance of that section, the steepest fall in pressure is in the arterioles (see Figure 16.2).

Although the various sizes of blood vessel are arranged in series, each organ or region of the body is supplied by its own major arteries which emerge from the aorta. The vascular beds for the various organs are therefore arranged in *parallel* with each other. Similarly, the vascular beds within each organ are mainly arranged into parallel subdivisions (e.g. the arteriolar resistances $R_{\text{arteriole}}$ are in parallel with each other). For 'n' vascular beds arranged in parallel:

$$1/R_{\text{total}} = 1/R_1 + 1/R_2 + 1/R_3 + 1/R_4 \ldots 1/R_n$$

An important consequence of this relationship is that the blood flow to a particular organ can be altered (by adjustments of the resistances of the arterioles in that organ) without greatly affecting pressures and flows in the rest of the system. This can be accomplished, as a consequence of Poiseuille's law, by relatively small dilatations or constrictions of the arterioles within an organ or vascular bed.

Because there are so many small blood vessels (e.g. millions of arterioles, billions of venules, trillions of capillaries), the overall cross-sectional area of the vasculature reaches its peak in the microcirculation. As the velocity of the blood at any level in the system is equal to the total flow (the cardiac output) divided by the cross-sectional area at that level, the blood flow is slowest in the capillaries (see Figure 16.2), favouring O_2/CO_2 exchange and tissue absorption of nutrients. The capillary transit time at rest is 0.5–2 s.

Blood viscosity

Very viscous fluids like motor oil flow more slowly than less viscous fluids like water. **Viscosity** is caused by frictional forces within a fluid which resist flow. Although the viscosity of plasma is similar to that of water, the viscosity of blood is normally three to four times that of water, because of the presence of blood cells, mainly erythrocytes. In **anaemia**, where the cell concentration (haematocrit) is low, viscosity and therefore vascular resistance decrease, and CO rises. Conversely, in the high-haematocrit condition **polycythaemia**, vascular resistance and blood pressure are increased.

Laminar flow

As liquid flows steadily through a long tube, frictional forces are exerted by the tube wall. These, in addition to viscous forces within the liquid, set up a *velocity gradient* across the tube (see Figure 16.1) in which the fluid adjacent to the wall is motionless, and the flow velocity is greatest at the centre of the tube. This is termed **laminar flow**, and occurs in the microcirculation, except in the smallest capillaries. One consequence of laminar flow is that erythrocytes tend to move away from the vessel wall and align themselves edgewise in the flow stream. This reduces the effective viscosity of the blood in the microcirculation (the **Fåhraeus–Lindqvist effect**), helping to minimize resistance.

Wall tension

In addition to the pressure gradient along the length of blood vessels, there exists a pressure difference across the wall of a blood vessel. This *transmural pressure* is equal to the pressure inside the vessel minus the interstitial pressure. The transmural pressure exerts a circumferential *tension* on the wall of the blood vessel that tends to distend it, much as high pressure within a balloon stretches it. According to the **Laplace/Frank law**:

wall tension $= P_t(r/\mu)$

where P_t is the transmural pressure, r is the vessel radius, and μ is the wall thickness. In the aorta, where P_t and r are high, atherosclerosis may cause thinning of the arterial wall, and the development of a bulge or **aneurysm** (see Chapter 36). This increases r and decreases μ, setting up a vicious cycle of increasing wall tension which, if not treated, may result in vessel rupture.

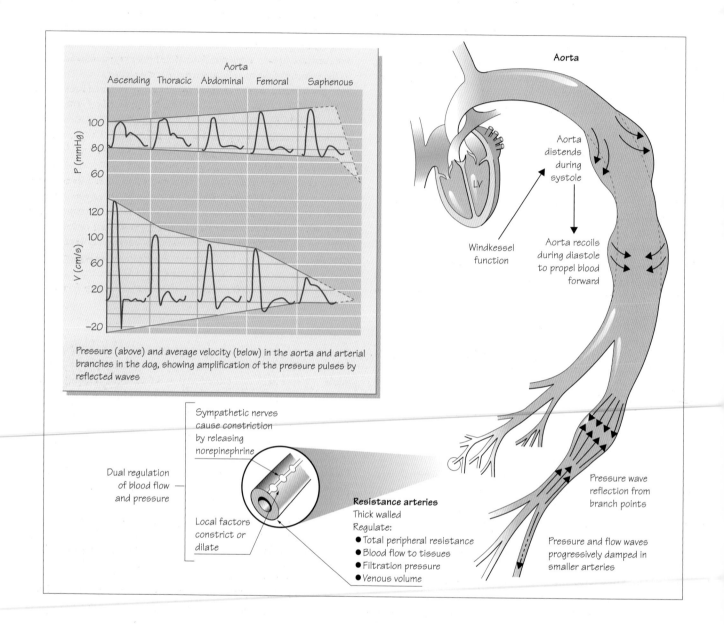

Pressure (above) and average velocity (below) in the aorta and arterial branches in the dog, showing amplification of the pressure pulses by reflected waves

Factors controlling arterial blood pressure

The mean arterial blood pressure is equal to the product of the cardiac output (about 5 L/min at rest) and the total peripheral resistance (TPR). Since the total drop of mean pressure across the systemic circulation is about 100 mmHg, TPR is calculated to be 100 mmHg/5000 mL/min, or 0.02 mmHg/mL/min. The unit mmHg/mL/min is referred to as a peripheral resistance unit (PRU), so that TPR is normally about 0.02 PRU.

Systolic pressure is mainly influenced by the stroke volume, the left ventricular ejection velocity and aortic/arterial stiffness, and rises when any of these increase. Conversely, diastolic pressure rises with an increase in TPR. Arterial pressure falls progressively during diastole (see figure in Chapter 14), so that a shortening of the diastolic interval associated with a rise in the heart rate also increases diastolic pressure.

Blood pressure and flow in the arteries

The blood flow in the aorta and the larger arteries is *pulsatile*, as a result of the rhythmic emptying of the left ventricle.

As blood is ejected from the left ventricle during systole, it hits the column of blood already present in the ascending aorta, creating a *pressure wave* in the aortic blood which is rapidly (at between 4 and 10 m/s) conducted towards the arterioles. As this pulse pressure wave passes each point along the aorta and the major arteries, it sets up a transient pressure gradient that briefly propels the blood at that point forward, causing a pulsatile *flow wave*. The blood in the arteries therefore moves forward in short bursts, separated by longer periods of stasis, so that its average velocity in the aorta is about 0.2 m/s.

The pressure wave also causes the elastic arterial wall to bulge out, thereby storing some of the energy of the wave. The arterial wall then rebounds, releasing part of this energy to drive the blood forward during diastole (*diastolic run-off*). This pumping mechanism of the elastic arteries is termed the **Windkessel** function (see figure).

The large arteries also absorb and dissipate some of the energy of the pressure wave. This progressively damps the oscillations in flow, as shown by the lower traces in the inset to the figure. However, as the upper traces illustrate, the pulse pressure wave becomes somewhat *larger* as it moves down the aorta and major arteries (e.g. the saphenous artery), before it then progressively dies out along the smaller arteries. This occurs in part because a fraction of the pressure wave is *reflected* back towards the heart at arterial branch points. In the aorta and large arteries, the reflected wave *summates* with the forward-moving pulse pressure wave, increasing its amplitude. Once the blood has entered the smaller arteries, however, the damping properties of the arterial wall predominate, and progressively depress the oscillations in flow and pressure, so that these die out completely by the time the blood reaches the microcirculation.

Arterioles and vascular resistance

The mean blood pressure falls progressively along the arterial system. The decline is particularly steep in the smallest arteries and the arterioles (diameter < 100 µm), because these vessels present the greatest resistance to flow (see figure). The walls of the arterioles are very thick in relation to the diameter of the lumen, and these vessels can therefore constrict powerfully, dramatically increasing this resistance. Because the arterioles are normally partially constricted, their resistance can also be decreased by vasodilating stimuli.

The role of the arterioles in setting the vascular resistance has several important implications.

1 Constriction or dilatation of all, or a large proportion, of the arterioles in the body will affect the TPR and the blood pressure.

2 Constriction of the arterioles in one organ or region will selectively direct the flow of blood away from that region, while dilatation will have the opposite effect.

3 Changes in arteriolar resistance in a region affect the 'downstream' hydrostatic pressure within the capillary beds and veins in that region. Changes in the pressure within the capillaries affect the movement of fluid from the blood to the tissues (see Chapter 19). Because the veins are very compliant, their volume is very sensitive to alterations in pressure (see Chapter 20). Thus, arteriolar constriction in a region of the body will both promote the movement of fluid from its tissue spaces into its exchange vessels, and also decrease its venous volume. Both effects work to increase the blood supply to other parts of the body.

Table 17.1 lists important endogenous substances and factors that affect arteriolar tone.

Table 17.1 Endogenous substances and other factors affecting arteriolar tone.

	Vasoconstrictors	Vasodilators

Neurotransmitters	Sympathetic
	  Norepinephrine
	ATP
	Neuropeptide Y
		Parasympathetic and sensory (limited distribution)
		  Acetylcholine (acts via NO)
		Substance P
		Calcitonin gene-related peptide
		Vasoactive intestinal peptide

Hormones	Epinephrine (most blood vessels) Angiotensin II Vasopressin (antidiuretic hormone)	Epinephrine (in skeletal muscle, coronary, hepatic arteries) Atrial natriuretic peptide
Endothelium-derived substances	Endothelin Endothelium-derived constricting factor (chemical identity unknown)	Endothelium-derived relaxing factor (NO) Prostaglandin I_2 (prostacyclin) Endothelium-derived hyperpolarizing factor (chemical identity unknown)
Metabolites and related factors	Hypoxia (pulmonary arteries only)	Hypoxia (other vessels) Adenosine, hyperosmolarity, H^+ ions, lactic acid, K^+ ions, CO_2
Other locally produced factors	Histamine (veins, pulmonary arteries) Prostaglandin $F_{2\alpha}$, thromboxane A_2 5-Hydroxytryptamine Growth factors (e.g. PDGF)	Histamine (arterioles) Prostaglandin E_2 Bradykinin
Other factors	Pressure (myogenic response) Moderate cold (skin)	Increased flow Heat (skin)

PDGF, platelet-derived growth factor

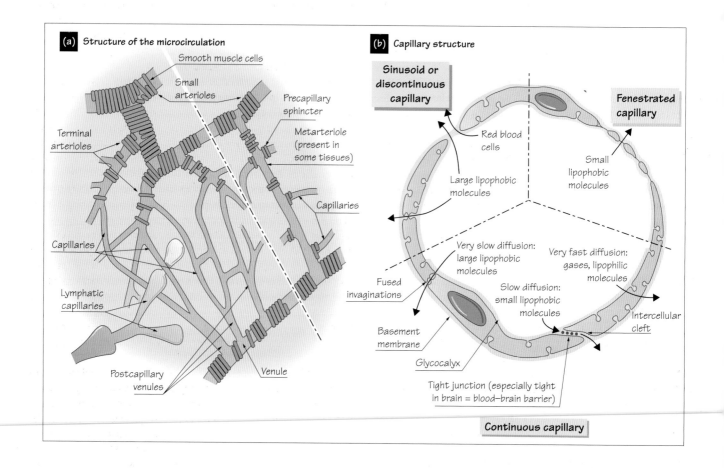

(a) Structure of the microcirculation

Smooth muscle cells
Small arterioles
Precapillary sphincter
Terminal arterioles
Metarteriole (present in some tissues)
Capillaries
Capillaries
Lymphatic capillaries
Postcapillary venules
Venule

(b) Capillary structure

Sinusoid or discontinuous capillary
Fenestrated capillary
Red blood cells
Large lipophobic molecules
Small lipophobic molecules
Very slow diffusion: large lipophobic molecules
Very fast diffusion: gases, lipophilic molecules
Fused invaginations
Slow diffusion: small lipophobic molecules
Intercellular cleft
Basement membrane
Glycocalyx
Tight junction (especially tight in brain = blood–brain barrier)
Continuous capillary

The **microcirculation** comprises the **smallest arterioles**, and the **exchange vessels**, including the **capillaries** and the **postcapillary venules**. The transfer of gases, water, nutrients, waste materials and other substances between the blood and body tissues carried out by the exchange vessels is the ultimate function of the cardiovascular system.

Organization of the microcirculation

Blood enters the microcirculation via small arterioles, the walls of which contain smooth muscle cells. These vessels are densely innervated by the sympathetic system, particularly in the splanchnic and cutaneous vascular beds. Sympathetically mediated constriction of each small arteriole reduces the blood flow to many capillaries.

In the vast majority of tissues, the smallest or **terminal** arterioles divide to give rise to sets of capillaries (Figure 18a, left). The terminal arteriole itself acts as a functional precapillary sphincter for its entire cluster of capillaries. Terminal arterioles are not innervated, and their tone is controlled by local metabolic factors (see Chapter 21). Under basal conditions, terminal arterioles constrict and relax periodically. This **vasomotion** causes the flow of blood through the cluster of capillaries to fluctuate.

In a few tissues, however (e.g. mesentery), capillaries branch from **thoroughfare vessels** which run from small arterioles to venules (Figure 18a, right). The proximal (arteriolar) end of such a vessel is termed

a **metarteriole**, and it is wrapped intermittently in smooth muscle cells. The capillaries have a ring of smooth muscle called a **precapillary sphincter** at their origin, but thereafter lack smooth muscle cells. Constriction of the precapillary sphincter controls the flow of blood through that capillary.

The capillaries join to form *postcapillary venules*, which also lack smooth muscle cells. These merge to form *venules*, which contain smooth muscle cells and are sympathetically innervated.

Movement of solutes across the capillary wall

Water, gases and solutes (e.g. electrolytes, glucose, proteins) cross the walls of exchange vessels mainly by **diffusion**, a passive process by which substances move down their concentration gradients. O_2 and CO_2 can diffuse through the lipid bilayers of the endothelial cells. These and other **lipophilic** substances (e.g. general anaesthetics) therefore cross the capillary wall very rapidly. However, the lipid bilayer is impermeable to electrolytes and small **hydrophilic** (lipid-insoluble) molecules such as glucose, which therefore cross the walls of **continuous** capillaries (Figure 18b, bottom) 1000–10 000 times more slowly than does O_2. Hydrophilic molecules cross the capillary wall mainly by diffusing between the endothelial cells. This process is slowed by *tight junctions* between the endothelial cells which impede diffusion through the intercellular clefts. Diffusion is also retarded by the **glycocalyx**, a dense network of fibrous macromolecules coating the luminal side of the endothelium. This tortuous diffusion pathway (the **small pore** system) acts as a sieve which admits molecules of molecular weight (MW) less than 10 000.

Even large proteins (e.g. albumin, MW 69 000) can cross the capillary wall, albeit very slowly. This suggests that the capillary wall also contains a small number of **large pores**, although these have never been directly visualized. It has been proposed that large pores exist transiently when membrane invaginations on either side of the endothelial cell fuse, temporarily creating a channel through which large molecules diffuse.

The endothelial cells of **fenestrated** capillaries (found in kidneys, intestines and joints) contain pores called **fenestrae** (Figure 18b, upper right). Fenestrated capillaries are about 10 times more permeable than are continuous capillaries to small hydrophilic molecules, because these can move through the fenestrae. **Sinusoidal** or **discontinuous** capillaries (liver, bone marrow, spleen) are very highly permeable, because they have wide spaces between adjacent endothelial cells through which proteins and even erythrocytes can pass (Figure 18b, upper left).

The blood–brain barrier

The composition of the extracellular fluid in the brain must be kept extremely constant in order to allow stable neuronal function. This is made possible by the existence of the **blood–brain barrier** (BBB), which tightly controls the movement of ions and solutes across the walls of the continuous capillaries within the brain and the choroid plexus. The BBB has two important features. First, the junctions between the endothelial cells of cerebral capillaries are extremely tight (resembling the *zonae occludens* of epithelia), preventing any significant movement of hydrophilic solutes. Second, specialized membrane transporters exist in cerebral endothelial cells which allow the controlled movement of inorganic ions, glucose, amino acids and other substances across the capillary wall. Thus, the relatively uncontrolled diffusion of solutes present in other vascular beds is replaced in the brain by a number of specific transport processes. This can present a therapeutic problem, as most drugs are excluded from the brain (e.g. many antibiotics).

The BBB is interrupted in the **circumventricular organs**, areas of the brain which need to be influenced by blood-borne factors, or to release substances into the blood. These include the *pituitary* and *pineal* glands, the *median eminence*, the *area postrema* and the *choroid plexus*. The BBB can break down with large elevations of blood pressure, osmolarity or P_{CO_2}, and in infected areas of the brain.

The lymphatic system

Approximately 8 L of fluid containing solutes and plasma proteins is filtered from the microcirculation into the tissue spaces each day. This returns to the blood via the **lymphatic system**. Most body tissues contain *lymphatic capillaries* (Figure 18a). These are blind-ended bulbous tubes 15–75 µm in diameter, with walls formed of a monolayer of endothelial cells. Interstitial fluid, plasma proteins and bacteria can easily enter the lymphatic capillaries via the gaps between these cells, the arrangement of which then prevents these substances from escaping. These vessels merge to form *collecting lymphatics*, the walls of which contain smooth muscle cells and one-way valves (as do the larger lymphatic vessels). The sections between these valves constrict strongly, forcing the lymph towards the blood. Lymph is also propelled by compression of the vessels by muscular contraction, body movement and tissue compression. Lymph then enters the larger *afferent lymphatics*, which flow into the **lymph nodes**. Here, foreign particles and bacteria are scavenged by phagocytes, and can initiate the production of activated lymphocytes. These enter the lymph fluid for transport into the circulation, where they mount an immune response.

Much of the lymph fluid is returned to the blood via capillary absorption in the lymph nodes. The remaining fluid enters *efferent lymphatics*, most of which eventually merge into the *thoracic duct*. This duct empties into the left subclavian vein in the neck. Lymphatics from parts of the thorax, the right arm, and the right sides of the head and neck merge forming the *right lymph duct*, which enters the right subclavian vein. The lymphatic system is also important in the absorption of lipids from the intestines. The *lacteal* lymphatics are responsible for transporting about 60% of digested fat into the venous blood.

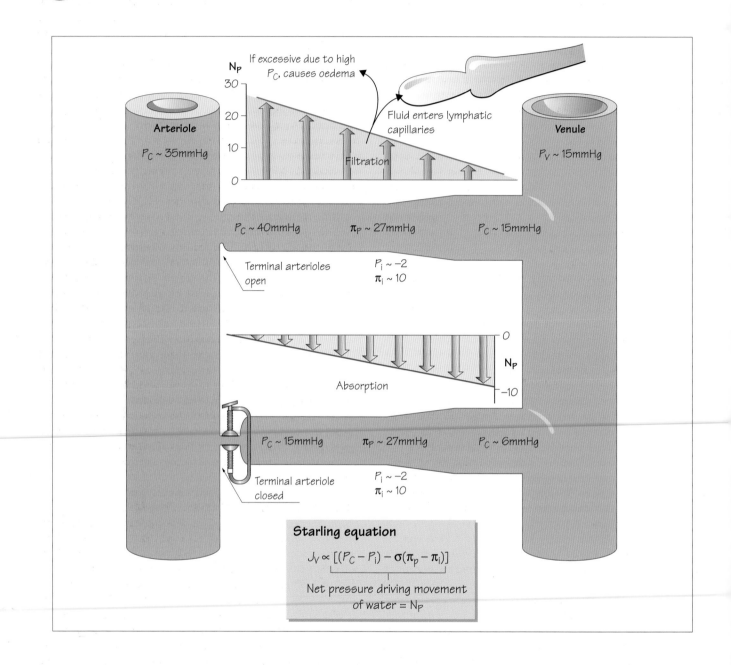

Starling equation

$$J_V \propto [(P_C - P_i) - \sigma(\pi_p - \pi_i)]$$

Net pressure driving movement of water = N_P

Movement of water across the capillary wall

The capillary wall (here taken to include also the wall of postcapillary venules) is very permeable to water molecules, which are able to pass easily in both directions through the plasma membranes of the endothelial cells. However, although individual water molecules can move freely between the plasma and the tissue spaces, the *net* flow of water across the capillary wall is quite small. This flow is determined by a balance between two forces or pressures which are exerted across the wall of the capillaries. These are a **hydrostatic pressure**, which tends to drive water out of the capillary, and a colloid **osmotic pressure**, which tends to draw water in from the surrounding tissue spaces. The sum of these two pressures at each point along the capillary is equal to a net pressure that will be directed either out of or into the capillary. The net flow of water is then proportional to this net pressure. The relationship between net flow (J_v) and the hydrostatic and osmotic pressures is described by the **Starling equation**:

$$J_v \propto [(P_c - P_i) - \sigma(\pi_p - \pi_i)]$$

The **hydrostatic force** ($P_c - P_i$) is equal to the difference between the blood pressure inside the capillary (P_c) and the pressure in the interstitium around the capillary (P_i). When capillaries are open (upper part of figure), P_c ranges from about 35 mmHg at the arteriolar end of the capillaries to about 15 mmHg in the venules. P_i is slightly subatmospheric in many tissues ($-5-0$ mmHg), due to a suction of fluid from the interstitium by the lymphatic capillaries. The greater pressure inside the capillary tends to drive water out into the tissues.

As described in Chapter 18, the capillary wall acts as a *semipermeable membrane* or barrier to free diffusion, across which electrolytes and small molecules pass with much greater ease than plasma proteins. A substance dissolved on one side of a semipermeable membrane exerts an osmotic pressure that draws water across the membrane from the other side. This osmotic pressure is proportional to the concentration of the substance in solution, and is also a function of its permeability. Substances that can easily permeate a barrier (in this case the capillary wall) exert little osmotic pressure across it, whereas those that permeate less readily exert a larger osmotic pressure. For this reason, the osmotic force across the capillary wall is largely a result of the relatively impermeant plasma proteins, in particular albumin. The osmotic pressure exerted by plasma proteins is referred to as the **oncotic** or **colloid osmotic** pressure.

The osmotic force across the capillary wall is equal to the difference between the oncotic pressure of the plasma (π_p) and that of the interstitium (π_i), multiplied by a factor, the **reflection coefficient** (σ), which is a measure of how difficult it for the proteins to cross the capillary wall. Substances that cannot cross the membrane at all have a reflection coefficient of 1, while those that pass freely have a reflection coefficient of zero. σ ranges from 0.8 to 0.95 for most plasma proteins, while ($\pi_p - \pi_i$) is typically about 13 mmHg.

Water filtration and absorption

Until recently, it was thought that the balance of forces described by the Starling equation was such that fluid tended to be *filtered* (i.e. to move out of the capillary) at the arteriolar end of the capillaries, and to be *absorbed* (move into the capillaries) at the venular end. However, the osmotic pressure term in the Starling equation is now thought to be somewhat smaller than previously estimated. Therefore, in most tissues, capillaries and venules that are being perfused with blood will be mainly filtering plasma (upper part of figure). On the other hand, certain sites such as the kidneys or the intestinal mucosa are specialized for water reabsorption. Here the osmotic pressure term is large, because plasma proteins are continually being washed out of the interstitium, so that net reabsorption occurs.

It is also the case that the balance between filtration and reabsorption is a dynamic one, mainly because the hydrostatic pressure within the capillaries is variable. Arteriolar vasodilatation, which increases intracapillary hydrostatic pressure, increases filtration, while arteriolar vasoconstriction favours absorption. For example, arterioles often demonstrate *vasomotion* (i.e. random opening and closing). During periods of arteriolar *constriction*, capillary pressure *falls*, favouring the *absorption* of interstitial fluid. The lower part of the figure illustrates this principle, showing that arteriolar constriction sufficient to reduce capillary hydrostatic pressure to the values shown would result in absorption of fluid, especially at the venous end of the capillary. This absorption tends to be transient, however, because as fluid moves into the capillaries P_i falls and π_i increases. Both effects progressively diminish absorption.

Assumption of the upright posture increases the transcapillary hydrostatic pressure gradient in the lower extremities, thereby immediately increasing filtration in these regions. However, this effect is partially compensated for by a rapid constriction of the arterioles of the leg, which is mediated by a local sympathetic axon reflex. This reduces blood flow and attenuates the rise in capillary hydrostatic pressure in these areas.

By the same token, fluid tends to accumulate in the tissue spaces of the upper body and face during the night, since assumption of the supine position increases capillary hydrostatic pressures above the heart. This causes morning 'puffiness'.

Normally, there is a slight predominance of filtration over absorption in the body as a whole. Of about 4000 L of plasma entering the capillaries daily as the blood recirculates, a *net* filtration of 8 L occurs. This fluid is returned to the vascular compartment through the lymphatic system.

Pulmonary and systemic oedema

The hydrostatic and osmotic pressures in the capillaries of the pulmonary circulation are atypical. Both P_c (~7 mmHg) and P_i (~8 mmHg) are low, while π_i is high (~18 mmHg), because these vessels are highly permeable to plasma proteins. The balance of forces slightly favours filtration. In **congestive heart failure**, the output of both the left and right ventricles is markedly reduced (see Chapter 46). Failure of the left ventricle results in an increase in left ventricular end-diastolic pressure. This pressure backs up into the lungs, causing increased pulmonary venular and capillary pressures. This promotes filtration in these vessels, causing an accumulation of fluid in the lungs (**pulmonary oedema**) which dramatically worsens the dyspnoea (breathlessness) and inadequate tissue oxygenation characteristic of congestive heart failure. Similarly, failure of the right ventricle increases systemic venous and therefore capillary pressure, leading to systemic oedema, particularly of the lower extremities.

Oedema of the legs is also caused by **varicose veins**, a condition in which the venous valves are unable to operate properly because the veins become swollen and overstretched. By interfering with the effectiveness of the skeletal muscle pump, the incompetence of the valves leads to increases in venous and capillary hydrostatic pressure, resulting in the rapid development of oedema during standing.

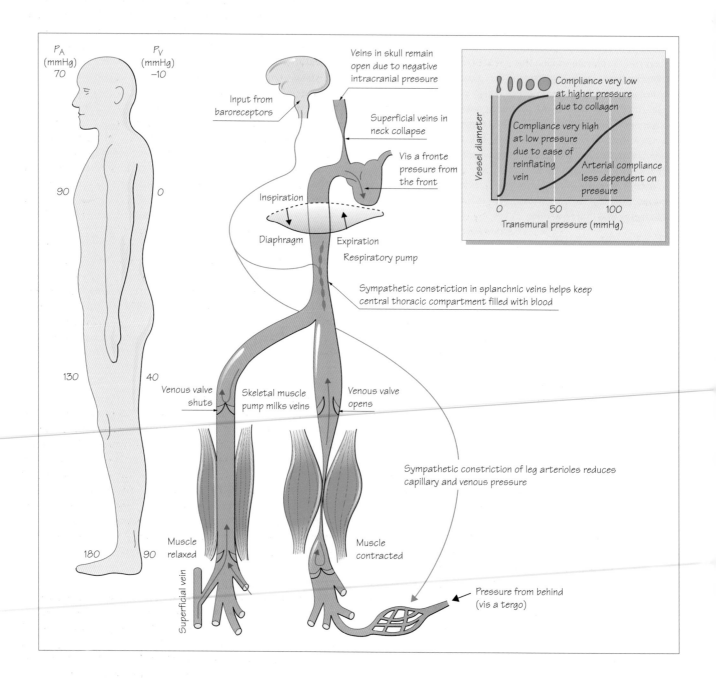

The venules and veins return the blood from the microcirculation to the right atrium. They do not, however, serve merely as passive conduits. Instead, they have a crucial active role in stabilizing and regulating the **venous return** of blood to the heart.

The venous system differs from the arterial system in two important respects. First, the total volume (and cross-sectional area) of the venous system is much greater than that of the arterial system. This is because there are many more venules than arterioles; venules also tend to have larger internal diameters than arterioles. Second, the veins are quite thin walled, and can therefore expand greatly to hold more blood if their internal pressure rises.

As a result of its large cross-sectional area, the venous system offers much less resistance to flow than the arterial system. The pressure gradient required to drive the blood through the venous system (15 mmHg) is therefore much smaller than the pressure needed in the arterial system (80 mmHg). The average pressure in the venae cavae at the level of the heart (the **central venous pressure**) is usually close to 0 mmHg (i.e. atmospheric pressure). The flow of blood back to the heart is aided by the presence of one-way **venous valves** in the arms and especially the legs, which prevent backflow.

Venous arterial compliance

The graph in the figure (upper right) illustrates the relationship between pressure and volume in a typical vein and artery. The slope of the volume/pressure curve is referred to as the **compliance**. Compliance is a measure of **expandability**. Veins are much more compliant than arteries at low pressures (0–10 mmHg). Small increases in venous pressure in this range therefore cause large increases in venous blood volume.

One reason for high venous compliance is that their thin walls allow veins to collapse at low internal pressures. Only small increases in pressure are needed to 'reinflate' a collapsed vein with blood until it has nearly rounded up. At higher pressures, however, venous compliance decreases dramatically (see graph) because the slack in rigid collagen fibres in the venous wall is rapidly taken up. This limit on the expandability of the veins is important in limiting the pooling of blood in the veins of the legs which occurs during standing.

The veins as capacitance vessels

Because of their large volumes and high compliance, the veins/venules accommodate a much larger volume of the blood (~70% of the total) than do the arteries/arterioles (~12%). They are therefore termed **capacitance vessels**, and are able to serve as *blood volume reservoirs*. During exercise, and in hypotensive states (e.g. during haemorrhage), sympathetically mediated constriction of the veins/venules, notably in the *splanchnic* (including the gastrointestinal tract and liver) and *cutaneous* circulations, displaces blood into the rest of the cardiovascular system. In particular, the resulting reduction of the venous volume increases the volume of blood in the *central thoracic compartment* (i.e. the heart and pulmonary circulation), thereby boosting cardiac output, assisting perfusion of other essential vascular beds, and helping to maintain the blood pressure.

Effects of posture

When the upright position is assumed, the pull of gravity increases the absolute pressures within *both* the arteries and veins of the lower extremities. The average arterial and venous blood pressures in a normal adult standing quietly are about 100 and 0 mmHg respectively at the level of the heart, while in the feet the pressures are about 190 and 90 mmHg, respectively. However, gravity does not affect the *pressure gradient* driving the blood circulation, because the *difference* between the arterial and venous pressures is similar (100 mmHg) at both levels. Therefore standing does not stop blood from flowing back to the heart.

The increased pressure within the veins of the lower extremities causes them to distend, so that about 500 mL of blood is shifted into this part of the circulation. The rise in hydrostatic pressure within the capillaries of the lower extremities increases fluid filtration, causing a progressive loss of plasma volume into the tissues of the legs and feet. The resulting loss of fluid from the central thoracic compartment lowers cardiac output.

These potentially harmful effects are limited by the baroreceptor and cardiopulmonary reflexes, which respond to a fall in the pulse pressure (see Chapter 25). These cause an *increased heart rate* and widespread *vasoconstriction*. This limits the loss of blood from the central thoracic compartment and slightly raises MABP and TPR. The cardiac output falls by about 20%. A local *sympathetic axon reflex* also reduces blood flow to the lower extremities, limiting fluid filtration.

In the upright position, the reduction of intravascular pressures above the heart causes the partial collapse of superficial veins, although the deeper veins remain partly open because their walls are anchored to surrounding tissues. Standing also causes a downward displacement into the spinal canal of the cerebrospinal fluid bathing the central nervous system (CNS), creating a negative pressure inside the rigid cranium that prevents cerebral veins from collapsing. Because cerebral venous pressure is not able to fall as much as arterial pressure, cerebral blood flow decreases by 10–20%.

The skeletal muscle pump

Even during quiet standing, the leg muscles are stimulated by reflexes to contract and relax rhythmically, causing swaying. During contraction, veins within the muscles are squeezed, forcing blood towards the heart, as the venous valves prevent retrograde flow. Upon relaxation, these veins expand, drawing in blood from venules and from superficial veins that communicate with the muscle veins via collaterals (see figure). This *skeletal muscle pump* thus 'milks' the veins, driving blood towards the heart to assist venous return. The skeletal muscle pump is greatly potentiated during walking and running, dramatically lowering the venous pressure in the foot to levels as low as 30 mmHg.

The respiratory pump

During inspiration, downward displacement of the diaphragm causes the intrathoracic pressure to fall and the intra-abdominal pressure to rise. This increases the pressure gradient favouring venous return, and vena caval flow rises. An opposite effect occurs during expiration. During straining movements in which there is forced expiration against a closed glottis (e.g. the Valsalva manoeuvre), the rise in intrathoracic pressure severely reduces venous return.

Effect of cardiac contraction

Downward displacement of the ventricles during systole pulls on the atria, expanding them and drawing in blood from the venae cavae and pulmonary veins. When the valves between the atria and ventricles then open during diastole, the blood is drawn in from these veins by the expansion of the ventricles, further aiding venous return. Venous return is therefore driven not only by the upstream pressure, but also (to a smaller extent) by downstream suction.

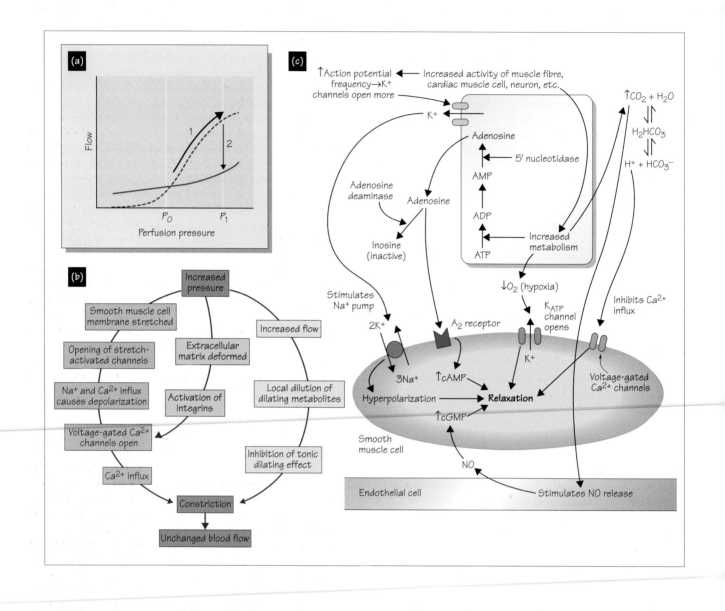

The activity of the sympathetic nervous system provides for centrally coordinated control of vascular tone (see Chapters 25, 26) and serves to maintain constant arterial blood pressure. There are, however, additional mechanisms that regulate vascular tone. Local mechanisms arise either from within the blood vessel itself, or from the surrounding tissue. These **local** mechanisms function primarily to regulate **flow**. Regulation tends to be most important in organs which require a constant blood supply, or in which metabolic needs may increase markedly (brain, kidneys, heart, skeletal muscles).

Local mechanisms have two main functions. First, under *basal conditions* they regulate local vascular resistance to maintain the blood flow in many types of vascular beds at a nearly constant level over a large range of arterial pressures (50–170 mmHg). This tendency to maintain a *constant flow* during variations in pressure is termed **autoregulation**. Autoregulation prevents major fluctuations in capillary pressure that would lead to uncontrolled movement of fluid into the tissues.

Second, when a tissue requires more blood to meet its metabolic needs, local mechanisms cause dilatation of resistance vessels and upregulate blood flow. This response is referred to as **metabolic vasodilatation**. Autoregulation may persist under these conditions, but is adjusted to maintain flow around the new set point.

Autoregulation

Figure (a) illustrates the phenomenon of autoregulation. When the upstream pressure driving blood through a resistance artery is suddenly increased to P_1 from its starting level P_0, the artery dilates passively and blood flow immediately rises as predicted by Poiseuille's law (arrow 1). Within a minute, however, the resistance artery responds to the increased pressure by *actively constricting* (arrow 2), thereby bringing blood flow back down towards its initial level (solid line). Similarly, decreases in upstream pressure cause rapid compensatory dilatations to maintain flow. Autoregulation ensures that under basal conditions blood flow remains nearly constant over a wide range of pressures, and is particularly important in the heart, the brain and the kidneys. Two homeostatic negative feedback mechanisms are involved, the **myogenic response** and the effect of **vasodilating metabolites** (Figure 21b).

The myogenic response is probably controlled by sensors in the plasma membrane of vascular smooth muscle cells which react to changes in pressure and/or stretch. There is increasing evidence that **integrins**, membrane-spanning proteins that act as adhesion molecules linking the extracellular matrix with the cytoskeleton (see Chapter 4), may constitute one class of such sensors. Integrins have two subunits (i.e. they are *dimers*), designated α and β, and there are multiple isoforms of each subunit. Recent studies indicate that integrins consisting of $\alpha_5\beta_1$ and $\alpha_v\beta_3$ dimers are necessary for the myogenic response. It is proposed that when pressure increases, changes in the conformation of extracellular matrix proteins occur, and activate the integrins. Integrin activation induces the opening of L-type voltage-gated Ca^{2+} channels, causing Ca^{2+} influx and vasoconstriction. Increased pressure may in addition stimulate **stretch-activated channels**, leading to Na^+ and Ca^{2+} influx, cell depolarization and an additional stimulus for opening L-type Ca^{2+} channels. The identities of the stretch-activated channels involved are uncertain, but there is evidence supporting the involvement of two types of **transient receptor potential** (TRP) channels, TRPC6 and TRPM4. The opposite processes (i.e. hyperpolarization, and closing of stretch-activated and voltage-gated Ca^{2+} channels) occur when pressure falls, causing vasodilatation.

Cellular metabolism results in the production of **vasodilating metabolites** or **factors** (Figure 21c) which diffuse into the tissue spaces and affect neighbouring arterioles. If blood flow increases, these substances tend to be washed out of the tissue, leading to an inhibition of vasodilatation that counteracts the rise in blood flow. Conversely, decreased blood flow causes a local accumulation of metabolites, leading to a homeostatic vasodilatation.

Metabolic and reactive hyperaemia

When metabolism in cardiac and skeletal muscle increases during exercise, tissue concentrations of vasodilating metabolites rise markedly. Similarly, focal changes in brain metabolism accompany diverse types of mental activity, causing enhanced local production of metabolites. The increased presence of such factors in the interstitium causes a powerful vasodilatation, termed **metabolic** or **functional hyperaemia**, allowing the rises in blood flow necessary to supply the increased metabolic demand.

An accumulation of vasodilating metabolites also occurs during flow occlusion (e.g. caused by thrombosis). Release of occlusion then results in **reactive hyperaemia**; this is a large increase in blood flow that hastens the re-establishment of cellular energy stores. This response is transient, persisting until levels of these metabolites fall back to normal.

Metabolic factors

Many factors contribute to metabolic vasodilatation. The most important factors are thought to be **adenosine**, K^+ **ions** and **hypercapnia** (increased P_{CO_2}). Local **hypoxia** (reduced P_{O_2}) can also relax vascular smooth muscle cells, partly by opening ATP-sensitive K^+ channels. **Inorganic phosphate**, **hyperosmolarity** and **lactic acid** may also act as metabolic vasodilators (not shown), although this is less well established.

Adenosine is a potent vasodilator that is released from the heart, skeletal muscles and brain during increased metabolism and hypoxia. It is thought to contribute to metabolic control of blood flow in these organs. Adenosine is produced when AMP, which accumulates as a result of increased ATP breakdown, is dephosphorylated by the cell membrane enzyme **5′-nucleotidase**. It passes into the extracellular space, dilating neighbouring arterioles before being broken down to inosine by **adenosine deaminase**. It causes vasodilatation by acting on A_2 **receptors** to increase cAMP levels in vascular myocytes. Adenosine also has other actions in the body (e.g. inhibiting conduction in the atrioventricular node), some of which are mediated by A_1 **receptors** (which lower cAMP).

Ischaemia or increased activation of muscles and nerves causes K^+ ions to move out of cells. Resulting increases in the extracellular K^+ concentration (up to 10–15 mM) dilate arterioles, partly by stimulating the Na^+–K^+-ATPase, during functional hyperaemia in skeletal muscle and brain tissue. **Hypercapnia** associated with **acidosis** occurs in brain tissue during stimulation of local metabolism, and also during **cerebral ischaemia** (stroke). These are thought to provide a powerful vasodilating stimulus, both by releasing **nitric oxide** from endothelial cells, and by directly inhibiting Ca^{2+} influx into arteriolar cells.

Other local mechanisms

There are also a number of mechanisms acting locally in selected vascular beds under specific circumstances. For example, during the inflammatory reaction, local infection or trauma causes the release of various **autocoids** (local hormones), including the arteriolar dilators **histamine**, **prostaglandin E$_2$**, **bradykinin** and **platelet activating factor**. These increase local blood flow and increase postcapillary venular permeability, thereby increasing the access of leucocytes and antibodies to damaged and infected tissues. The generation of **bradykinin** by sweat glands during sweating promotes cutaneous vasodilatation. **Prostaglandin I$_2$** (PGI$_2$, prostacyclin) is synthesized and released in the renal cortex under conditions where renal blood flow is reduced by vasoconstrictors. Prostacyclin has a vasodilating action that helps to maintain renal blood flow. Conversely, the release of **serotonin** (5-hydroxytryptamine) and **thromboxane A$_2$** from platelets during haemostasis causes vasospasm, which helps to reduce bleeding (see Chapter 7).

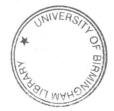

22 Regulation of the vasculature by the endothelium

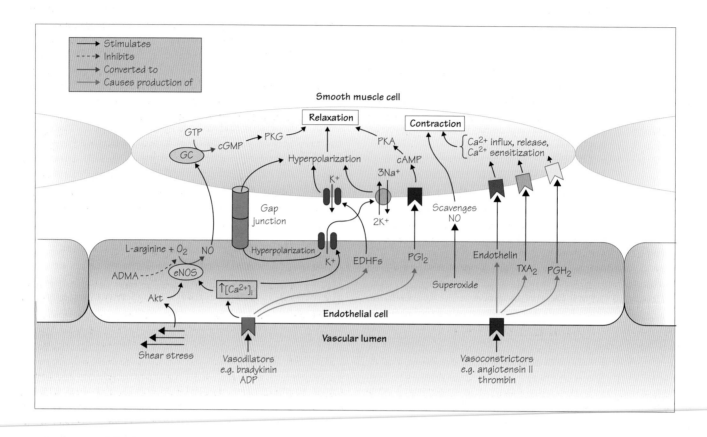

The entire vascular lumen is lined by a monolayer of endothelial cells which are crucial in regulating vascular tone. Endothelial cells can release both constricting and dilating substances when stimulated by blood-borne substances or by shear stress associated with the flow of blood (see figure). Important endothelial vasodilators include **endothelium-derived relaxing factor** (EDRF, now known to be **nitric oxide** or a closely related nitroso-containing compound), **prostacyclin** (PGI$_2$), and **endothelium-derived hyperpolarizing factor** (EDHF). The major endothelial vasoconstrictors are **endothelin-1, thromboxane A$_2$ (TXA$_2$)**, and **prostaglandin H$_2$**.

Endothelial cells also play a crucial role in suppressing platelet aggregation and thereby regulating haemostasis (see Chapter 7), and, as the major constituents of the capillary wall, control vascular permeability to many substances (see Chapter 18).

Nitric oxide

Nitric oxide (chemical formula NO) is the major vasodilator released by endothelial cells. NO is synthesized from the amino acid L-arginine and O$_2$ by nitric oxide synthase (NOS). The most important form of NOS in the cardiovascular system is **endothelial NOS** (eNOS), which is responsible for a continual basal production and release of NO by endothelial cells (also by platelets and the heart). eNOS is further activated by a variety of substances that act on their receptors to increase the endothelial cell intracellular Ca^{2+} [Ca^{2+}]$_i$, leading to raised levels of the Ca^{2+}–calmodulin complex that stimulates the enzyme. The rise in [Ca^{2+}]$_i$ is initiated by Ca^{2+} release from the endoplasmic reticulum, and

is subsequently sustained at a lower but still elevated level by Ca^{2+} influx via store-operated Ca^{2+} channels (see Chapter 13). Substances that cause vasodilatation in this way include locally released factors such as bradykinin, adenine, adenosine nucleotides, histamine, serotonin and the neurotransmitter substance P. Acetylcholine has a similar effect, although this probably has little physiological importance.

Shear forces exerted on the endothelium by the flow of blood also activate eNOS, and this is thought to contribute to both basal NO release and local regulation of blood flow. This effect is not caused by a rise in [Ca^{2+}]$_i$, but by cellular pathways activated by shear force-induced deformation of the endothelial cell cytoskeleton. One such pathway involves the sequential activation of the enzymes **phosphatidylinositol 3-kinase (PI3K)** and **Akt**, the latter of which stimulates eNOS via phosphorylation.

Once released from the endothelium, NO diffuses through the vascular wall and into the smooth muscle cells, where it activates the cytosolic enzyme **guanylyl cyclase**. This increases levels of cellular cyclic GMP, which causes relaxation as described in Chapter 13.

NO is a free radical (i.e. it contains an unpaired electron), and is therefore very reactive. In particular, upon its release NO reacts very rapidly with **superoxide**, another free radical which is continually being produced by a variety of enzymes (including eNOS). This results in the formation of **peroxynitrite**, a substance that does not cause vasodilatation, and which in excess may damage cells. Any given molecule of NO therefore survives for only a few seconds, meaning that the effects of NO are exerted locally, and depend upon its continued production.

Inducible NOS (iNOS) is expressed in macrophages, lymphocytes, vascular smooth muscle and many other types of cells during inflammation. iNOS is capable of producing much greater amounts of NO, and probably contributes to the destruction of foreign organisms by the immune system. An overproduction of NO by iNOS in septic shock is thought to contribute to the severe hypotension characterizing this condition.

The formation of NO can be competitively antagonized by artificial L-arginine analogues such as L-nitro arginine methyl ester (L-NAME) which are useful experimental tools for evaluating the roles of NO *in vitro* and *in vivo*. It has been shown, for example, that infusion of L-NAME into the human forearm causes a fall in blood flow, suggesting that a tonic basal release of NO is acting to reduce the total peripheral resistance. Remarkably, there is also an *endogenous* competitive inhibitor of NO production, **ADMA** (asymmetrical dimethyl arginine). ADMA has a normal plasma concentration of ~1 µmol/L, and is formed by *protein arginine methyltransferases*, enzymes in the nucleus that attach methyl groups to arginine residues in proteins. Subsequent protein hydrolysis then releases ADMA. ADMA is metabolized by the ubiquitous enzyme *dimethylarginine dimethylaminohydrolase*, and is also excreted by the kidneys. Elevated plasma levels of ADMA are a cardiovascular risk factor, and occur in diabetes mellitus, hyperhomocysteinaemia and pre-eclampsia.

Other endothelium-derived relaxing mechanisms

Many of the factors that evoke endothelial NO production also stimulate the endothelial release of prostacyclin and EDHF. Prostacyclin promotes vasodilatation by increasing smooth muscle cell cyclic AMP levels, but its most important role is in limiting platelet attachment and aggregation. EDHF is thought to be particularly important in causing dilatation of arterioles, where its influence may exceed that of NO. Its identity remains controversial, and it is generally defined as a substance or substances released from the endothelium which cause(s) smooth muscle hyperpolarization (and therefore relaxation, see Chapter 13) by opening K^+ channels and/or stimulating the activity of the Na^+ pump. Proposed EDHFs include arachidonic acid metabolites, hydrogen peroxide and K^+ ions. However, in many types of arterioles, EDHF is probably not only or primarily a chemical factor, but represents a process by which endothelial hyperpolarization caused by substances such as bradykinin is transmitted directly to the surrounding smooth muscle cells through **myoendothelial gap junctions** which connect these two types of cells and allow current to flow between them.

Endothelium-derived constricting factors

Endothelin-1 is a 21 amino acid peptide that is released from the endothelium by many vasoconstrictors, including angiotensin, vasopressin, thrombin and epinephrine. Endothelin is a potent vasoconstricting agent, particularly in veins and arterioles, and stimulates two subtypes of receptor on vascular smooth muscle cells, designated ET_A and ET_B. Endothelin causes vasoconstriction via G-protein-linked mechanisms similar to those activated by norepinephrine. The infusion of endothelin receptor antagonists into humans causes a sustained fall in total peripheral resistance, implying that ongoing endothelin release contributes to maintaining the blood pressure.

Endothelial cells can also release other vasoconstricting substances, including **prostanoids** (thromboxane A_2 and prostaglandin H_2), and superoxide anions which may enhance constriction by breaking down NO. In addition, **angiotensin-converting enzyme** (ACE) present on the surface of endothelial cells is responsible for both the production of the vasoconstrictor angiotensin II (see Chapter 27) and the breakdown of the potent vasodilator bradykinin.

The endothelium in cardiovascular disease

Many diseases that disturb vascular function are associated with abnormalities of the endothelium. Dysfunction of the endothelium is thought to contribute to the early stages of **atherosclerosis**, while damage to the endothelium is a crucial factor leading to thrombus formation in the advanced atherosclerotic lesion (see Chapter 36). Plasma from patients with **diabetes mellitus** contains abnormally high levels of biochemical markers indicative of endothelial damage, and there is evidence, both in animal models of insulin-dependent diabetes and in patients with this disorder, for blunted endothelium-dependent relaxation. This deficit in endothelial function is thought to contribute to the increased risks of atherosclerosis, neuropathy and hypertension that are associated with diabetes. The mechanisms leading to diabetes-associated endothelial dysfunction remain incompletely defined, but may include damage by raised levels of glucose and/or oxidized low-density lipoproteins.

Endothelial dysfunction may also be important in causing **pre-eclampsia**, a disorder of pregnancy characterized by hypertension and increased blood clotting, which is the leading cause of maternal mortality. The endothelium is thought to play an important role in causing the fall in maternal blood pressure that normally occurs during pregnancy. This protective function may, however, be disrupted in patients suffering from pre-eclampsia, possibly due to the release of substances from the placenta that damage the endothelial cells.

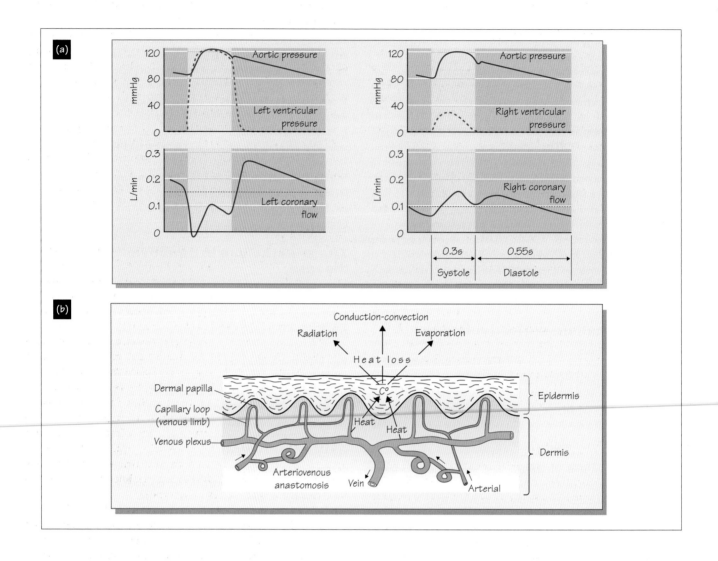

The vascular beds supplying the different organs of the body are structurally and functionally specialized, allowing an optimal matching of blood flow with their individual requirements.

Coronary circulation

The **left** and **right coronary** arteries branch from the aorta just above the aortic valve. The left coronary artery gives rise to **left circumflex** and **anterior descending** branches which supply mainly the left ventricle and septum. The right coronary artery supplies mainly the right ventricle. Venous drainage of the heart occurs mainly (95%) into the right atrium via the **coronary sinus** and **anterior cardiac vein**. A small amount of venous blood also enters all cardiac chambers through **thebesian** and **anterior coronary** veins.

The *high capillary density* of the myocardium (~1 capillary per muscle cell), allows it to extract an unusually large fraction (about 70%) of the oxygen from its blood supply. The resting blood flow to the heart is relatively high, and moreover increases approximately fivefold during strenuous exercise.

Figure (a) shows left and right coronary blood flow during the cardiac cycle at a resting heart rate of 70 beats/min. During systole, the branches of the left coronary artery that penetrate the myocardial wall to supply the subendocardium of the left ventricle are strongly compressed by the high pressure within the ventricle and its wall. Left coronary blood flow is therefore almost abolished during systole, so that 85% of flow occurs during diastole. Conversely, right coronary arterial flow rate is highest during systole, because the aortic pressure driving flow increases more during systole (from 80 to 120 mmHg) than the right ventricular pressure which opposes flow (from 0 to 25 mmHg).

With a heart rate of 70 beats/min, systole and diastole last 0.3 and 0.55 s, respectively. As the heart rate increases during exercise or excitement, however, the duration of diastole shortens more than that of systole. At 200 beats/min, for example, systole and diastole both last for 0.15 s. In order to cope with the greatly increased oxygen demand of the heart, which occurs simultaneously with a marked reduction in the time available for left coronary perfusion, the coronary arteries/arterioles dilate dramatically to allow for a pronounced rise in blood flow. Dilatation is caused by *vasodilating factors*, including **adenosine**, **hypoxia** and K^+, which are generated as a result of *increased cardiac metabolism. The heart therefore regulates its own blood supply via a well-developed **metabolic hyperaemia*** (see Chapter 21).

Skeletal muscle circulation

The skeletal muscles comprise about 50% of body weight, and at rest receive 15–20% of cardiac output. At rest, skeletal muscle arterioles have a high basal tone as a result of tonic sympathetic vasoconstriction. At any one time, most muscle capillaries are not perfused, due to intermittent constriction of precapillary sphincters (vasomotion).

Because the muscles form such a large tissue mass, their arterioles make a major contribution to total peripheral resistance. Sympathetically mediated alterations in their arteriolar tone therefore play a crucial role in regulating total peripheral resistance and blood pressure during operation of the baroreceptor reflex. The muscles thus serve as a '*pressure valve*' which can be closed to increase blood pressure and opened to lower it.

With *rhythmic exercise*, compression of blood vessels during the contraction phase causes the blood flow to become intermittent. However, increased muscle metabolism causes the generation of *vasodilating factors*; these factors cause an enormous increase in blood flow during the relaxation phase, especially to the white or *phasic* fibres involved in movement. With maximal exercise, the skeletal muscles receive 80–90% of cardiac output. Vasodilating factors include K^+ **ions**, CO_2 and **hyperosmolarity**. In working muscle their effects completely *override* sympathetic vasoconstriction, while arterioles in non-working muscle remain sympathetically constricted so that their blood flow does not increase.

Sustained compression of blood vessels during *static* (isometric) muscle contractions causes an occlusion of flow that rapidly results in muscle fatigue.

Cutaneous circulation

Apart from supplying the relatively modest metabolic requirements of the skin, the main function of the cutaneous vasculature is to maintain a constant body temperature. **Thermoregulation** is aided by the presence of **arteriovenous anastomoses** (AVAs). AVAs are coiled, thick-walled thoroughfare blood vessels, which connect arterioles and veins directly, bypassing the capillaries. AVAs are located mainly in the skin of the *hands, feet, lips, nose* and *ears*. When open, AVAs allow a high-volume blood flow into a cutaneous venous *plexus* (network) from which heat can be radiated to the environment (Figure 23b).

The sympathetic nervous system acts through α_1-*receptors* to control the resistance of AVAs and also cutaneous arterioles and veins. A fall in temperature, sensed by peripheral and hypothalamic thermoreceptors, causes a hypothalamically mediated increase in sympathetic outflow to the skin. This causes the AVAs and cutaneous arterioles and veins to constrict. This minimizes the loss of body heat by producing a pronounced decrease in cutaneous blood flow, which can fall to one-tenth of its thermoneutral level of 10–20 mL/min/100 g.

With an increased temperature, decreased sympathetic outflow allows the AVAs and other cutaneous blood vessels to open, bringing blood to the skin to increase sweating and heat loss. High temperatures also activate **cholinergic sympathetic fibres** innervating these areas of the skin. These stimulate sweating, leading to the local formation of **bradykinin**, which further promotes vasodilatation. The flow of blood to the skin can increase up to 30-fold with increases in temperature.

Local skin temperature also directly affects cutaneous blood vessels, which dilate with heat and constrict as temperature falls. Prolonged cold, however, causes a paradoxical vasodilatation. Cutaneous vessels are also constricted by the baroreceptor reflex, helping to increase TPR and shift blood to the vital organs during haemorrhage or shock.

Cerebral circulation

The brain receives about 15% of cardiac output. The **basilar** and **internal carotid arteries** entering the cranium join to form an arterial ring, the **circle of Willis**, from which arise the **anterior**, **middle** and **posterior cerebral arteries** that supply the cranium. This arrangement helps to defend the cerebral blood supply, which if occluded causes immediate unconsciousness and irreversible tissue damage within minutes.

The brain, especially the neuronal grey matter, has a very high capillary density (~3000–4000 capillaries/mm^3), and *arteriolar autoregulation* is highly developed, allowing cerebral blood flow to be maintained constant at arterial pressures between about 50 and 170 mmHg. Autoregulation is both myogenic and metabolic; the K^+ and CO_2 concentrations in the surrounding brain are particularly important in causing functional hyperaemia (see Chapter 21). The effect of CO_2 is in part caused by NO release from endothelial cells. Hyperventilation, which reduces arterial CO_2, can cause a marked cerebral vasoconstriction and temporary unconsciousness. Sympathetic regulation of the blood flow to the brain is probably of minor importance.

The brain and spinal cord float in the **cerebrospinal fluid** (CSF), which is contained within the rigid cranium and the spinal canal. Because the cranium is rigid and its contents are incompressible, the volume of blood within the brain remains roughly constant, and increases in arterial inflow are compensated for by decreases in venous volume. By increasing the tissue mass, brain tumours increase the intracerebral pressure and reduce cerebral blood flow. Increased intracerebral pressure is partially compensated for by the **Cushing reflex**, a characteristic rise in arterial pressure associated with a reflex bradycardia.

The pulmonary and fetal circulations

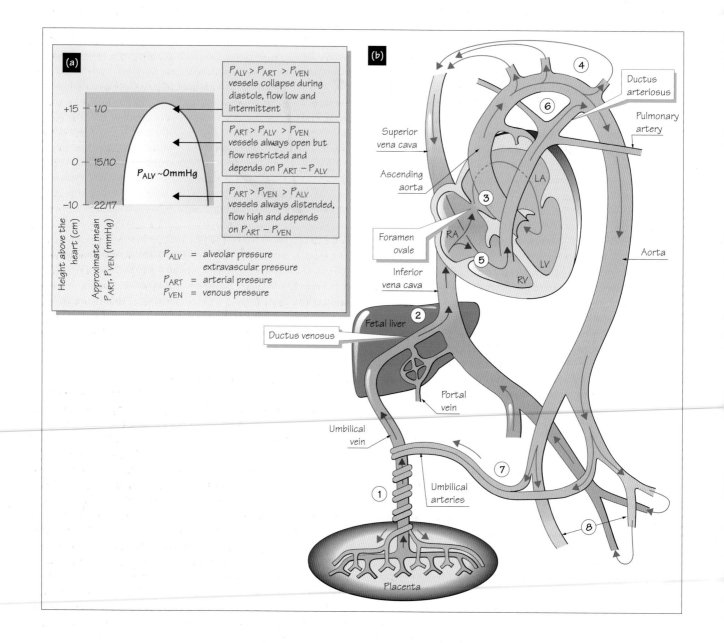

(a)

$P_{ALV} > P_{ART} > P_{VEN}$ vessels collapse during diastole, flow low and intermittent

$P_{ART} > P_{ALV} > P_{VEN}$ vessels always open but flow restricted and depends on $P_{ART} - P_{ALV}$

$P_{ART} > P_{VEN} > P_{ALV}$ vessels always distended, flow high and depends on $P_{ART} - P_{VEN}$

+15   1/0

0   15/10

−10   22/17

$P_{ALV} \sim 0$ mmHg

Height above the heart (cm)

Approximate mean P_{ART}, P_{VEN} (mmHg)

P_{ALV} = alveolar pressure extravascular pressure
P_{ART} = arterial pressure
P_{VEN} = venous pressure

(b)

Ductus arteriosus

Pulmonary artery

4

6

Superior vena cava

Ascending aorta

LA

3

Foramen ovale

RA

Aorta

5

Inferior vena cava

LV

RV

Ductus venosus

Fetal liver

2

Portal vein

Umbilical vein

Umbilical arteries

7

1

8

Placenta

The lungs contain two circulations. The **bronchial circulation** arises from the aorta, comprises about 1% of cardiac output, and supplies the metabolic needs of the airways. It drains partly into the superior vena cava through bronchial veins, and partly into pulmonary veins. The **pulmonary circulation** receives the entire output of the right ventricle. Its high-density capillary network surrounds the lung alveoli, allowing the O_2-poor blood from the pulmonary arteries to exchange CO_2 for O_2. The pulmonary veins return highly oxygenated blood to the left atrium. The pulmonary circulation contains about 800 mL of blood in recumbent subjects, falling to about 450 mL during quiet standing.

The pulmonary circulation

Mean pulmonary arterial pressure is ~15 mmHg, and left atrial pressure is ~5 mmHg. The right ventricle is able to drive its entire output through the pulmonary circulation utilizing a pressure head of only 10 mmHg because the resistance of the pulmonary circulation is only 10–15% that of the systemic circulation. This arises because the vessels of the pulmonary microcirculation are short and of relatively wide bore, with little resting tone. They are also very numerous, so that their total cross-section is similar to that of the systemic circulation. The walls of both arteries and veins are thin and distensible, and contain comparatively little smooth muscle.

The low pressure within the pulmonary circulation means that regional perfusion of the lungs in the upright position is greatly affected by gravity (Figure 24a). The extravascular pressure throughout the lungs is similar to the alveolar pressure (~ 0 mmHg). However, the intravascular pressure is low in the lung apices, which are above the heart, and high in the lung bases, which are below the heart. Pulmonary vessels in the lung apices therefore collapse during diastole, causing intermittent flow. Conversely, vessels in the bases of the lungs are perfused throughout the cardiac cycle, and are distended. A small increase in pulmonary arterial pressure during exercise is sufficient to open up apical capillaries, allowing more O_2 uptake by the blood.

The low hydrostatic pressure in pulmonary capillaries (mean of 7–10 mmHg) does not lead to net fluid resorption, because it is balanced by a low extravascular hydrostatic pressure and an unusually high interstitial plasma protein oncotic pressure (~18 mmHg). The lung capillaries therefore produce a small net flow of lymph, which is drained by an extensive pulmonary lymphatic network. During left ventricular failure or mitral stenosis, however, the increased left atrial pressure backs up into the pulmonary circulation, increasing fluid filtration and leading to **pulmonary oedema**.

Neither the sympathetic nervous system nor myogenic/metabolic autoregulation play a role in regulating pulmonary vascular resistance or flow. The pulmonary vasculature is, however, well supplied with sympathetic nerves. When stimulated, these decrease the compliance of the vessels, limiting the pulmonary blood volume so that more blood is available to the systemic circulation.

The most important mechanism regulating pulmonary vascular tone is **hypoxic pulmonary vasoconstriction** (HPV), a process by which pulmonary vessels *constrict* in response to alveolar **hypoxia**. This unique mechanism (*systemic* vessels typically *dilate* to hypoxia) diverts blood away from poorly ventilated regions of the lungs, thereby maximizing the **ventilation-perfusion ratio**. HPV is probably caused by the release of an unidentified endothelium-derived constricting factor. Hypoxia-mediated inhibition of smooth muscle K^+-channel activity, resulting in membrane depolarization, may also be involved.

The fetal circulation

A diagram of the fetal circulation is shown in Figure 24b. The fetus receives O_2 and nutrients from, and discharges CO_2 and metabolic waste products into, the maternal circulation. This exchange occurs in the **placenta**, a thick spongy pancake-shaped structure lying between the fetus and the uterine wall. The placenta is composed of a space containing maternal blood, which is packed with **fetal villi**, branching tree-like structures containing fetal arteries, capillaries and veins. They receive the fetal blood from branches of the two **umbilical arteries**, and drain back into the fetus via the **umbilical vein**. Gas and nutrient exchange occurs between the fetal capillaries in the villi and the maternal blood surrounding and bathing the villi.

The fetal circulation differs from that of adults in that *the right and left ventricles pump the blood in parallel rather than in series.* This arrangement allows the heart and head to receive more highly oxygenated blood, and is made possible by three structural *shunts* unique to the fetus: the **ductus venosus**, the **foramen ovale** and the **ductus arteriosus** (highlighted in Figure 24b).

Blood leaving the placenta (**1**) via the umbilical vein is 80% saturated with O_2. About half of this flows into the fetal liver. The rest is diverted into the inferior vena cava via the **ductus venosus** (**2**), mixing with poorly oxygenated venous blood returning from the fetus' lower body. When the resulting relatively oxygen-rich mixture (about 67% saturated) enters the right atrium, most of it does not pass into the right ventricle as it would in the adult, but is directed into the left atrium via the **foramen ovale**, an opening between the fetal atria (**3**). Blood then flows into the left ventricle, and is pumped into the ascending aorta, from which it perfuses the head, the coronary circulation and the arms (**4**). Venous blood from these areas re-enters the heart via the superior vena cava. This blood, now about 35% saturated with O_2, mixes with the fraction of blood from the inferior vena cava not entering the foramen ovale (**5**), and flows into the right ventricle, which pumps it into the pulmonary artery. Instead of then entering the lungs, as it would in the adult, about 90% of the blood leaving the right ventricle is diverted into the descending aorta through the **ductus arteriosus** (**6**). This occurs because pressure in the pulmonary circulation is higher than that in the systemic circulation, as a result of pulmonary vasoconstriction and the collapsed state of the lungs. About 60% of blood entering the descending aorta then flows back to the placenta for oxygenation (**7**). The rest, now 58% saturated with O_2, supplies the fetus' trunk and legs (**8**).

Circulatory changes at birth

Two events at birth quickly cause the fetal circulation to assume a quasi-adult pattern. First, the pulmonary vascular pressure falls well below the systemic pressure because of the initiation of breathing and the resulting pulmonary vasodilatation. Together with constriction of the ductus arteriosus caused by increased blood O_2 levels, this reversal of the pulmonary–systemic pressure gradient, which is aided by the loss of the low-resistance placental circulation, abolishes the blood flow from the pulmonary artery into the aorta within 30 min after delivery.

Second, tying off the umbilical cord stops venous return from the placenta, abruptly lowering inferior vena caval pressure. Together with the fall in pulmonary resistance, this lowers right atrial pressure, causing within hours functional closure of the foramen ovale. The ductus venosus also closes with the abolition of venous return from the placenta.

Although these fetal circulatory shunts are *functionally* closed soon after birth, complete *structural* closure only occurs after several months. In 20% of adults, the structural closure of the foramen ovale remains incomplete, although this is of no haemodynamic consequence.

25 Cardiovascular reflexes

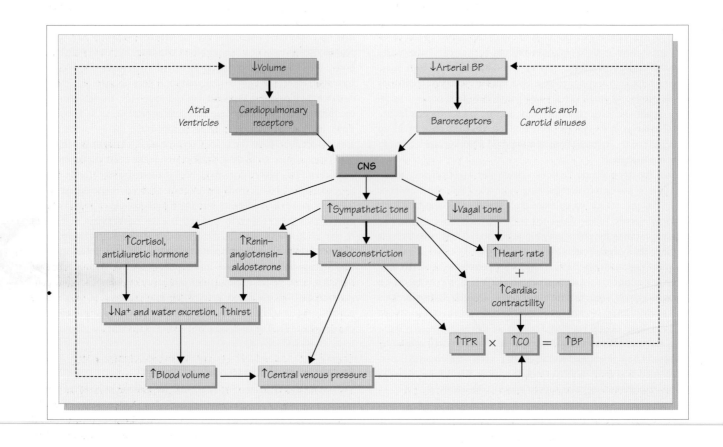

The cardiovascular system is centrally regulated by **autonomic reflexes**. These work with local mechanisms (see Chapter 21) to minimize fluctuations in the mean arterial blood pressure (MABP) and volume, and to maintain adequate cerebral and coronary perfusion. **Intrinsic** reflexes, including the **baroreceptor**, **cardiopulmonary** and **chemoreceptor** reflexes, respond to stimuli originating within the cardiovascular system. Less important **extrinsic** reflexes mediate the cardiovascular response to stimuli originating elsewhere (e.g. pain, temperature changes). The figure illustrates the responses of the baroreceptor and cardiopulmonary reflexes to reduced blood pressure and volume, as would occur, for example, during haemorrhage.

Cardiovascular reflexes involve three components:

1 afferent nerves ('receptors') sense a change in the state of the system, and communicate this to the brain, which

2 processes this information and implements an appropriate response, by

3 altering the activity of efferent nerves controlling cardiac, vascular and renal function, thereby causing homeostatic responses which reverse the change in state.

Intrinsic cardiovascular reflexes
The baroreceptor reflex

This reflex acts rapidly to minimize moment-to-moment fluctuations in the MABP. **Baroreceptors** are afferent (sensory) nerve endings in the walls of the **carotid sinuses** (thin-walled dilatations at the origins of the internal carotid arteries) and the **aortic arch**. These **mechanoreceptors** sense alterations in wall stretch caused by pressure changes, and respond by modifying the frequency at which they fire action potentials. Pressure elevations increase impulse frequency; pressure decreases have the opposite effect.

When MABP decreases, the fall in baroreceptor impulse frequency causes the brain to reduce the firing of vagal efferents supplying the sinoatrial node, thus causing tachycardia. Simultaneously, the activity of sympathetic nerves innervating the heart and most blood vessels is increased, causing increased cardiac contractility and constriction of arteries and veins. Stimulation of renal sympathetic nerves increases renin release, and consequently angiotensin II production and aldosterone secretion (see Chapter 27). The resulting tachycardia, vasoconstriction and fluid retention act together to raise MABP. Opposite effects occur when arterial blood pressure rises.

There are two types of baroreceptors. *A fibres* have large, myelinated axons and are activated over lower levels of pressure. *C fibres* have small, unmyelinated axons and respond over higher levels of pressure. Together, these provide an input to the brain which is most sensitive to pressure changes between 80 and 150 mmHg. The brain is able to reset the baroreflex to allow increases in MABP to occur, e.g. during exercise and the defence reaction. Ageing, hypertension and atherosclerosis decrease arterial wall compliance, reducing baroreceptor reflex sensitivity.

The baroreceptors quickly show partial *adaptation* to new pressure levels. Therefore alterations in frequency are greatest while pressure is changing, and tend to moderate when a new steady-state pressure level is established. If unable to prevent a change in MABP, the reflex will within several hours become *reset* to maintain pressure around the new level. This finding, together with studies by Cowley and coworkers in the 1970s showing that destroying baroreceptor function increased the variability of MABP but had little effect on its average value measured over a long time, led to general acceptance of the idea that baroreceptors play no role in long-term regulation of MABP. However, recent evidence that baroreceptor resetting is incomplete and that electrical stimulation of baroreceptors causes reductions in MABP that are sustained over many days has led some experts to re-evaluate this issue.

Cardiopulmonary reflexes

Diverse intrinsic cardiovascular reflexes originate in the heart and lungs. Cutting the vagal afferent fibres mediating these **cardiopulmonary reflexes** causes an increased heart rate and vasoconstriction, especially in muscle, renal and mesenteric vascular beds. Cardiopulmonary reflexes are therefore thought to exert a *net tonic depression of the heart rate and vascular tone*. Receptors for these reflexes are located mainly in *low-pressure regions* of the cardiovascular system, and are well placed to sense the *blood volume* in the central thoracic compartment. These reflexes are thought to be particularly important in controlling blood volume, as well as vascular tone, and act together with the baroreceptors to stabilize the MABP. However, these reflexes have been studied mainly in animals, and their specific individual roles in humans are incompletely understood.

Specific components of the cardiopulmonary reflexes include the following.

1 Atrial mechanoreceptors with non-myelinated vagal afferents which respond to increased atrial volume/pressure by causing bradycardia and vasodilatation.

2 Mechanoreceptors in the left ventricle and coronary arteries with mainly non-myelinated vagal afferents which respond to increased ventricular diastolic pressure and afterload by causing a vasodilatation.

3 Ventricular chemoreceptors which are stimulated by substances such as bradykinin and prostaglandins released during cardiac ischaemia. These receptors activate the **coronary chemoreflex**. This response, also termed the **Bezold–Jarisch effect**, occurs after the intravenous injection of many drugs, and involves marked bradycardia and widespread vasodilatation.

4 Pulmonary mechanoreceptors, which when activated by marked lung inflation, especially if oedema is present, cause tachycardia and vasodilatation.

5 Mechanoreceptors with myelinated vagal afferents, located mainly at the juncture of the atria and great veins, which respond to increased atrial volume and pressure by causing a sympathetically mediated tachycardia (the **Bainbridge reflex**). This reflex also helps to control blood volume; its activation decreases the secretion of **antidiuretic hormone** (vasopressin), **cortisol** and **renin**, causing a diuresis. Although powerful in dogs, this reflex has been difficult to demonstrate in humans.

Chemoreceptor reflexes

Chemoreceptors activated by **hypoxia**, **hypocapnia** and **acidosis** are located in the aortic and carotid bodies. These are stimulated during asphyxia, hypoxia and severe hypotension. The resulting **chemoreceptor reflex** is mainly involved in stimulating breathing, but also has cardiovascular effects. These include sympathetic constriction of (mainly skeletal muscle) arterioles, splanchnic venoconstriction and a tachycardia resulting indirectly from the increased lung inflation. This reflex is important in maintaining blood flow to the brain at arterial pressures too low to activate the baroreceptors.

The CNS ischaemic response

Brainstem hypoxia stimulates a powerful generalized peripheral vasoconstriction. This response develops during severe hypotension, helping to maintain the flow of blood to the brain during shock. It also causes the **Cushing reflex**, in which vasoconstriction and hypertension develop when increased cerebrospinal fluid pressure (e.g. due to a brain tumour) produces brainstem hypoxia.

Extrinsic reflexes

Stimuli that are external to the cardiovascular system also exert effects on the heart and vasculature via extrinsic reflexes. Moderate pain causes tachycardia and increases MABP; however, severe pain has the opposite effects. Cold causes cutaneous and coronary vasoconstriction, possibly precipitating angina in susceptible individuals.

Central regulation of cardiovascular reflexes

The afferent nerves carrying impulses from cardiovascular receptors terminate in the **nucleus tractus solitarius** (NTS) of the medulla. Neurons from the NTS project to areas of the brainstem that control both parasympathetic and sympathetic outflow, influencing their level of activation. The **nucleus ambiguus** and **dorsal motor nucleus** contain the cell bodies of the preganglionic vagal parasympathetic neurons, which slow the heart when the cardiovascular receptors report an increased blood pressure to the NTS. Neurons from the NTS also project to areas of **ventrolateral medulla**; from these descend bulbospinal fibres which influence the firing of the sympathetic preganglionic neurons in the intermediolateral (IML) columns of the spinal cord.

These neural circuits are capable of mediating the basic cardiovascular reflexes. However, the NTS, the other brainstem centres and the IML neurons receive descending inputs from the hypothalamus, which in turn is influenced by impulses from the limbic system of the cerebral cortex. Input from these higher centres modifies the activity of the brainstem centres, allowing the generation of integrated responses in which the functions of the cardiovascular system and other organs are coordinated in such a way that the appropriate responses to changing conditions can be orchestrated.

26 Autonomic control of the cardiovascular system

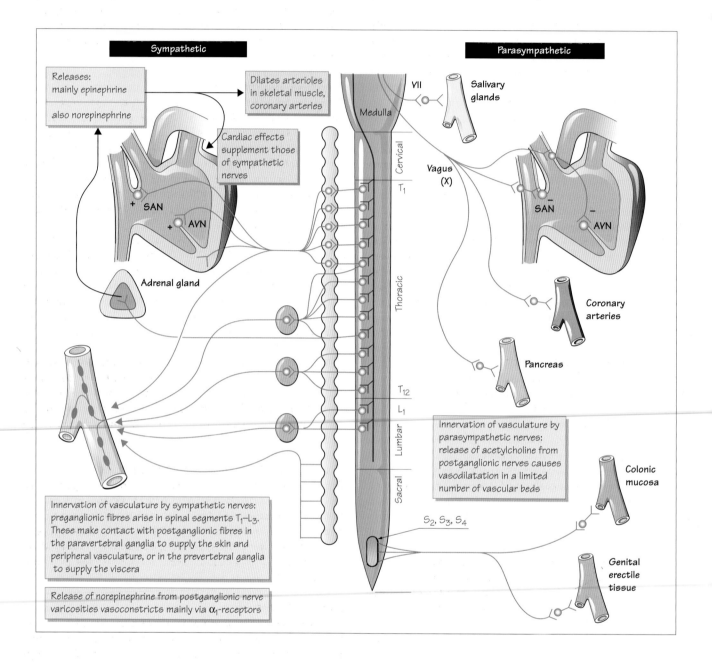

Sympathetic

Releases:
mainly epinephrine

also norepinephrine

Dilates arterioles
in skeletal muscle,
coronary arteries

Cardiac effects
supplement those
of sympathetic
nerves

+ SAN

+ AVN

Adrenal gland

Medulla

Cervical

T₁

Thoracic

T₁₂

L₁

Lumbar

Sacral

Parasympathetic

VII

Salivary
glands

Vagus
(X)

— SAN

— AVN

Coronary
arteries

Pancreas

Colonic
mucosa

S₂, S₃, S₄

Genital
erectile
tissue

Innervation of vasculature by
parasympathetic nerves:
release of acetylcholine from
postganglionic nerves causes
vasodilatation in a limited
number of vascular beds

Innervation of vasculature by sympathetic nerves:
preganglionic fibres arise in spinal segments T₁–L₃.
These make contact with postganglionic fibres in
the paravertebral ganglia to supply the skin and
peripheral vasculature, or in the prevertebral ganglia
to supply the viscera

Release of norepinephrine from postganglionic nerve
varicosities vasoconstricts mainly via α₁-receptors

The **autonomic nervous system** (ANS) comprises a *system of efferent nerves* that regulate the involuntary functioning of most organs, including the heart and vasculature. The cardiovascular effects of the ANS are deployed for two purposes.

First, the ANS provides the effector arm of the cardiovascular *reflexes*, which respond mainly to activation of receptors in the cardiovascular system (see Chapter 25). They are designed to maintain an *appropriate blood pressure*, and play a crucial role in homeostatic adjustments to *postural changes* (see Chapter 20), *haemorrhage* (see Chapter 29) and *changes in blood gases*. The autonomic circulation is able to override local vascular control mechanisms in order to serve the needs of the body as a whole.

Second, ANS function is also regulated by signals initiated within the brain as it reacts to *environmental stimuli* or *emotional stress*. The brain can selectively modify or override the cardiovascular reflexes, producing specific patterns of cardiovascular adjustments, which are sometimes coupled with behavioural responses. Complex responses of this type are involved in *exercise* (see Chapter 28), *thermoregulation* (see Chapter 23), the *'fight or flight' (defence) response*, and *'playing dead'*.

The ANS is divided into **sympathetic** and **parasympathetic** branches. The nervous pathways of both branches of the ANS consist of two sets of neurons arranged in series. **Preganglionic neurons** originate in the central nervous system and terminate in peripheral **ganglia**, where they synapse with **postganglionic neurons** innervating the target organs.

The sympathetic system

Sympathetic preganglionic neurons originate in the **intermediolateral** (IML) columns of the spinal cord. These neurons exit the spinal cord through ventral roots of segments T_1–L_2, and synapse with the postganglionic fibres in either *paravertebral* or *prevertebral* ganglia. The paravertebral ganglia are arranged in two sympathetic chains, one of which is shown in the figure. These are located on either side of the spinal cord, and usually contain 22 or 23 ganglia. The prevertebral ganglia, shown to the left of the sympathetic chain, are diffuse structures which form part of the visceral autonomic plexuses of the abdomen and pelvis. The ganglionic neurotransmitter is **acetylcholine**, and it activates postganglionic **nicotinic cholinergic** receptors.

The postganglionic fibres terminate in the effector organs, where they release **norepinephrine**. Preganglionic sympathetic fibres also control the **adrenal medulla**, which releases **epinephrine** and norepinephrine into the blood. Under physiological conditions, the effect of neuronal norepinephrine release is more important than that of epinephrine and norepinephrine released by the adrenal medulla.

Epinephrine and norepinephrine are **catecholamines**, and activate **adrenergic** receptors in the effector organs. These receptors are *G-protein linked* and exist as three types.

1 α_1-**receptors** are linked to G_q and have subtypes α_{1A}, α_{1B} and α_{1D}. Epinephrine and norepinephrine activate α_1-receptors with similar potencies.
2 α_2-**receptors** are linked to $G_{i/o}$ and have subtypes α_{2A}, α_{2B} and α_{2C}. Epinephrine activates α_2-receptors more potently than does norepinephrine.
3 β-**receptors** are linked to G_s and have subtypes β_1, β_2 and β_3. Norepinephrine is more potent than epinephrine at β_1- and β_3-receptors, while epinephrine is more potent at β_2-receptors.

Effects on the heart

Catecholamines acting via cardiac β_1-**receptors** have positive inotropic and chronotropic effects via mechanisms described in Chapters 10 and 11. At rest, cardiac sympathetic nerves exert a tonic accelerating influence on the sinoatrial node, which is, however, overshadowed in younger people by the opposite and dominant effect of parasympathetic vagal tone. Vagal tone decreases progressively with age, causing a rise in the resting heart rate as the sympathetic influence becomes more dominant.

Effects on the vasculature

At rest, vascular sympathetic nerves fire impulses at a rate of 1–2 impulses/s, thereby tonically vasoconstricting the arteries, arterioles and veins. Increasing activation of the sympathetic system causes further vasoconstriction. Vasoconstriction is mediated mainly by α_1-**receptors** on the vascular smooth muscle cells. The arterial system, particularly the arterioles, is more densely innervated by the sympathetic system than is the venous system. Sympathetic vasoconstriction is particularly marked in the splanchnic, renal, cutaneous and skeletal muscle vascular beds.

The vasculature also contains both β_1- and β_2-receptors, which when stimulated exert a *vasodilating* influence, especially in the *skeletal* and *coronary* circulations. These may play a limited role in dilating these vascular beds in response to epinephrine release, for example during mental stress. In some species, sympathetic *cholinergic* fibres innervate skeletal muscle blood vessels and cause vasodilatation during the defence reaction. A similar but minor role for such nerves in humans has been proposed, but is unproven.

It is a common fallacy that the sympathetic nerves are always activated *en masse*. In reality, changes in sympathetic vasoconstrictor activity can be limited to certain regions (e.g. to the skin during thermoregulation). Similarly, a sympathetically mediated tachycardia occurs with no change in inotropy or vascular resistance during the Bainbridge reflex (see Chapter 25).

The parasympathetic system

The parasympathetic preganglionic neurons involved in regulating the heart have their cell bodies in the **nucleus ambiguus** and the **dorsal motor nucleus** of the medulla. Their axons run in the **vagus** nerve (cranial nerve X) and release acetylcholine onto nicotinic receptors on short postganglionic neurons originating in the cardiac plexus. These innervate the *sinoatrial node (SAN)*, the *atrioventricular node (AVN)* and the *atria*.

Effects on the heart

Basal acetylcholine release by vagal nerve terminals acts on muscarinic receptors to slow the discharge of the SAN. Increased vagal tone further decreases the heart rate and the speed of impulse conduction through the AVN and also decreases the force of atrial contraction when activated.

Effects on the vasculature

Although vagal slowing of the heart can decrease the blood pressure by lowering cardiac output, the parasympathetic system has no effect on total peripheral resistance, because it innervates only a limited number of vascular beds. In particular, activation of parasympathetic fibres in the pelvic nerve causes **erection** by vasodilating arterioles in the erectile tissue of the genitalia. Parasympathetic nerves also cause vasodilatation in the pancreas and salivary glands.

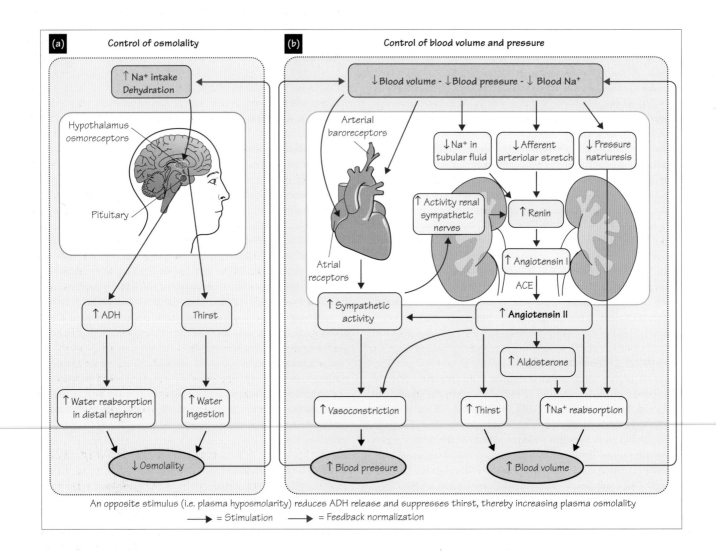

(a) Control of osmolality

↑ Na⁺ intake Dehydration

Hypothalamus osmoreceptors

Pituitary

↑ ADH

Thirst

↑ Water reabsorption in distal nephron

↑ Water ingestion

↓ Osmolality

(b) Control of blood volume and pressure

↓ Blood volume - ↓ Blood pressure - ↓ Blood Na⁺

Arterial baroreceptors

↓ Na⁺ in tubular fluid

↓ Afferent arteriolar stretch

↓ Pressure natriuresis

↑ Activity renal sympathetic nerves

↑ Renin

↑ Angiotensin I

ACE

Atrial receptors

↑ Sympathetic activity

↑ **Angiotensin II**

↑ Aldosterone

↑ Vasoconstriction

↑ Thirst

↑ Na⁺ reabsorption

↑ Blood pressure

↑ Blood volume

An opposite stimulus (i.e. plasma hyposmolarity) reduces ADH release and suppresses thirst, thereby increasing plasma osmolality

⟶ = Stimulation   ⟶ = Feedback normalization

The baroreceptor system effectively minimizes short-term fluctuations in the arterial blood pressure. Over the longer term, however, the ability to sustain a constant blood pressure depends on maintenance of a *constant blood volume*. This dependency arises because alterations in blood volume affect central venous pressure and therefore cardiac output. Changes in cardiac output also ultimately lead to adaptive effects of the vasculature which increase peripheral resistance, and therefore blood pressure (see Chapter 38).

Blood volume is affected by changes in total body Na⁺ and water, which are mainly controlled by the kidneys. Maintenance of blood pressure therefore involves mechanisms that adjust renal excretion of Na⁺ and water.

Plasma volume: the role of sodium and osmoregulation

Alterations in body water content, caused for example by variations in fluid intake or perspiration, result in changes in plasma **osmolality** (see Chapter 5). Any deviation of plasma osmolality from its normal value of *~300 mosmol/kg* is sensed by *hypothalamic osmoreceptors*, which activate the homeostatic feedback control system illustrated in Figure 27a. Osmoreceptors regulate both thirst and the release from the posterior pituitary of **antidiuretic hormone** (**ADH**, also **vasopressin**), a peptide that suppresses renal water excretion. For example, dehydration raises plasma osmolality, resulting in increased thirst and enhanced release of ADH. ADH acts on the distal nephron to increase reabsorption of water, thereby reducing its loss in the urine. Both effects act to bring plasma osmolality back to its set point by restoring the water content of the body. Opposite effects are stimulated by an excess of body water, which reduces plasma osmolality.

An important consequence of this osmoregulatory mechanism is that the plasma volume is primarily controlled by the Na⁺ content of the extracellular fluid (ECF). Na⁺ and its associated anions Cl⁻ and HCO₃⁻ account for about 95% of the osmotic solute present in the ECF, of which the plasma is a part. Any change in the Na⁺ content of the body (e.g. after eating a salty meal) will quickly affect plasma osmolality. This will cause the osmoregulatory system to readjust the body water content (and therefore the plasma volume) in order to restore plasma osmolality. Under normal conditions, therefore, alterations in body Na⁺

lead to changes in plasma volume. It follows that the maintenance of a stable plasma volume requires tight regulation of total body (and therefore ECF) Na^+ content, a function mainly carried out by the kidneys.

Control of total body Na^+ content and plasma volume by the kidneys

Total body Na^+ content is maintained within narrow limits. The body apparently has a set point for total Na^+ content, and is able to sense when deviations from this set point occur. This is referred to as 'sodium memory'. As shown in Figure 27b, changes in vascular volume, pressure and body Na^+ activate mechanisms that cause compensatory alterations in renal Na^+ excretion which return these parameters back to their original levels. Only effects of decreases in vascular volume and pressure are illustrated; increases cause opposite responses.

Pressure natriuresis is an intrinsic renal homeostatic process whereby decreases in blood volume and pressure strongly inhibit diuresis and **natriuresis** (Na^+ excretion in the urine). Although its mechanisms remain mysterious, a leading hypothesis is that decreases in renal perfusion pressure cause a fall in blood flow within the renal medulla. This then reduces the hydrostatic pressure within the renal interstitium, promoting reabsorption of fluid from the nephron and acting to restore blood volume. Opposite effects occur during volume expansion.

The **renin–angiotensin–aldosterone system** responds to stimuli associated with reductions in vascular volume and pressure by inhibiting Na^+ excretion, increasing thirst and causing vasoconstriction. **Renin** is a proteolytic enzyme stored in the *granular cells* of the renal juxtaglomerular apparatus. Renin release into the blood is increased by:
1 activation of the baroreceptor reflex by a reduction of vascular pressure, which increases firing of sympathetic nerves innervating the granular cells
2 decreased atrial stretch/pressure, sensed by cardiac mechanoreceptors
3 decreased stretch of renal afferent arterioles caused by a fall in renal perfusion pressure
4 the release of prostacyclin (PGI_2) by the *macula densa cells* of the early distal tubule and juxtaglomerular apparatus, stimulated by a fall in NaCl content of the tubular fluid.

Renin cleaves a plasma α_2-globulin, **angiotensinogen**, to the decapeptide **angiotensin I**. Plasma angiotensin I is converted by **angiotensin-converting enzyme** (ACE) on the surface of endothelial cells to the octapeptide **angiotensin II**. Angiotensin II has a variety of effects, which raise blood pressure and volume. These include increasing Na^+ reabsorption by the proximal tubule, stimulating thirst, promoting ADH release, increasing activation of the sympathetic nervous system, and causing a direct vasoconstriction. ACE, also called **kininase II**, has the additional function of breaking down bradykinin, a vasodilating local hormone.

Angiotensin II also promotes release of the steroid hormone **aldosterone** from the zona glomerulosa cells of the adrenal cortex. Aldosterone increases Na^+ retention by acting on principal cells of the distal nephron to enhance Na^+ reabsorption. It does so by increasing synthesis of both Na^+ pumps in the basolateral membrane and Na^+ channels in the apical membrane of these cells. In addition, aldosterone conserves body Na^+ by enhancing reabsorption from several types of glands, including salivary and sweat glands. Aldosterone secretion is also increased by decreased stimulation of the atrial volume/pressure mechanoreceptors.

Atrial natriuretic peptide (ANP) is a 28-amino-acid peptide released from atrial myocytes when these are stretched by increased atrial volume. ANP can cause both diuresis and natriuresis by increasing glomerular filtration rate, decreasing renin and aldosterone secretion, and reducing Na^+ reabsorption throughout the nephron. ANP also dilates arterioles and increases capillary permeability. On a cellular level, ANP stimulates a membrane-associated guanylyl cyclase, raising the intracellular cyclic GMP concentration.

Although pressure natriuresis has long been thought to be the main mechanism controlling total body Na^+, this concept has been challenged recently by studies in dogs which suggest that the renin–angiotensin–aldosterone system is of predominant importance in controlling total body Na^+, and therefore long-term blood pressure. ANP and other mechanisms such as changes in renal nitric oxide and prostaglandins seem to have a more limited role, and may be involved chiefly in the response to volume overload.

Antidiuretic hormone in volume regulation

Under emergency conditions, plasma volume is maintained at the expense of osmoregulation. For example, a fall in blood volume sensed by atrial pressure/stretch mechanoreceptors causes an increased ADH release, leading to water retention by the kidneys. In addition, the ADH system is rendered more sensitive to increases in plasma osmolality by a fall in vascular volume, so that ADH release is promoted even at normal plasma osmolality. Increases in plasma volume have the opposite effect on ADH release.

28 Cardiovascular effects of exercise

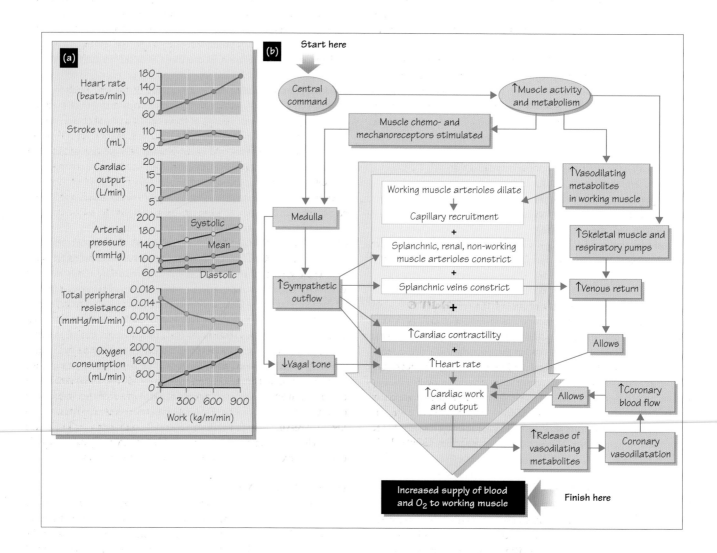

Figure (a) summarizes important cardiovascular adaptations that occur at increasing levels of dynamic (rhythmic) exercise, thereby allowing working muscles to be supplied with the increased amount of O_2 they require. By far the most important of these adaptations is an increase in cardiac output (CO), which rises almost linearly with the rate of muscle O_2 consumption (level of work) as a result of increases in both **heart rate** and to a lesser extent **stroke volume**. The heart rate is accelerated by a reduction in vagal tone, and by increases in sympathetic nerve firing and circulating catecholamines. The resulting stimulation of cardiac β-adrenoceptors increases stroke volume by *increasing myocardial contractility* and enabling more complete systolic emptying of the ventricles. CO is the limiting factor determining the maximum exercise capacity.

Table 28.1 shows that the increased CO is channelled mainly to the active muscles, which may receive 85% of CO against about 15–20% at rest, and to the heart. This is caused by a profound arteriolar vasodilatation in these organs. Dilatation of terminal arterioles causes **capillary recruitment**, a large increase in the number of open capillaries, which shortens the diffusion distance between capillaries and muscle fibres.

Table 28.1 Cardiac output and regional blood flow in a sedentary man. Values are mL/min.

	Quiet standing	Exercise
Cardiac output	5900	24 000
Blood flow to:		
Heart	250	1000
Brain	750	750
Active skeletal muscle	650	20 850
Inactive skeletal muscle	650	300
Skin	500	500
Kidney, liver, gastrointestinal tract, etc.	3100	600

This, combined with increases in $P\text{CO}_2$, temperature and acidity, promotes the release of O_2 from haemoglobin, allowing skeletal muscle to increase its O_2 extraction from the basal level of 25–30% to about 90% during maximal exercise.

Increased firing of sympathetic nerves and levels of circulating catecholamines constrict arterioles in the *splanchnic* and *renal* vascular beds, and in *non-exercising muscle*, reducing the blood flow to these organs. Cutaneous blood flow is also initially reduced. As core body temperature rises, however, cutaneous blood flow increases as autonomically mediated vasodilatation occurs to promote cooling (see Chapter 23). With very strenuous exercise, cutaneous perfusion again falls as vasoconstriction diverts blood to the muscles. The increased CO necessitates a rise in venous return. This is enhanced by increased activity of skeletal muscle and respiratory pumps, and is also transiently promoted by splanchnic constriction, which reduces the capacitance of the venous system. Blood flow to the crucial cerebral vasculature remains constant.

Vasodilatation of the skeletal and cutaneous vascular beds decreases total peripheral resistance. This is sufficient to balance the effect of the increased CO on diastolic blood pressure, which rises only slightly and may even fall, depending on the balance between skeletal muscle vasodilatation and splanchnic/renal vasoconstriction. Significant rises in the systolic and pulse pressures are, however, caused by the more rapid and forceful ejection of blood by the left ventricle, leading to some elevation of the mean arterial blood pressure.

Effects of exercise on plasma volume

Arteriolar dilatation in skeletal muscles increases capillary hydrostatic pressure, while capillary recruitment vastly increases the surface area of the microcirculation available to exchange fluid. These effects, coupled with a rise in interstitial osmolarity caused by an increased production of metabolites within the muscle fibres, lead via the Starling mechanism to *extravasation of fluid into muscles*. Taking into account also fluid losses caused by sweating, plasma volume may decrease by 15% during strenuous exercise. This fluid loss is partially compensated by enhanced fluid reabsorption in the vasoconstricted vascular beds, where capillary pressure decreases.

Regulation and coordination of the cardiovascular adaptation to exercise

In anticipation of exercise, and during its initial stages, a process termed **central command** (Figure 28b, upper left) causes the cardiovascular adaptations necessary for increased effort. Impulses from the cerebral cortex act on the medulla to suppress vagal tone, thereby increasing the heart rate and CO. Central command is also thought to raise the set point of the baroreceptor reflex. This allows the blood pressure to be regulated around a higher set point, resulting in an increased sympathetic outflow which contributes to the rise in CO and causes constriction of the splanchnic and renal circulations. An increase in circulating epinephrine also vasodilates skeletal muscle arterioles via β_2-receptors. The

magnitude of these anticipatory effects increases in proportion to the degree of perceived effort.

As exercise continues, cardiovascular regulation by central command is supplemented by two further control systems which are activated and become crucial. These involve: (i) autonomic reflexes (Figure 28b, left); and (ii) direct effects of metabolites generated locally in working skeletal and cardiac muscle (right).

Systemic effects mediated by autonomic reflexes

Nervous impulses originating mainly from receptors in working muscle which respond to contraction (mechanoreceptors) and locally generated metabolites and ischaemia (chemoreceptors) are carried to the CNS via afferent nerves. CNS autonomic control centres respond by suppressing vagal tone and causing graded increases in sympathetic outflow which are matched to the ongoing level of exercise. An increased release of epinephrine and norepinephrine from the adrenal glands causes plasma catecholamines to rise by as much as 10–20-fold.

Effects of local metabolites on muscle and heart

The autonomic reflexes described above are responsible for most of the cardiac and vasoconstricting adaptations to exercise. However, the marked vasodilatation of coronary and skeletal muscle arterioles is almost entirely caused by *local metabolites* generated in the heart and working skeletal muscle. This **metabolic hyperaemia** (see Chapter 21) causes decreased vascular resistance and increased blood flow. Capillary recruitment (see above) is an important consequence of metabolic hyperaemia.

Static exercises such as lifting and carrying involve maintained muscle contractions with no joint movement. This results in vascular compression and a decreased muscle blood flow, leading to a build-up of muscle metabolites. These activate muscle chemoreceptors, resulting in a **pressor reflex** involving *tachycardia*, and *increases* in *CO* and *TPR*. The resulting rise in blood pressure is much greater than in dynamic exercise causing the same rise in O_2 consumption.

Effects of training

Athletic training has effects on the cardiovascular system that improve delivery of O_2 to muscle cells, allowing them to work harder. The ventricular walls thicken and the cavities become larger, increasing the stroke volume from about 75 to 120 mL. The resting heart rate may fall as low as 45 beats/min, due to an increase in vagal tone, while the maximal rate remains near 180 beats/min. These changes allow CO, the crucial determinant of exercise capacity, to increase more during strenuous exercise, reaching levels of 35 L/min or more. TPR falls, in part due to a decreased sympathetic outflow. The capillary density of skeletal muscle increases, and the muscle fibres contain more mitochondria, promoting oxygen extraction and utilization.

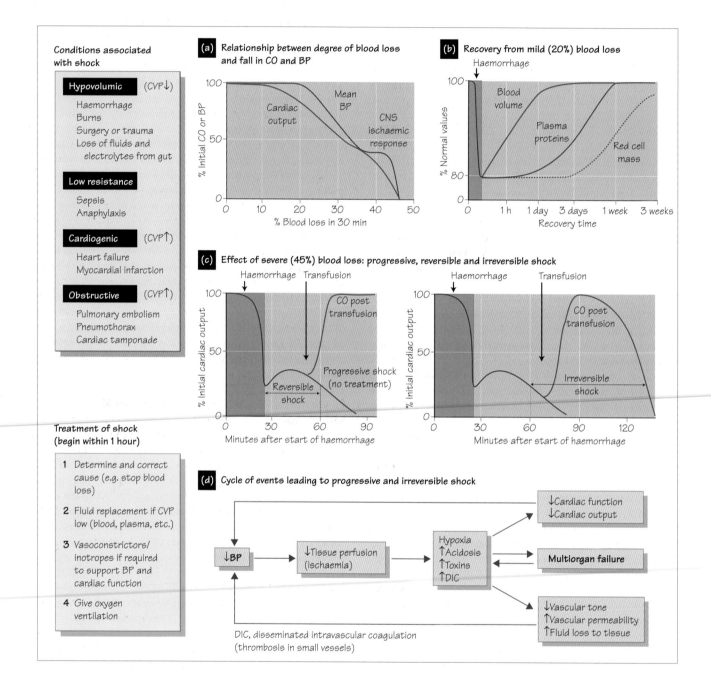

Conditions associated with shock

Hypovolumic   (CVP↓)

Haemorrhage
Burns
Surgery or trauma
Loss of fluids and
    electrolytes from gut

Low resistance

Sepsis
Anaphylaxis

Cardiogenic   (CVP↑)

Heart failure
Myocardial infarction

Obstructive   (CVP↑)

Pulmonary embolism
Pneumothorax
Cardiac tamponade

Treatment of shock (begin within 1 hour)

1 Determine and correct
   cause (e.g. stop blood
   loss)

2 Fluid replacement if CVP
   low (blood, plasma, etc.)

3 Vasoconstrictors/
   inotropes if required
   to support BP and
   cardiac function

4 Give oxygen
   ventilation

(a) Relationship between degree of blood loss and fall in CO and BP

% Initial CO or BP
Cardiac output
Mean BP
CNS ischaemic response
% Blood loss in 30 min

(b) Recovery from mild (20%) blood loss

Haemorrhage
% Normal values
Blood volume
Plasma proteins
Red cell mass
Recovery time
1 h   1 day   3 days   1 week   3 weeks

(c) Effect of severe (45%) blood loss: progressive, reversible and irreversible shock

Haemorrhage   Transfusion
% Initial cardiac output
CO post transfusion
Reversible shock
Progressive shock (no treatment)
Minutes after start of haemorrhage

Haemorrhage   Transfusion
% Initial cardiac output
CO post transfusion
Irreversible shock
Minutes after start of haemorrhage

(d) Cycle of events leading to progressive and irreversible shock

↓BP → ↓Tissue perfusion (ischaemia) → Hypoxia ↑Acidosis ↑Toxins ↑DIC

↓Cardiac function
↓Cardiac output

Multiorgan failure

↓Vascular tone
↑Vascular permeability
↑Fluid loss to tissue

DIC, disseminated intravascular coagulation
(thrombosis in small vessels)

Cardiovascular or circulatory shock refers to an acute condition where there is a generalized inadequacy of blood flow throughout the body. The patient appears pale, grey or cyanotic, with cold clammy skin, a weak, rapid pulse, and rapid shallow breathing. Urine output is reduced, and blood pressure (BP) is generally low. Conscious patients may suffer from intense thirst. Cardiovascular shock may be caused by a reduced blood volume (**hypovolumic shock**), profound vasodilatation (**low-resistance shock**), acute failure of the heart to maintain output (**cardiogenic shock**), or blockage of the cardiopulmonary circuit (e.g. pulmonary embolism).

Haemorrhagic shock

Blood loss (**haemorrhage**) is the most common cause of **hypovolumic** shock. Loss of up to ~20% of total blood volume is unlikely to elicit shock in a fit person. If 20–30% of blood volume is lost, shock is normally induced and blood pressure may be depressed, although death is not common. Loss of 30–50% of volume, however, causes a profound reduction in BP and cardiac output (Figure 29a), with severe shock which may become **irreversible** or **refractory** (see below). Severity is related to amount and rate of blood loss—a very rapid loss of 30% can be fatal, whereas 50% over 24 h may be survived. Above 50% death is generally inevitable.

Immediate compensation

The initial fall in BP is detected by the **baroreceptors**, and reduced blood flow activates peripheral **chemoreceptors**. These cause a reflex increase in sympathetic and decrease in parasympathetic drive, with a subsequent increase in heart rate, venoconstriction (which restores CVP) and vasoconstriction of the splanchnic, cutaneous, renal and skeletal muscle circulations which helps restore BP. Vasoconstriction leads to pallor, reduced urine production and lactic acidosis. Increased sympathetic discharge also results in sweating, and characteristic clammy skin. Sympathetic vasoconstriction of the renal artery plus reduced renal artery pressure stimulates the **renin–angiotensin system** (see Chapter 27), and production of **angiotensin II**, a powerful vasoconstrictor. This plays an important role in the recovery of BP and stimulates thirst. In more severe blood loss, reduction in atrial stretch receptor output stimulates production of **vasopressin** (antidiuretic hormone, **ADH**) and adrenal production of **epinephrine**, both of which contribute to vasoconstriction. These initial mechanisms may prevent any significant fall in BP or cardiac output following moderate blood loss, even though the degree of shock may be serious. If BP falls below 50 mmHg the **CNS ischaemic response** is activated, with powerful sympathetic activation (Figure 29a).

Medium- and long-term mechanisms

The vasoconstriction and/or fall in BP decreases capillary hydrostatic pressure, resulting in fluid movement from the interstitium back into the vasculature (see Chapter 19). This 'internal transfusion' may increase blood volume by ~0.5 L and takes hours to develop. Increased glucose production by the liver may contribute by raising plasma and interstitial fluid osmolarity, thus drawing water from intracellular compartments. This process results in haemodilution, and patients with severe shock often present with a reduced haematocrit. Fluid volume is brought back to normal over days by increased fluid intake (thirst), decreased urine production (**oliguria**) due to renal vasoconstriction, increased Na^+ reabsorption caused by the production of **aldosterone** (stimulated by

angiotensin II) and a fall in **ANP** (atrial natriuretic peptide), and increased water reabsorption caused by vasopressin (Figure 29b). The liver replaces plasma proteins within a week, and haematocrit returns to normal within 6 weeks due to stimulation of **erythropoiesis** (Figure 29b, see Chapter 6).

Other responses to haemorrhage are: *increased ventilation* due to reduced flow through **chemoreceptors** (carotid body) and/or acidosis; *decreased blood coagulation time* due to an increase in platelets and fibrinogen that occurs within minutes (see Chapter 7); and *increased white cell (neutrophil) count* after 2–5 h.

Complications and irreversible (refractory) shock

When blood loss exceeds 30%, cardiac output may temporarily improve before continuing to decline (**progressive shock**; Figure 29c). This is due to a vicious circle initiated by circulatory failure and tissue hypoxia/ischaemia, leading to acidosis, toxin release and eventually **multiorgan failure**, including **depression of cardiac muscle function**, acute respiratory distress syndrome (**ARDS**), **renal failure**, disseminated intravascular coagulation (**DIC**), **hepatic failure** and damage to **intestinal mucosa**. Increased vascular permeability further decreases blood volume due to fluid loss into the tissues, and vascular tone is depressed. These complications lead to further tissue damage, impairment of tissue perfusion and gas exchange (Figure 29d). Rapid treatment (e.g. transfusion) is essential; after 1 h ('the golden hour') mortality increases sharply if the patient is still in shock, as transfusion and vasoconstrictor drugs may then cause only a temporary respite before cardiac output falls irrevocably. This is called **irreversible** or **re-fractory** shock (Figure 29c), and is primarily related to irretrievable damage to the heart.

Other types of hypovolumic shock

Severe burns result in a loss of plasma in exudate from damaged tissue. As red cells are not lost, there is **haemoconcentration**, which will increase blood viscosity. Treatment of burns-related shock therefore involves infusion of plasma rather than whole blood. **Traumatic and surgical shock** can occur after major injury or surgery. Although this is partly due to external blood loss, blood and plasma can also be lost into the tissues, and there may be dehydration. **Other conditions** include severe diarrhoea or vomiting and loss of Na^+ (e.g. **cholera**) with a consequent reduction in blood volume even if water is given, unless electrolytes are replenished.

Low-resistance shock

Unlike hypovolumic shock, low-resistance shock may present with warm skin due to profound peripheral vasodilatation.

Septic shock is caused by a profound vasodilatation due to endotoxins released by infecting bacteria, partly via induction of inducible nitric oxide synthase (see Chapter 22). Capillary permeability and cardiac function may be impaired, with consequent loss of fluid to the tissues and depressed cardiac output.

Anaphylactic shock is a rapidly developing and life-threatening condition resulting from presentation of antigen to a sensitized individual (e.g. bee stings or peanut allergy). A severe **allergic reaction** may result, with release of large amounts of histamine. This causes profound vasodilatation, and increased microvasculature permeability, leading to protein and fluid loss to tissues (oedema). Rapid treatment with antihistamines and glucocorticoids is necessary, but immediate application of a vasoconstrictor (epinephrine) may be required to save the patient's life.

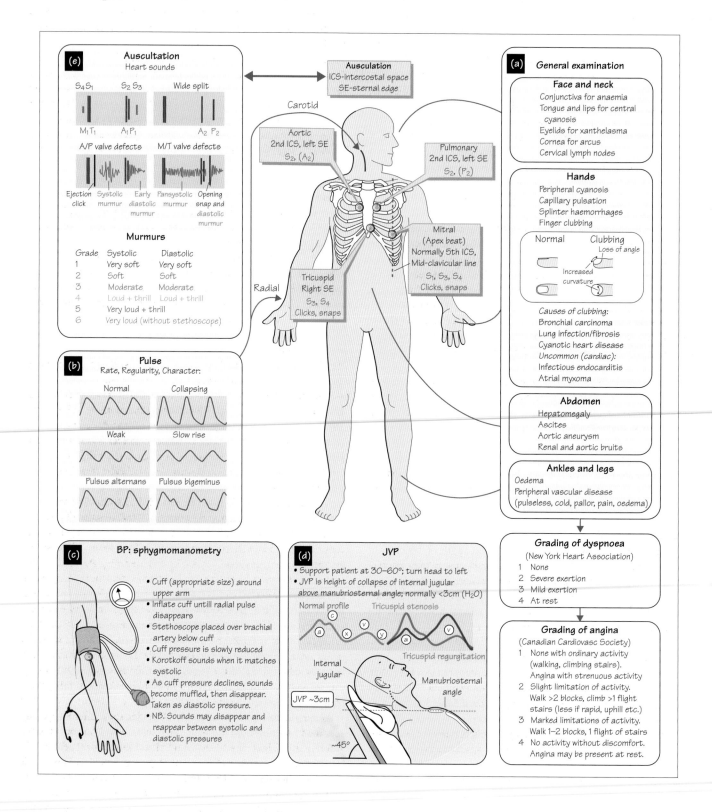

(e) Auscultation
Heart sounds

$S_4 S_1$ $S_2 S_3$ Wide split

$M_1 T_1$ $A_1 P_1$ $A_2 P_2$

A/P valve defects   M/T valve defects

Ejection click   Systolic murmur   Early diastolic murmur   Pansystolic murmur   Opening snap and diastolic murmur

Murmurs

Grade	Systolic	Diastolic
1	Very soft	Very soft
2	Soft	Soft
3	Moderate	Moderate
4	Loud + thrill	Loud + thrill
5	Very loud + thrill	
6	Very loud (without stethoscope)	

Auscultation
ICS-intercostal space
SE-sternal edge

Carotid

Aortic
2nd ICS, left SE
S_2, (A_2)

Pulmonary
2nd ICS, left SE
S_2, (P_2)

Mitral
(Apex beat)
Normally 5th ICS,
Mid-clavicular line
S_1, S_3, S_4
Clicks, snaps

Tricuspid
Right SE
S_3, S_4
Clicks, snaps

Radial

(a) General examination

Face and neck
Conjunctiva for anaemia
Tongue and lips for central cyanosis
Eyelids for xanthelasma
Cornea for arcus
Cervical lymph nodes

Hands
Peripheral cyanosis
Capillary pulsation
Splinter haemorrhages
Finger clubbing

Normal   Clubbing
Loss of angle
Increased curvature

Causes of clubbing:
Bronchial carcinoma
Lung infection/fibrosis
Cyanotic heart disease
Uncommon (cardiac):
Infectious endocarditis
Atrial myxoma

Abdomen
Hepatomegaly
Ascites
Aortic aneurysm
Renal and aortic bruits

Ankles and legs
Oedema
Peripheral vascular disease
(pulseless, cold, pallor, pain, oedema)

(b) Pulse
Rate, Regularity, Character:

Normal   Collapsing

Weak   Slow rise

Pulsus alternans   Pulsus bigeminus

(c) BP: sphygmomanometry

- Cuff (appropriate size) around upper arm
- Inflate cuff untill radial pulse disappears
- Stethoscope placed over brachial artery below cuff
- Cuff pressure is slowly reduced
- Korotkoff sounds when it matches systolic
- As cuff pressure declines, sounds become muffled, then disappear. Taken as diastolic pressure.
- NB. Sounds may disappear and reappear between systolic and diastolic pressures

(d) JVP

- Support patient at 30–60°; turn head to left
- JVP is height of collapse of internal jugular above manubriosternal angle; normally <3cm (H_2O)

Normal profile   Tricuspid stenosis

Tricuspid regurgitation

Internal jugular

Manubriosternal angle

JVP ~3cm

~45°

Grading of dyspnoea
(New York Heart Association)
1   None
2   Severe exertion
3   Mild exertion
4   At rest

Grading of angina
(Canadian Cardiovasc Society)
1   None with ordinary activity (walking, climbing stairs). Angina with strenuous activity
2   Slight limitation of activity. Walk >2 blocks, climb >1 flight stairs (less if rapid, uphill etc.)
3   Marked limitations of activity. Walk 1–2 blocks, 1 flight of stairs
4   No activity without discomfort. Angina may be present at rest.

History

Presenting complaint Most common in cardiovascular disease are breathlessness, chest pain, palpitations, and dizziness or syncope.

History of presenting complaint Explore features of the main symptoms (e.g. onset, progression, grading; see Figure 30a).

- **Breathlessness (dyspnoea)** The most common symptom of heart disease. Establish whether it occurs at rest, on exertion (walking, climbing stairs), when lying down (**orthopnoea**; relieved by extra pillows) or at night. Determine rate of onset (sudden, gradual). Is it a recent development? Dyspnoea due to pulmonary oedema (heart failure) may cause sudden wakening (**paroxysmal nocturnal dyspnoea; PND**).

- **Chest pain** SOCRATES – **S**ite: where is it? **O**nset: gradual, sudden? **C**haracter: sharp, gripping, crushing? **R**adiation: does it spread to arm, neck, jaw? **A**ssociations: associated with nausea, dizziness or palpitations? **T**iming: does it vary during the day? **E**xacerbating and relieving factors: is it worse/better with breathing, posture? **S**everity: does it interfere with daily activities or sleep? **Angina** is described as crushing or gripping pain in the centre of the chest, radiating to left arm/shoulder, neck or jaw. Pain due to **pericarditis** is sharp and severe, aggravated by breathing, relieved by leaning forward.
- **Palpitations** Increased awareness of heart beat, thumping sensation. Get patient to tap out rhythm; is it constant or intermittent? Premature beats and extrasystoles give sensation of **missed beats**.
- **Dizziness/headache** **Postural hypotension**, paroxysmal arrhythmias and cerebrovascular disease. Common in hypertension and heart failure.
- **Syncope** Commonly **vasovagal**, provoked by e.g. anxiety. Cardiovascular syncope is usually due to sudden changes in heart rhythm, e.g. heart block, paroxysmal arrhythmias (**Stokes–Adams attacks**).
- **Others** Fatigue – heart failure, arrhythmias and drugs (e.g. β-blockers). Oedema and abdominal discomfort – raised CVP, heart failure. Leg pain on walking may be due to **claudication** and vascular disease.

Past medical history Previous (including childhood) and current conditions, such as myocardial infarction (MI), hypertension, diabetes, rheumatic fever. Determine prescribed and other medications, and compliance. Review previous blood pressures, lipids, chest X-rays and ECGs.

Family, occupational and social history Family history of hypertension, diabetes, stroke or early death? **Smoking** including duration and amount (1 pack/day for 1 year = 1 pack-year) and alcohol consumption. **Occupation**: stress, sedentary or active.

Examination

General examination (Figure 30a):
Note general features including anxiety, obesity, cachexia (wasting), jaundice, anaemia and any discomfort. Assess breathlessness.

- **Hands** Tremor; peripheral cyanosis (blue colouration, deoxy-haemoglobin > 5 g/dL, e.g. vasoconstriction, shock, heart failure; not seen in anaemia); nail-bed capillary pulsation (*Quincke's sign*; aortic regurgitation, thyrotoxicosis); splinter haemorrhages under nails (trauma, infective endocarditis); finger clubbing (Figure 30a).
- **Face and neck** Examine conjunctivae for anaemia; tongue (lips) for central cyanosis; eyelids for xanthelasma (yellow plaques: hyperlipidaemia); retina for hypertensive damage. Check for enlarged lymph nodes or thyroid, and signs of systemic disease.
- **Abdomen** Palpate for liver enlargement/tenderness (**hepatomegaly**), ascites (raised CVP, heart failure), splenomegaly (infective endocarditis).
- **Lower limbs, ankles** Assess for oedema, signs of peripheral vascular disease.

Pulse (Figure 30b)
Resting rate 60–90 beats/min, slows with age and in atheletes.

Compare radial with apex beat (delay: e.g. atrial fibrillation) and femoral/lower limbs (delay: atherosclerosis, aortic stenosis). Changes in rate with breathing are normal (**sinus arrhythmia**).

- **Irregular beats** *Regularly irregular*: e.g. extrasystoles (disappear on exertion), second-degree heart block. *Irregularly irregular*: e.g. atrial fibrillation (unchanged by exertion).
- **Character** (carotid) *Thready or weak*: heart failure, shock, valve disease; with *slow rise*: aortic stenosis. *Strong/bounding*: high output; followed by *sharp fall* (**collapsing**, *water hammer*): very high output, aortic valve regurgitation. *Alternating weak/strong* (**pulsus alternans**): left heart failure; distinguish from **pulsus bigeminus**, normal beat followed by weak premature beat. *Pulsus paradoxus, accentuated weakening of pulse on inspiration*: cardiac tamponade, severe asthma, restrictive pericarditis.

Blood pressure (Figure 30c)
At rest, adult arterial systolic pressure is normally < 150 mmHg, diastolic < 90 mmHg. Systolic rises with age. May be elevated due to anxiety ('white coat syndrome').

- **Jugular venous pressure** (JVP) (Figure 30d) Indirect measure of right atrial pressure. Raised in heart failure and volume overload. Large 'a' wave (see Chapter 14): pulmonary hypertension, pulmonary valve stenosis, tricuspid stenosis; large 'v' wave: tricuspid regurgitation. Absent 'a': atrial fibrillation.

Chest examination
Position patient comfortably on couch with chest at ~45°. Examine for surgical scarring, and deformities (e.g. funnel chest).

- **Palpation; Apex beat**, usually at 5th intercostal space, midclavicular line (mitral area). *Missing*: obesity, hyperinflation, pleural effusion. *Displacement*: cardiomegaly, pneumothorax. *Tapping*: mitral stenosis. *Double*: ventricular hypertrophy. *Heaving* (forceful and sustained): pressure overload – hypertension, aortic stenosis. *Parasternal heave*: right ventricular hypertrophy. **Thrills** are palpable (therefore strong) murmurs (see below).
- **Auscultation** (Figure 30e; see Chapters 14, 52, 53) Correlate with pulse. **First heart sound** (S_1): closure of mitral (M_1) and tricuspid (T_1) valves. *Loud*: AV valve stenosis, short PR interval; *soft*: mitral regurgitation, long PR, heart failure. **Second heart sound** (S_2): closure of aortic (A_2) and pulmonary (P_2) valves, A_2 louder and preceding P_2. *Loud A_2/P_2*: systemic/pulmonary hypertension. *Splitting*: normal during inspiration or exercise, particularly in young. *Wide splitting*: delayed activation (e.g. right bundle branch block) or termination (pulmonary hypertension, stenosis) of RV systole. *Reverse splitting*: delayed activation (e.g. left bundle branch block) or termination (hypertension, aortic stenosis) of LV systole. **Others**: S_3 – rapid ventricular filling, common in young but may reflect heart failure in patients > 30 years. S_4 – precedes S_1, due to ventricular stiffness and abnormal filling during atrial systole. Presence of S_3 and/or S_4 gives a **gallop rhythm**. **Ejection click**: after S_1, opening of stenotic semilunar valve. **Opening snap**: after S_2, opening of stenotic AV valve. Mitral sounds best heard when lying on left side.
- **Murmurs** (Figure 30e) Due to turbulent blood flow. Soft systolic murmurs are common and innocent in young (~40% children 3–8 years) and in exercise; all **diastolic murmurs** are pathological. Most non-benign murmurs are due to **valve defects** (see Chapters 52, 53). Others include a hyperdynamic circulation and atrial or ventricular septal defects. Vascular murmurs (**bruits**) may indicate stenosis, e.g. carotid, abdominal (aorta, renal artery).

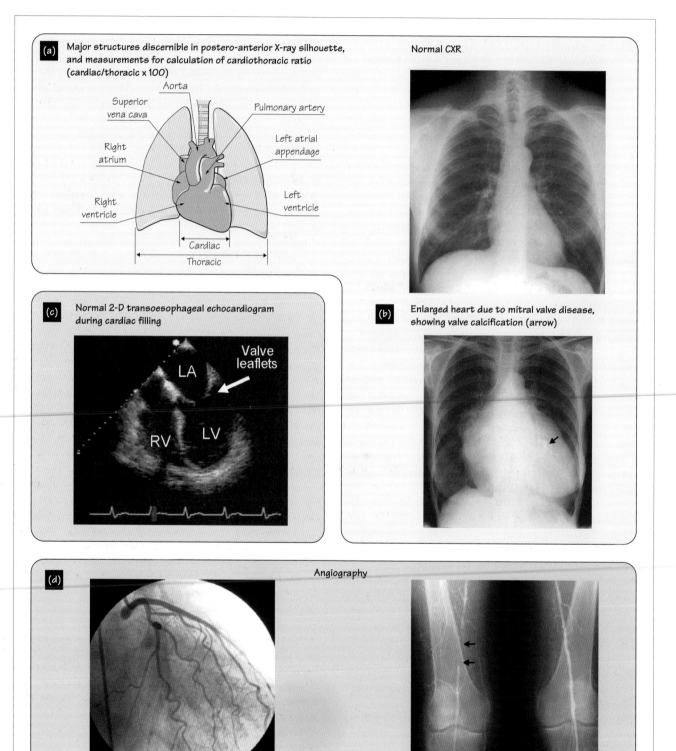

(a) Major structures discernible in postero-anterior X-ray silhouette, and measurements for calculation of cardiothoracic ratio (cardiac/thoracic x 100)

Aorta
Superior vena cava
Right atrium
Right ventricle
Pulmonary artery
Left atrial appendage
Left ventricle
Cardiac
Thoracic

Normal CXR

(c) Normal 2-D transoesophageal echocardiogram during cardiac filling

Valve leaflets
LA
RV
LV

(b) Enlarged heart due to mitral valve disease, showing valve calcification (arrow)

Angiography

Normal left coronary angiogram

Occluded segment in right femoral (arrowed)

Key investigations for cardiovascular disease are electrocardiogram (ECG; see Chapter 32), chest X-ray and echocardiogram. Others include exercise ECG testing, ambulatory blood pressure monitoring, lipid profile, cardiac enzyme assays, and catheterization with coronary or pulmonary angiography.

X-rays (chest radiography)

The chest X-ray (CXR) is an essential diagnostic tool. The initial CXR is taken in the postero-anterior (PA) direction, with the patient upright and at full inspiration. Figure (a) shows diagrammatically the major structures in which gross abnormalities can be detected, such as enlargement of the heart chambers and major vessels, and a normal PA CXR. Heart size and **cardiothoracic ratio** (size of heart relative to thoracic cavity) can also be estimated. This ratio is normally < 50%, except in neonates, infants and athletes, but may be greatly increased in heart failure (see Chapter 46). Calcification due to tissue damage and necrosis may be detected by CXR if significant (Figure 31c). Enlargement of the main pulmonary arteries coupled with pruning of the peripheral arteries suggests pulmonary hypertension, whereas haziness of the lung fields is indicative of pulmonary venous hypertension and fluid accumulation in the tissues.

Echocardiography and Doppler ultrasound

Echocardiography can be used to detect enlarged hearts and abnormal cardiac movement, and to estimate the ejection fraction. An ultrasound pulse of ~2.5 MHz is generated by a piezoelectric transmitter–receiver on the chest wall, and is reflected back by internal structures. As sound travels through fluid at a known velocity, the time taken between transmission and reception is a measure of distance. This allows a picture of internal structure to be built up. In an M-mode echocardiogram the transmitter remains static, and the trace shows changes in reflections with time. In two-dimensional (2D) echocardiograms the transmitter scans backwards and forwards, so that a 2D picture is built up. Echocardiography is non-invasive and quick. However, when imaging the heart it is restricted by the presence of the rib cage and air in the lungs, which reflect or absorb the ultrasound. This interference can be minimized by using specific locations on the chest. Alternatively, the probe can be placed in the oesophagus (**transoesophageal echocardiography**; TOE). Although more invasive, this provides greater resolution (Figure 31b), and improved access to pulmonary artery, aorta and atria.

Sound reflected back from a moving target shows a shift in frequency; for example if the target is moving towards the source, the frequency is increased. This **Doppler** effect can be used to calculate the *velocity* of blood movement from the frequency shift in the ultrasound pulse caused by reflection from red cells, and the *pressure gradient* across obstructions from the Bernoulli equation: $P = 4 \times (velocity)^2$. Blood flow can be calculated if the cross-sectional area of the vessel is estimated using echocardiography.

Catheterization and angiography

Radiopaque catheters (opaque to X-rays) are introduced into the heart or blood vessels via peripheral veins or arteries. Catheters with small balloons at the tip (**Swan–Ganz** catheters) assist placement from the venous side as the tip moves with the flow. Placement can be ascertained from the pressure wave-form and X-rays. Catheters are used for measurement of pressures or cardiac output, for **angiography**, or to take samples for estimating metabolites and Po_2. Left atrial pressure cannot be measured directly as it requires access via the mitral valve. Instead, a Swan–Ganz catheter is passed through the right heart, and is wedged in a distal pulmonary artery. As there is thus no flow through that artery, the pressure is the same throughout the capillaries to the pulmonary vein. This **pulmonary wedge pressure** is an estimate of left atrial pressure.

Angiography A radiopaque **contrast medium** is introduced into the lumen of cardiac chambers, and coronary (Figure 31d), pulmonary or other blood vessels. This allows direct visualization of the blood and vessels with X-rays, and can be used to examine cardiac pumping function and to locate blockages (e.g. emboli) in the vasculature (Figure 31d).

Imaging

Advances in medical imaging techniques have provided several powerful diagnostic aids, of particular use in cardiac disease.

Nuclear imaging Radiopharmaceuticals introduced into the heart or circulation are detected by a gamma camera, and their distribution (depending on type) can be used to measure or detect cardiac muscle perfusion, damage and function. Three-dimensional information can be obtained in a similar fashion using single photon emission computed tomography (**SPECT**). The most common tracers used are thallium-201 (^{201}Tl), and technetium-99m (^{99m}Tc)-labelled sestamibi (a large synthetic molecule of the isonitrile family), which are distributed according to blood flow and taken up by living cardiac muscle cells. These therefore show up brightly immediately after infusion; ischaemic and infarcted areas remain dark because of poor perfusion. Whereas over time ^{201}Tl will redistribute into ischaemic areas as well, ^{99m}Tc-sestamibi will not, so a delayed ^{201}Tl image will show infarcted areas only. This is useful for determining savable areas of the heart prior to angioplasty or coronary bypass. Technetium-99m, however, has a higher photon energy and shorter half-life, allowing lower radionucleotide doses with better images. It is therefore better for SPECT, and the higher energy allows **gated acquisition** (sequential images taken during a cardiac cycle), and evaluation of resting left and right ventricular function in combination with either resting or exercise myocardial perfusion.

Magnetic resonance imaging (MRI) Radiofrequency stimulation of hydrogen atoms held in a high magnetic field emits energy, which can be used to generate a high-fidelity image that reflects tissue density. MRI is useful for the location of masses and malformations, including aneurysms. It is entirely non-invasive and uses no damaging radiations.

32 The electrocardiogram

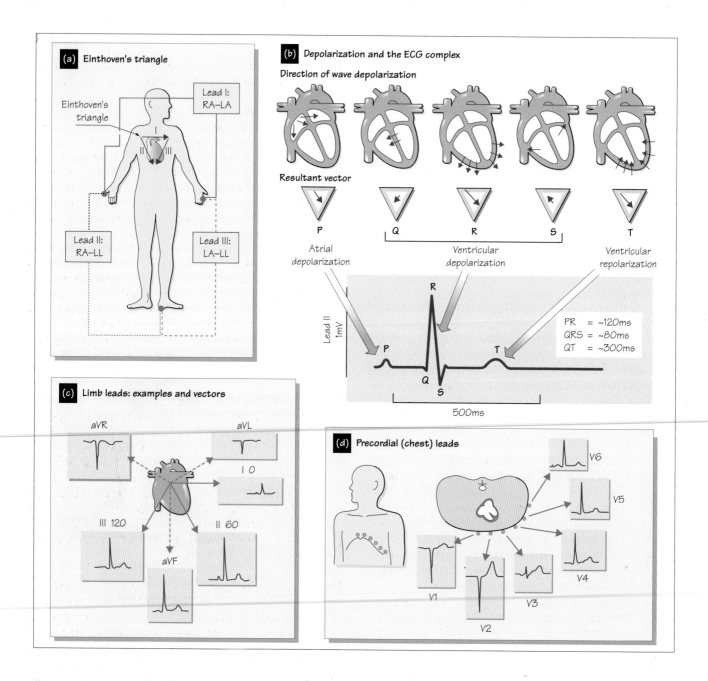

(a) Einthoven's triangle

Einthoven's triangle

Lead I: RA–LA

Lead II: RA–LL

Lead III: LA–LL

(b) Depolarization and the ECG complex

Direction of wave depolarization

Resultant vector

P   Q   R   S   T

Atrial depolarization

Ventricular depolarization

Ventricular repolarization

Lead II 1mV

R
P   T
Q
S

PR = ~120ms
QRS = ~80ms
QT = ~300ms

500ms

(c) Limb leads: examples and vectors

aVR

aVL

I 0

III 120

II 60

aVF

(d) Precordial (chest) leads

V6

V5

V4

V1

V2

V3

The extracellular fluids contain salts, and therefore conduct electricity. As these fluids are distributed throughout the body, the body acts as a **volume conductor**. When cardiac muscle depolarizes, extracellular currents between depolarized and resting cells cause potentials that can be measured at the body surface. These form the basis of the **electrocardiogram** (ECG).

Recording the ECG

The ECG is based around the concept of an equilateral triangle (**Einthoven's triangle**), with the heart as the current source at its centre (Figure 32a). The points of the triangle are approximated by the limb leads, connected to the right arm, left arm and left leg. The potential difference between two leads will depend on the amplitude of the current, related to muscle mass, and the direction of current flow. There is a directional component because maximum potential occurs in line with the maximum current flowing between depolarized and resting tissue. The ECG thus has both amplitude and direction, and is a **vector quantity** (Figure 32b).

By convention, the ECG is connected in such a way that a positive voltage causes an upward deflection, and the paper speed of the recorder is normally 25 or 50 mm/s. Note that the term **lead**, when used for the ECG, refers to a measurement made for a particular configuration, not to the wires connected to the patient.

The **classic bipolar leads** of the ECG approximate the potential difference across the sides of Einthoven's triangle, and are essentially looking at electrical activity in the heart from three different directions, separated by 60°. They are **lead I**, measured as the potential difference between the right and left arm; **lead II**, right arm and left leg; and **lead III**, left leg and left arm. Lead II normally has the largest deflections, as it lies closest to the direction of ventricular depolarization. As the ventricles have the largest muscle mass, they give the largest current and thus voltage.

The **unipolar leads** use a single sensing electrode, and the voltage measured is the potential difference between this and an estimate of zero potential. Practically, the latter is obtained by connecting the limb leads together via a resistor. This approximates to the centre of the current source and hence Einthoven's triangle, i.e. the heart. Nine unipolar leads are commonly used clinically, consisting of six chest (**precordial**) leads, V1–V6, and the **augmented** leads **aVR**, **aVL**, and **aVF**. The chest leads use a separate sensing electrode placed on the chest (Figure 32d), whereas the augmented leads use a limb lead as a sensing electrode (right arm, aVR; left arm, aVL; left leg, aVF), with the remaining two limb leads connected together to give the zero potential estimate. As the augmented leads measure between one point of Einthoven's triangle and the centre, they are seeing the heart at an angle rotated by 30° compared to the bipolar leads. The six limb leads together therefore give a view of the electrical activity of the heart every 30° (Figure 32c).

General features of the ECG

The ECG trace has three main components that are related to the amplitude and direction of the wave of depolarization (vector) at that moment (Figure 32b). The **P wave** is a small deflection due to depolarization of the atria. This is followed by the **QRS complex**, which is generally ~0.08 s in duration and reflects ventricular depolarization. It is the largest deflection because of the large ventricular muscle mass. The relative size of the Q, R and S components varies between leads, and is dependent on the orientation of the heart. In lead II the Q wave is seen as a small downward deflection, correlating to the left to right depolarization of the interventricular septum. The R wave is a strong upwards deflection, corresponding to depolarization of the main mass of the ventricles. The S wave is a small downward deflection in lead II, and relates to depolarization of the last part of the ventricles close to the base of the heart. The **T wave** corresponds to ventricular repolarization. Note that atrial repolarization is too diffuse to be seen. As the mass of the conducting system (sinoatrial and atrioventricular node, bundle of His) is very small, the associated currents are too small to cause any appreciable deflection in the ECG.

The **PR** and **ST segments** are normally **isoelectric**, i.e. at zero potential. There is no potential because no current is flowing; the relevant tissue (atria or ventricles) is either all depolarized or all at rest. The nonconducting *annulus fibrosus* prevents current flow between the atria and ventricles during the PR segment. The **PR interval** reflects the delay between atrial and ventricular depolarization, and is largely related to delay in the atrioventricular node. It is measured from the beginning of the P wave to the beginning of the QRS, and ranges from 0.12 to 0.20 s. It shortens as heart rate increases.

The **ST segment** approximates to the plateau of the ventricular muscle action potential (AP), and is ~0.25 s. When the myocardium is injured, e.g. during ischaemia, some cells will be partially depolarized causing **injury currents** between them and undamaged tissue. This can either depress or elevate the ECG baseline. However, during the ST segment all cells are completely depolarized. This gives rise to an apparent elevation or depression of the ST segment, although it is actually the baseline that has altered. This is a common indication for acute myocardial damage such as a **myocardial infarction**.

Why the T wave is positive The QRS complex in lead II is positive because the wave of depolarization progresses from the apex and endocardium towards the base and epicardium. As the T wave reflects repolarization it might be expected to be negative, because polarity is reversed. However, because the AP is shorter in the base and epicardium they repolarize first, and the wave of repolarization moves towards the apex and endocardium. The change in both polarity and direction cancel out, and the T wave is upwards. In pathological conditions where the AP is prolonged, or conduction from apex to base is slow, repolarization at the base may be delayed until after that at the apex. Under these conditions the T wave will be *inverted*.

The electrical axis of the heart The angle of the ECG vector at its maximum amplitude is called the electrical axis of the heart. It corresponds to the point of maximum current developed during the heart beat, and hence depolarization of the main mass of the ventricles. It can be calculated from the three bipolar leads, which are at 60° to each other, and normally lies closest to lead II. Changes in the position of the heart will alter the axis, e.g. during breathing. An increase in mass of one of the ventricles will shift the axis in that direction. Thus left ventricular hypertrophy will cause **left axis deviation**, and right ventricular hypertrophy **right axis deviation**.

ECG investigations

The standard, short, resting 12-lead ECG test detects conduction blocks and changes due to muscle damage (e.g. post-MI). It is unlikely to detect intermittent events such as paroxysmal arrhythmias, which require continuous monitoring with a **Holter** test (ambulatory ECG recording for 24 h). In the **exercise tolerance test** workload is progressively increased, and the ECG monitored for ST depression and arrhythmias caused by ischaemia related to coronary artery disease.

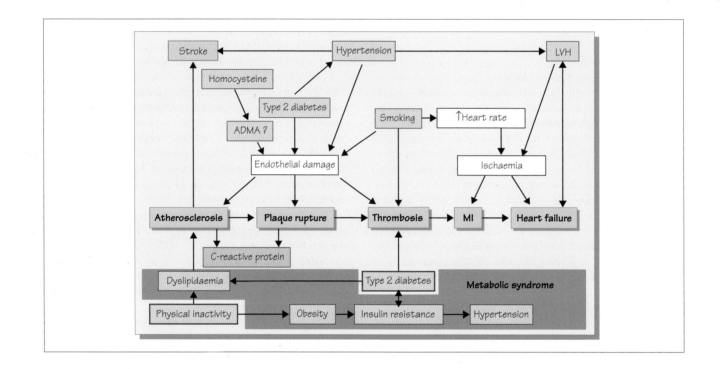

Numerous factors or conditions are known to increase the probability that cardiovascular disease (CVD) will develop. The presence in an individual of these **cardiovascular risk factors** can be used to assess the likelihood that overt cardiovascular morbidity and death will occur in the medium term. Table 33.1 presents an abbreviated summary of the impact of major risk factors on coronary heart disease as determined by the Framingham Heart Study.

Although some risk factors such as *age*, *male sex* and *family history of CVD* are **fixed**, others, including *smoking, dyslipidaemias, hypertension, diabetes mellitus, obesity* and *physical inactivity*, are **modifiable** and can be targeted in order to ameliorate CVD progression. This approach has been shown to reduce the occurrence and severity of CVD, and is particularly justified because overt CVD is typically both irreversible and ultimately lethal. Patients often have multiple modifiable risk factors, in which case all of these should be simultaneously addressed.

The figure illustrates the main mechanisms by which major risk factors are thought to promote the development of atherosclerosis and its most important consequence, **coronary heart disease**. Additional aspects of dyslipidaemias and hypertension are described in Chapters 35–38.

Modifiable risk factors

Dyslipidaemias are a heterogeneous group of conditions characterized by abnormal levels of one or more **lipoproteins**. Lipoproteins are blood-borne particles that contain cholesterol and other lipids. They function to transfer lipids between the intestines, liver and other organs (see Chapter 35).

Dyslipidaemias involving excessive plasma concentrations of **low-density lipoprotein (LDL)**, are associated with rises in plasma cholesterol levels, because LDL contains 70% of total plasma cholesterol. As the level of plasma cholesterol rises, particularly above 240 mg/dL (6.2 mmol/L), there is a progressive increase in the risk of CVD due to the attendant rise in LDL levels. LDL plays a pivotal role in causing atherosclerosis because it can be converted to an oxidized form, which damages the vascular wall (see Chapter 36). Drugs that lower plasma LDL (and therefore oxidized LDL) slow the progression of atherosclerosis and reduce the occurrence of CVD. Elevated levels of **lipoprotein (a)**, a form of LDL containing the unique protein **apo(a)**, have been reported to confer additional cardiovascular risk. Apo(a) contains a structural component closely resembling plasminogen, and it may inhibit fibrinolysis (see Chapter 7) by competing with plasminogen for endogenous activators.

Table 33.1 Major modifiable risk factors: effects on the risk of coronary heart disease in men and women aged 35–64 years.

Risk factors	Age-adjusted relative risk*	
	Men	Women
Cholesterol > 240 mg/dL	1.9	1.8
Hypertension > 140/90 mmHg	2.0	2.2
Diabetes	1.5	3.7
Left ventricular hypertrophy	3.0	4.6
Smoking	1.5	1.1

* Indicates relative risk for individuals with a given factor vs those without it.

On the other hand, the risk of CVD is *inversely* related to the plasma concentration of **high-density lipoprotein (HDL)**, possibly because HDL functions to remove cholesterol from body tissues, and may act to inhibit lipoprotein oxidation. The ratio of total to HDL cholesterol is therefore a better predictor of risk than cholesterol levels *per se*. Low HDL levels often coexist with high levels of plasma *triglycerides*, which are also correlated with CVD. This is probably due to the atherogenicity of the triglyceride-rich **very low density lipoprotein (VLDL)** and **intermediate-density lipoprotein (IDL)**.

Hypertension, defined as a blood pressure above 140/90 mmHg, occurs in ~25% of the population. Hypertension promotes atherogenesis, probably by damaging the endothelium and causing other deleterious effects on the walls of large arteries. Hypertension damages blood vessels of the brain and kidneys, increasing the risk of stroke and renal failure. The higher cardiac workload imposed by the increased arterial pressure also causes a thickening of the left ventricular wall. This process, termed **left ventricular hypertrophy (LVH)**, is both a cause and harbinger of more serious cardiovascular damage. LVH predisposes the myocardium to arrhythmias and ischaemia, and is a major contributor to heart failure, myocardial infarction and sudden death.

Physical inactivity promotes CVD via multiple mechanisms. Low fitness is associated with reduced plasma HDL, higher levels of blood pressure and insulin resistance, and **obesity**, itself a CVD risk factor. Studies show that a moderate to high level of fitness is associated with a halving of CVD mortality.

Diabetes mellitus is a metabolic disease present in approximately 5% of the population. Diabetics either lack the hormone *insulin* entirely, or become resistant to its actions. The latter condition, which usually develops in adulthood, is termed type2 diabetes mellitus (DM2), and accounts for 95% of diabetics. Diabetes causes progressive damage to both the microvasculature and larger arteries over many years. Approximately 75% of diabetics eventually die from CVD.

There is evidence that DM2 patients have both endothelial damage and increased levels of oxidized LDL. Both effects may be a result of mechanisms associated with the hyperglycaemia characteristic of this condition. Also, blood coagulability is increased in DM2 because of elevated plasminogen activator inhibitor 1 (PAI-1) and increased platelet aggregability.

A set of cardiovascular risk factors including high plasma triglycerides, low plasma HDL, hypertension, elevated plasma glucose and obesity (particularly abdominal) are often associated with each other. This combination of risk factors is closely linked to, and could arise as a result of, **insulin resistance**. Individuals with three or more of these risk factors are said to have **metabolic syndrome**.

Atherosclerosis can be viewed as a chronic low-grade inflammation which is localized to certain sites of the vascular wall. This causes the release into the plasma of numerous inflammatory mediators and related substances. Many studies have shown that an elevated serum level of one of these, the acute phase reactant **C-reactive protein (CRP)**, is predictive of future CVD. CRP is a **risk marker** rather than a risk factor, because although it indicates that atherosclerosis is present, it is unlikely to play a causal part in its development. Although it was initially seen as a potentially crucial marker because it seemed able to predict CVD even in those with low LDL, recent epidemiological studies are increasingly questioning whether CRP levels are truly independent of other established risk factors (e.g metabolic syndrome).

Tobacco smoking causes CVD by lowering HDL, increasing blood coagulability and damaging the endothelium, thereby promoting atherosclerosis. In addition, nicotine-induced cardiac stimulation and a carbon monoxide-mediated reduction of the oxygen-carrying capacity of the blood also occur. These effects, coupled with an increased occurrence of coronary spasm, set the stage for cardiac ischaemia and myocardial infarction. Epidemiological evidence suggests that CVD risk is not reduced with low tar cigarettes.

High plasma levels of **homocysteine**, a metabolite of the amino acid methionine, are proposed to be a CVD risk factor, although the evidence for this association is controversial. Hyperhomocysteinaemia may increase cardiovascular risk by causing overproduction of the endogenous eNOS inhibitor **ADMA** (see Chapter 22), since homocysteine can serve as a donor of methyl groups which are enzymatically transferred to arginine to form ADMA.

Fixed risk factors
Family history of CVD
Numerous epidemiological surveys have shown the existence of a familial predisposition to CVD. This arises in part because many CVD risk factors (e.g. hypertension) have a *multifactorial genetic basis* (are due to multiple abnormal genes interacting with environmental influences). Additional deleterious genetic influences are also probably involved, because the familial predisposition remains if epidemiological data are corrected for known risk factors. For example, the angiotensin-converting enzyme (ACE) gene can exist in two forms, characterized by the insertion/deletion of a 287-base-pair DNA segment within intron 16. Those homozygous for the deletion polymorphism have higher plasma ACE concentrations, which may modestly increase the risk of myocardial infarction.

Male sex
Middle-aged women are much less likely than men to develop CVD. This difference progressively narrows after the menopause, and is mainly oestrogen mediated. Oestrogen's potentially beneficial actions include acting as an antioxidant, lowering LDL and raising HDL, stimulating the expression and activity of nitric oxide synthase, causing vasodilatation and increasing the production of plasminogen.

Beta-blockers, angiotensin-converting enzyme inhibitors, angiotensin receptor blockers, and Ca²⁺-channel blockers

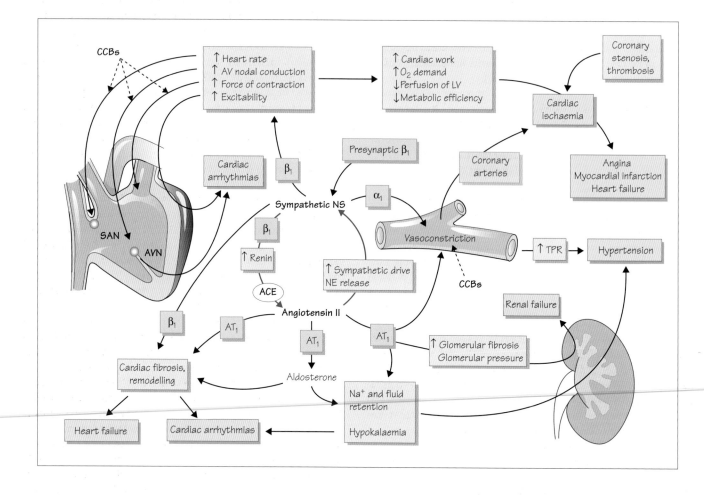

The four classes of drugs described in this chapter each stand out as being useful in treating multiple disorders of the cardiovascular system. Core aspects of their mechanisms of action and properties are described here and further details on their use are presented in chapters dealing specifically with these disorders.

Beta-adrenoceptor antagonists (β-blockers)

Beta-blockers (βB) are used to treat hypertension, angina, supraventricular cardiac arrhythmias, myocardial infarction and chronic heart failure. Their usefulness derives mainly from their blockade of cardiac *β₁-receptors* (see figure). When stimulated by norepinephrine released from sympathetic nerves, and by blood-borne epinephrine, these receptors increase the rate and force of cardiac contraction, thereby increasing the output, work and O_2 requirement of the heart. Although these responses are important for the normal physiological response to stress, they have the undesirable effect of promoting cardiac ischaemia and its downstream effects if coronary blood flow is compromised by atherosclerotic stenosis or thrombosis (see Chapters 39 and 44). Activation of β₁-receptors also increases AV nodal conduction and the excitability of the heart, effects which can sometimes cause or promote cardiac arrhythmias (see Chapters 44, 48–51). Chronic activation of the

sympathetic system, as in congestive heart failure, causes cardiac fibrosis and remodelling, leading to a progressive deterioration of cardiac function and increasing the occurrence of life-threatening arrhythmias (see Chapter 47).

Beta-blockers have additional useful effects. Importantly, renal afferent arterioles contain *renin-producing granular cells* which are stimulated by sympathetic nerves to release renin via their β₁ receptors. Thus, the renin–angiotensin–aldosterone (RAA) axis (see Chapter 28) can be stimulated by the sympathetic system, an effect that βB inhibit. Beta-blockers also inhibit the release of norepinephrine from sympathetic nerves by inhibiting presynaptic β-receptors on sympathetic varicosities which act to facilitate its release.

Propranolol, a 'first-generation' βB, acts on both β₁- and β₂-receptors, whereas second-generation βB (e.g. **atenolol, metoprolol, bisoprolol**) selectively antagonize β₁-receptors. Third-generation βB also cause vasodilatation; for example **carvidelol** does this by blocking α-receptors and by releasing nitric oxide. **Pindolol** belongs to a fourth group of βB with *intrinsic sympathomimetic activity*; it antagonizes β₁-receptors but stimulates β₂-receptors, thereby causing vasodilatation. Although in all cases the main therapeutic effect of these drugs lies in their effect on β₁-receptors, these various properties, as well as differences between βB with respect to their pharmacokinetics and adverse effects mean that specific βB may be more or less appropriate for individual patients. Adverse effects of βB as a class include exercise intolerance, excessive bradycardia and negative inotropy, all due to their cardiosuppressive effects. Their block of vascular β-receptors, which promote blood flow to skeletal muscle by causing vasodilatation, can also cause fatigue and cold/tingling extremities. Beta-blockers can also cause bronchospasm, and are contraindicated in asthma. These drugs can also have the potentially dangerous effect of masking the perception of hypoglycaemia in diabetics.

Angiotensin-converting enzyme inhibitors (ACEI) and angiotensin II receptor blockers (ARBs)

The RAA system, acting through its effectors angiotensin II and aldosterone, plays a crucial role in conserving body Na^+ and fluid, thereby acting to maintain blood volume and pressure (see Chapter 27). However, even this normal functioning of the RAA system contributes to raised blood pressure in many hypertensives (see Chapters 37, 38), and abnormal activation of this system in those with heart failure (see Chapter 46) leads to additional adverse effects shown in the lower part of the figure. Angiotensin II also enhances sympathetic neurotransmission by promoting norepinephrine release and by stimulating the CNS to increase sympathetic drive, leading to further increases in blood pressure. The activity of angiotensin II can be suppressed either with ACEI, which block its synthesis by ACE (see Chapter 27), or by ARBs that inhibit its action at **AT1 receptors**, which mediate its various deleterious effects.

Because both block RAA system function, ACEI and ARBs suppress the various vasoconstricting effects of angiotensin II on the vasculature, thereby reducing total peripheral resistance and blood pressure. Both cause natriuresis and diuresis which contribute to their blood pressure-lowering effects and also help to reverse the pulmonary and systemic oedema and cardiac remodelling that contribute to the symptoms and progression of chronic heart failure. ACEI have the additional effect of preventing the breakdown of the peptide *bradykinin*, which is synthesized in the plasma by ACE and causes *vasodilatation* by releasing nitric oxide, prostacyclin and EDHF from the endothelium. Increases in bradykinin may contribute to the ability of ACEI to reduce blood pressure and possibly to prevent cardiac remodelling, but may also cause the chronic cough which ACEI evoke in ~10% of people. ARBs differ from ACEI in that they do not increase bradykinin, and also in that they may cause a greater functional suppression of the RAA system because ACEI do not block *chymase*, another enzyme that synthesizes angiotensin II. Excepting the fact that ARBs cause less cough than do ACEI, the extent to which these mechanistic differences between the two types of drug are therapeutically relevant remains to be fully elucidated. At present, both ACEI and ARBs are used to treat hypertension and heart failure, and to protect against renal complications in diabetes. ACEI are additionally used to treat myocardial infarction.

The vast majority of ACEI (e.g. **enalapril, ramipril, trandolapril**; class II) are administered orally as inactive *prodrugs* which, being lipophilic, are processed in the liver to produce an active metabolite (e.g. enalapril yields *enaloprilat*). **Captopril** (class I), the oldest ACEI, is itself active, but is also acted on by the liver to give active metabolites. **Lisinopril** (class III) is active, and being water soluble, is excreted by the kidneys rather than being metabolized in the liver. Examples of ARBs include **losartan** and **candesartan**. Apart from cough, ACEI and ARBs share common contraindications and side effects. They should not be used by pregnant women since they retard fetal growth, or by those with bilateral renal stenosis, since in these individuals decreased renal blood flow typically leads to a powerful activation of the RAA system which is crucial for maintaining kidney function. Because they diminish levels of aldosterone, which promotes renal K^+ excretion, both can also elevate the plasma K^+ concentration (hyperkalaemia).

Ca^{2+}-channel blockers (CCBs)

CCBs inhibit the influx of Ca^{2+} into cells through L-type Ca^{2+} channels. The interaction of blocker and Ca^{2+} channel is best understood for the *dihydropyridines* (DHPs), which include **nifedipine, amlodipine** and **felodipine**. The affinity of DHPs for the channel increases enormously when the channel is in its *inactivated* state (see Chapter 10). Channel inactivation is favoured by a less negative membrane potential (E_m). DHPs therefore have a relatively selective effect on vascular muscle (E_m ~−55) compared to cardiac muscle (E_m ~−90). This functional selectivity is further enhanced because DHP-mediated vasodilatation stimulates the baroreceptor reflex and increases sympathetic drive, overcoming any direct negative inotropic effects of these drugs. This sympathetic activation is thought to be particularly marked with rapidly acting DHPs, and may lead to cardiac ischaemia and unstable angina. Thus, the DHPs in current use have a slow onset and prolonged effect.

The phenylalkylamine **verapamil** interacts preferentially with the channel in its *open* state. Verapamil binding is therefore less dependent on E_m; thus both cardiac and vascular Ca^{2+} channels are blocked. In addition to its vasodilating properties, verapamil therefore has negative inotropic effects and severely depresses AV nodal conduction. The benzothiazepine **diltiazem** has similar properties; at therapeutic doses it vasodilates but also depresses AV conduction and has negative inotropic/chronotropic effects.

The DHPs are currently first-line agents for treating hypertension (see Chapter 37) and also all forms of angina pectoris (see Chapters 39, 41). The non-DHPs (verapamil and diltiazem) are also used for these conditions, and are additionally used for *supraventricular cardiac arrhythmias*, based on their ability to suppress AV nodal conduction (see Chapters 49, 50). Adverse effects of the DHPs are due to their profound vasodilating properties, and include headache, flushing and oedema. The non-DHPs can cause powerful negative inotropic and chronotropic effects, and verapamil can cause constipation.

35 Hyperlipidaemias

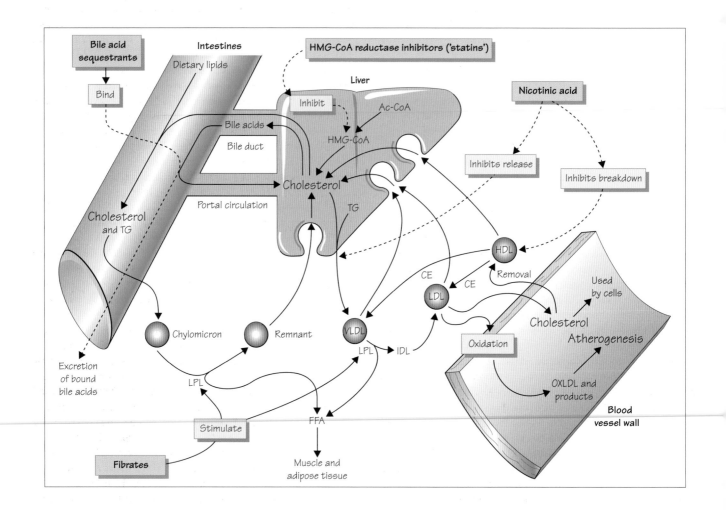

All cells require **lipids** (fats) to synthesize membranes and provide energy. Lipids are transported in the blood as **lipoproteins**. These small particles consist of a core of **triglycerides** and **cholesteryl esters**, surrounded by a coat of **phospholipids, cholesterol** and proteins, termed **apolipoproteins** or **apoproteins**. Apoproteins stabilize the lipoprotein particles and help target specific types of lipoproteins to various tissues. **Hyperlipidaemias** are abnormalities of lipoprotein levels, which promote the development of *atherosclerosis* (see Chapter 36) and *coronary heart disease* (CHD; see Chapters 39–41).

Lipoproteins and lipid transport

The figure illustrates pathways of lipid transport in the body. The **exogenous** pathway (left side of the figure) delivers ingested lipids to the body tissues and liver. Ingested triglycerides and cholesterol are combined with apoproteins in the intestinal mucosa to form **chylomicrons**. Passing into the bloodstream via the lymphatic system, chylomicrons bind to the capillary endothelium in muscle and adipose tissue. Here, their triglycerides are hydrolysed by the enzyme **lipoprotein lipase** (LPL), yielding fatty acids which enter the tissues. The liver takes up the residual **chylomicron remnants**. These are broken down to yield cholesterol, which the liver also synthesizes. The rate-limiting

enzyme in cholesterol synthesis is **hydroxy-methylglutaryl coenzyme A reductase** (HMG-CoA reductase). The liver uses cholesterol to make bile acids and membrane components.

The **endogenous** pathway cycles lipids between the liver and peripheral tissues. The liver forms **very low density lipoproteins** (VLDLs), consisting mainly of triglycerides, with some cholesterol. VLDL triglycerides are hydrolysed by LPL, providing fatty acids to body tissues. As it is progressively drained of triglycerides, VLDL becomes **intermediate-density lipoprotein** (IDL) and then **low-density lipoprotein** (LDL), losing all of its apoproteins except for **apo B100** in the process. Most of the LDL, which contains mainly cholesteryl esters, is taken up by the liver. The remaining LDL serves to distribute cholesterol to the peripheral tissues. Cells regulate their cholesterol uptake by expressing more *LDL receptors* (which bind LDL via its apo B100) when their cholesterol requirement increases.

Cholesterol is removed from tissues by **high-density lipoprotein** (HDL), which is initially assembled in the plasma from lipids and apoproteins (particularly **apo A1**) lost by other lipoproteins. It accumulates cholesterol from cell membranes and transfers it (as cholesterol esters) to VLDL, IDL and LDL, which return it to the liver.

Hyperlipidaemias: types and treatments

Primary hyperlipidaemias are caused by genetic abnormalities affecting apoproteins, apoprotein receptors or enzymes involved in lipoprotein metabolism. *Secondary* hyperlipidaemias are caused by conditions or drugs (e.g. diabetes, renal disease, alcohol abuse, thiazide diuretics) affecting lipoprotein metabolism. Diets high in saturated fats also cause hypercholesterolaemia, probably by decreasing hepatic lipoprotein clearance. The **Frederickson/WHO classification** identifies six hyperlipidaemic phenotypes. Type IIa involves **hypercholesterolaemia** with elevated LDL cholesterol but normal triglycerides. Types I, IV and V involve mainly **hypertriglyceridaemia**, in which VLDL and/or chylomicron levels are raised. In **hypercholesterolaemia with hypertriglyceridaemia** (types IIb and III) both cholesterol and triglycerides are elevated.

The treatment of hyperlipidaemias aims to lower LDL cholesterol (LDL) and/or triglycerides and to raise HDL cholesterol. There is evidence that both effects may slow or even reverse the progression of atherosclerotic lesions. Target LDL levels in individuals at high risk of suffering a myocardial infarction (MI) or other serious cardiovascular event are set lower than for those who are at little risk. For example, current US guidelines state that LDL should be less than 160 mg/dL (4.1 mmol/L) for those in the lowest risk category, whereas for high-risk patients with existing CHD, diabetes or a 10-year risk of developing CHD of > 20%, LDL should be less than 100 mg/dL (2.6 mmol/L), with consideration given to a target of less than 70 mg/dL (1.8 mmol/L).

Treatment often begins with a low-fat, high-carbohydrate diet. If this fails to normalize hyperlipidaemia adequately after 3 months, therapy with a lipid-lowering drug is considered. Most of those with high cholesterol are treated with 'statins', since these have been consistently shown to reduce CHD and the mortality it causes. It is increasingly appreciated, however, that in addition to elevated LDL, high levels of triglycerides (reflected by high VLDL) and low levels of HDL promote the development of atherosclerosis. This combination of factors is common in those with *metabolic syndrome*, and the use with statins of 'fibrates' and nicotinic acid, which cause large increases in HDL levels, will probably increase in these individuals.

HMG-CoA reductase inhibitors or '**statins**' include **simvastatin, lovastatin, pravastatin, fluvastatin, mevastatin, atorvastatin** and **rosuvastatin**. The landmark **Scandinavian Simvastatin Survival Study** (4S) reported in 1994 that treatment with simvastatin of patients with high LDL levels and CHD reduced the incidence of cardiovascular mortality by 42% over a 6-year period. Statins act by reducing hepatic synthesis of cholesterol, causing an upregulation of hepatic receptors for B and E apoproteins. This increases the clearance of LDL, IDL and VLDL from the plasma. Statins also modestly increase plasma HDL levels by an unknown mechanism. Although the main benefits of statins are a result of their lipid-lowering effects, results from a number of clinical trials (e.g. AFCAPS/TEXCAPS; MIRACL) imply that statins may also reduce CHD through additional mechanisms. These have been proposed to include an enhancement of nitric oxide release, possibly due to activation of the PI3K/Akt pathway (see Chapter 22), as well as anti-inflammatory and antithrombotic effects. At least some of these effects may occur because the inhibition of HMG-CoA reduces cellular concentrations of lipids required for the functioning of G-proteins and other signalling intermediates. Serious statin-associated adverse effects are rare. They include *hepatoxicity* and *rhabdomyolysis* (destruction of skeletal muscle), the risk of which is increased with concomitant use of nicotinic acid or a fibric acid derivative.

Bile acid sequestrants. Bile acids are synthesized from cholesterol in the liver, and cycle between the liver and intestine (enterohepatic recirculation). **Cholestyramine** and **cholestipol** are exchange resins that bind and trap bile acids in the intestine, increasing their excretion. This enhances hepatic bile acid synthesis and cholesterol utilization. The resulting depletion of hepatic cholesterol causes an upregulation of LDL receptors, increasing the clearance of LDL cholesterol from the plasma. The bile acid sequestrants cause little systemic toxicity because they are not absorbed. They are, however, taken in large amounts (e.g. up to 30 g/day), and cause gastrointestinal side effects such as emesis, diarrhoea and reflux oesophagitis.

Nicotinic acid (niacin) is a B vitamin that has lipid-lowering effects at high doses. It inhibits the synthesis and release of VLDL by the liver. Because VLDL gives rise to IDL and LDL, plasma levels of these lipoproteins also fall. Conversely, HDL levels rise significantly as a result of decreased breakdown, an effect which the 2004 ARBITER 2 study indicates may slow the progression of atherosclerotic plaque in patients with low HDL. Nicotinic acid can cause a number of adverse effects, including hepatotoxicity, palpitations, impaired glucose tolerance, hyperuricaemia, hypotension and amblyopia. Most patients experience flushing with nicotinic acid therapy. This is caused by vasodilatation, which is secondary to prostaglandin release from the endothelium. This can be prevented by non-steroidal anti-inflammatory drugs.

Fibric acid derivatives ('fibrates') include **gemfibrazole, clofibrate, bezafibrate, ciprofibrate** and **fenofibrate**. These stimulate the activity of lipoprotein lipase, thereby reducing VLDL triglycerides by increasing their hydrolysis. They also promote changes in LDL composition, which render it less atherogenic, and enhance fibrolysis. Fibrates are mainly used with types IIb and III hyperlipidaemias. They cause mild gastrointestinal disorders in 5–10% of patients, and can potentially cause muscle toxicity and renal failure if combined with HMG-CoA reductase inhibitors or excessive alcohol use.

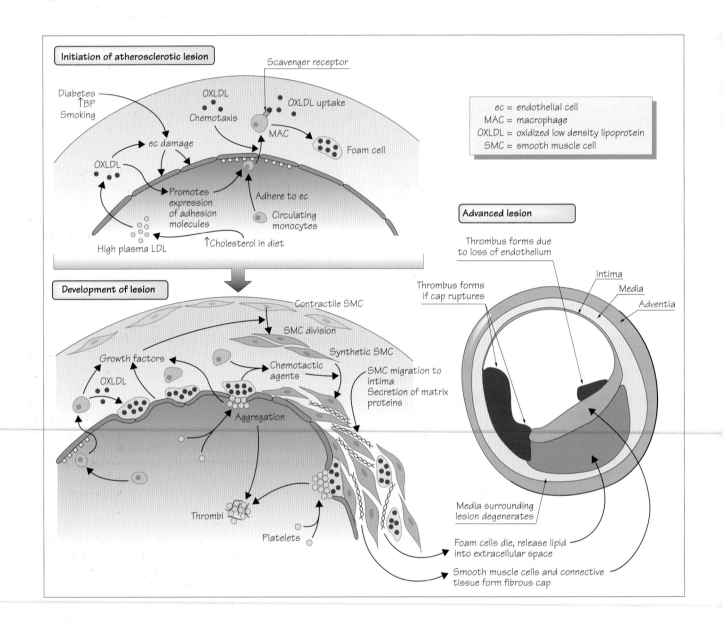

Initiation of atherosclerotic lesion

Scavenger receptor

Diabetes
↑BP
Smoking

OXLDL
Chemotaxis

OXLDL uptake

ec damage

MAC

Foam cell

OXLDL

Promotes
expression
of adhesion
molecules

Adhere to ec

Circulating
monocytes

High plasma LDL

↑Cholesterol in diet

ec = endothelial cell
MAC = macrophage
OXLDL = oxidized low density lipoprotein
SMC = smooth muscle cell

Advanced lesion

Thrombus forms due
to loss of endothelium

Intima

Media

Adventia

Development of lesion

Contractile SMC

SMC division

Synthetic SMC

Thrombus forms
if cap ruptures

Growth factors

Chemotactic
agents

SMC migration to
intima
Secretion of matrix
proteins

OXLDL

Aggregation

Thrombi

Platelets

Media surrounding
lesion degenerates

Foam cells die, release lipid
into extracellular space

Smooth muscle cells and connective
tissue form fibrous cap

Atherosclerosis is a disease of the larger arteries. It begins in childhood with localized accumulations of lipid within the arterial intima, termed **fatty streaks**. By middle age some of these develop into **atherosclerotic plaques**, focal lesions where the arterial wall is grossly abnormal. Plaques may be several centimetres across, and are most common in the *aorta*, the *coronary* and *internal carotid arteries*, and the *circle of Willis*. An advanced atherosclerotic plaque, illustrated on the right of the diagram, demonstrates several features.

1 The arterial wall is focally thickened by intimal smooth muscle cell proliferation and the deposition of fibrous connective tissue, forming a hard **fibrous cap**. This projects into the vascular lumen, restricting the flow of blood, and often causes ischaemia in the tissue region served by the artery.

2 A soft pool of extracellular lipid and cell debris accumulates beneath the fibrous cap (*athera* is Greek for gruel or porridge). This weakens the

arterial wall, so that the fibrous cap may fissure or tear away. As a result, blood enters the lesions and **thrombi** (blood clots) are formed. These thrombi, or the material leaking from the ruptured lesion, may be carried to the upstream vascular bed to *embolize* (plug) smaller vessels. A larger thrombus may totally occlude (block) the artery at the site of the lesion. This causes myocardial infarction or stroke if it occurs in a coronary or cerebral artery, respectively.

3 The endothelium over the lesion is partially or completely lost. This can lead to ongoing formation of thrombi, causing intermittent flow occlusion as in unstable angina.

4 The medial smooth muscle layer under the lesion degenerates. This weakens the vascular wall, which may distend and eventually rupture (an **aneurysm**). Aneurysms are especially common in the abdominal aorta.

Atherosclerotic arteries may also demonstrate spasms or reduced vasodilatation. This worsens the restriction of the blood flow and promotes thrombus formation (see Chapters 40, 43).

Pathogenesis of atherosclerosis

The risk of developing atherosclerosis is in part genetically determined. The incidence of clinical consequences of atherosclerosis such as ischaemic heart disease rises with age, especially after age 40. Atherosclerosis is much more common in men than in women. This difference is probably due to a protective effect of oestrogen, and progressively disappears after menopause. Important risk factors that predispose towards atherosclerosis include smoking, hypertension, diabetes and high serum cholesterol.

The most widely accepted hypothesis for the pathogenesis of atherosclerosis proposes that it is initiated by *endothelial injury or dysfunction*. Plaques tend to develop in areas of variable haemodynamic shear stress (e.g. where arteries branch or bifurcate). The endothelium is especially vulnerable to damage at such sites, as evidenced by increased endothelial cell turnover and permeability. Endothelial dysfunction promotes the adhesion of **monocytes**, white blood cells which burrow beneath the endothelial monolayer and become **macrophages**. Macrophages normally play an important role during inflammation, the body's response to injury and infection. They do so by acting as scavenger cells to remove dead cells and foreign material, and also by subsequently releasing *cytokines* and *growth factors* to promote healing. As described below, however, macrophages in the arterial wall can be abnormally activated, causing a type of slow inflammatory reaction, which eventually results in advanced and clinically dangerous plaques.

Oxidized low-density lipoprotein, macrophages and atherogenesis

Lipoproteins transport cholesterol and other lipids in the bloodstream (see Chapter 35). Elevated levels of one type of lipoprotein, low-density lipoprotein (LDL), are associated with atherosclerosis. Native LDL is not atherogenic. However, oxidative modification of LDL by oxidants derived from macrophages and endothelial and smooth muscle cells can lead to the generation of highly atherogenic **oxidized LDL** within the vascular wall.

Oxidized LDL is thought to promote atherogenesis through several mechanisms (upper panel of figure). Oxidized LDL is chemotactic for (i.e. attracts) circulating monocytes, and increases the expression of endothelial cell adhesion molecules to which monocytes attach. The monocytes then penetrate the endothelial monolayer, lodge beneath it, and mature into macrophages. Cellular uptake of native LDL is normally highly regulated. However, certain cells, including macrophages, are unable to control their uptake of oxidized LDL, which occurs via **scavenger receptors**. Once within the vascular wall, macrophages therefore accumulate large quantities of oxidized LDL, eventually becoming the cholesterol-laden **foam cells** forming the fatty streak.

As shown in the lower left of the figure, stimulation of macrophages and endothelial cells by oxidized LDL causes these cells to release cytokines. T-lymphocytes may also enter the vascular wall and release cytokines. Additional cytokines are released by platelets aggregating on the endothelium at the site at which it has been damaged by oxidized LDL and other toxic substances released by the foam cells. The cytokines act on the vascular smooth muscle cells of the media, causing them to *migrate into the intima*, to *proliferate*, and to *secrete abnormal amounts of collagen and other connective tissue proteins*. Over time, the intimal accumulation of smooth muscle cells and connective tissue forms the fibrous cap on the inner arterial wall. Underneath this, ongoing foam cell formation and deterioration forms a layer of extracellular lipid (largely cholesterol and cholesteryl esters) and cellular debris. Still-viable foam cells often localize at the edges or shoulders of the lesion. Underneath the lipid, the medial layer of smooth muscle cells is weakened and atrophied.

Clinical consequences of advanced atherosclerosis

Atherosclerotic lesions are of most clinical consequence when they occur in the coronary arteries. Lesions in which the fibrous cap becomes thick tend to cause a significant **stenosis**, or narrowing of the vascular lumen, which gradually comes to cause cardiac ischaemia, especially when myocardial oxygen demand rises. This leads to **stable** or **exertional angina** (see Chapter 39). Advanced plaques often have large areas of endothelial denudation, which serve as sites for thrombus formation. In addition, lipid- and foam-cell-rich lesions are particularly unstable and prone to tearing open. This **plaque rupture** may be favoured by the presence in the lesion of T-lymphocytes, as these produce interferon gamma which inhibits matrix formation, and of macrophages, which produce proteases that degrade the connective tissue matrix. Plaque rupture allows blood to enter the lesion, causing thrombi to form on the surface and/or within the lesion, often resulting in an acute coronary syndrome such as unstable angina (see Chapter 40) or myocardial infarction (see Chapter 43). Non-fatal chronic thrombi may gradually be replaced by connective tissue and incorporated into the lesion, a process termed **organization**. Atherosclerosis of cerebral arteries is the major cause of **stroke** (cerebral infarction). Atherosclerotic stenosis of the renal arteries causes about two-thirds of cases of **renovascular hypertension**.

37 Treatment of hypertension

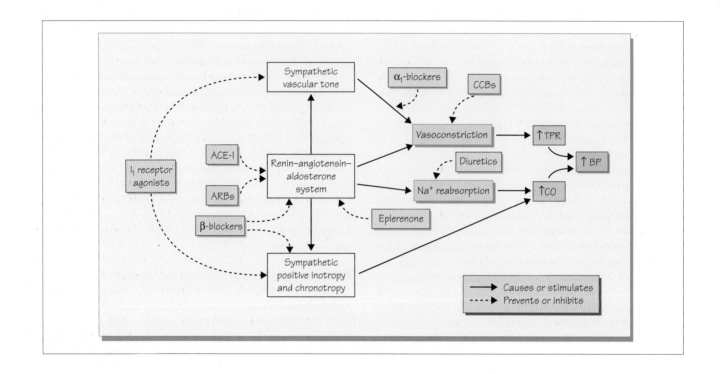

Hypertension is defined pragmatically as the level of blood pressure above which therapeutic intervention can be shown to reduce the risk of developing cardiovascular disease (Table 37.1). Risk increases progressively with *both* systolic and diastolic blood pressure levels. However, rises in systolic pressure are now given more emphasis and **isolated systolic hypertension** (ISH), which often develops in the elderly, is particularly deleterious. Individual blood pressure measurements can vary significantly, necessitating confirmation of all but severe hypertension by repeated measurements made on at least two separate occasions.

Epidemiological studies predict that a long-term 5–6-mmHg diminution of diastolic blood pressure (DBP) should reduce the incidence of stroke and CHD by about 40 and 25%, respectively. The World Health Organization recommends considering drug treatment when the DBP remains between 95 and 105 mmHg for more than 6 months, or if the DBP remains between 90 and 95 mmHg and certain risk factors are present. These include overt cardiovascular disease, diabetes, obesity, dyslipidaemia, a family history of cardiovascular disease, or disease of target organs vulnerable to hypertension (e.g. kidneys and brain). There is an emerging consensus that mild hypertension should be treated if a patient's overall risk of cardiovascular events (e.g. MI), as estimated using risk tables derived from the Framingham study (see Chapter 33), exceeds 2% per year. The goal of antihypertensive therapy is to reduce the blood pressure to below 140/90 mmHg (or to below 130/80 mmHg in diabetics and those with renal disease).

Lifestyle modifications such as *weight reduction*, *regular aerobic exercise* and *limitation of dietary sodium* and *alcohol intake* can often normalize pressure in mild hypertensives. They are also useful adjuncts to pharmacological therapy of more severe disease, and have the important added bonus of reducing overall cardiovascular risk.

Antihypertensive drugs act to reduce cardiac output and/or total peripheral resistance. There are multiple classes of such drugs, leading to an ongoing debate concerning which type is best. The results of recent large clinical trials have led to suggestions that low-dose thiazide diuretics and dihydropyridine Ca^{2+}-channel blockers are the most suitable for initiating therapy. However, other types of antihypertensive drugs can often exert beneficial actions on coexisting conditions (e.g. ACE inhibitors in heart failure, diabetes), so that these drugs may be more appropriate for many patients. However, no class of drug is effective in more than ~50% of patients, and in the majority of cases, combinations of two or three drugs are needed to achieve adequate blood pressure control.

Thiazide diuretics cause an initial increased Na^+ excretion by the kidneys, which is due to inhibition of Na^+/Cl^- symport in the distal nephron. This leads to a fall in blood volume and cardiac output.

Table 37.1 Classification of adult blood pressure by the US Joint National Committee on Detection, Evaluation and Treatment of High Blood Pressure. HT, hypertension.

Classification	Systolic (mmHg)		Diastolic (mmHg)
Normotension	< 130	*and/or*	< 85
High normal	130–139	*and/or*	85–89
Stage 1 HT	140–159	*and/or*	90–99
Stage 2 HT	160–179	*and/or*	100–109
Stage 3 HT	> 180	*and/or*	> 110

Subsequently, blood volume recovers, but total peripheral resistance falls due to an unknown mechanism. Thiazide diuretics can be combined with vasodilators (e.g. α_1-blockers, Ca^{2+}-channel antagonists), in order to ameliorate the volume expansion and oedema that vasodilating drugs may cause by activating the renin-angiotensin-aldosterone system. These diuretics cause hypokalaemia by promoting Na^+/K^+ exchange in the collecting tubule (see Chapter 47). This can be prevented by giving K^+ supplements, or also by combining thiazide diuretics with K^+-sparing diuretics (e.g. amiloride) to reduce Na^+ reabsorption and therefore K^+ secretion by blocking Na^+ channels in the collecting duct. Additional side effects can include increases in plasma insulin, glucose or cholesterol, as well as hypersensitivity reactions and impotence. In the 2002 ALLHAT study, the diuretic chlorthalidone lowered blood pressure as well as amlodipine and lisinopril (see below), and was superior to both at preventing major cardiovascular disease.

Angiotensin-converting enzyme inhibitors (ACEI) such as **captopril**, **enalopril** and **lisinopril** block the conversion of angiotensin I into angiotensin II. This reduces total peripheral resistance because angiotensin II stimulates the sympathetic system centrally, promotes release of norepinephrine from sympathetic nerves, and vasoconstricts directly. The fall in plasma angiotensin II, and consequently in aldosterone, also promotes diuresis/natriuresis, because both hormones cause renal Na^+ and water retention (see Chapter 27). ACE also metabolizes the vasodilator bradykinin, and part of the beneficial action of ACEI may be due to elevated levels of bradykinin. Increases in bradykinin may also, however, be responsible for the chronic cough which is the most common adverse effect of ACEI. This effect does not occur with **angiotensin II receptor (AT_1) blockers** (ARBs) such as **losartan** and **valsartan**, which selectively inhibit the effects of angiotensin II on its AT_1 subtype without affecting bradykinin levels. Both ACEI and ARBs have few side effects, leading to their increasing popularity. However, they are contraindicated in pregnancy, renovascular disease and aortic stenosis. **Eplerenone**, a selective *aldosterone receptor antagonist*, has recently been approved for treatment of hypertension (see also Chapter 47).

Calcium-channel blockers (CCBs) such as **nifedipine**, **verapamil** and **diltiazem** are commonly used to treat hypertension due to their vasodilating properties, as described in Chapter 34. The dihydropyridine CCBs, which are selective for vascular smooth muscle over the heart, are used most widely, and also have a useful diuretic effect. The 2005 ASCOT trial showed that the long-acting dihydropyridine **amlodipine** (with the ACEI perindopril added in if required to meet blood pressure targets) reduced cardiovascular morbidity and mortality more effectively than the β-blocker atenolol (with the diuretic bendroflumethiazide if required). DHPs have been shown to be especially effective in the elderly, and are safe in pregnancy.

Beta-receptor blockers antagonize sympathetic nervous system stimulation of cardiac β-receptors (mainly β_1), thereby reducing cardiac output through negative inotropic and chronotropic effects. They also block β-receptors on juxtaglomerular granule cells in the kidney, thus inhibiting renin release and reducing plasma levels of angiotensin II and aldosterone. During treatment, total peripheral resistance rises initially and then returns to the predrug level via an unknown mechanism, while cardiac output remains depressed. Some β-blockers are selective for the β_1 subtype (atenolol), while others block both β_1 and β_2 subtypes (propranolol), and several (pindolol) are partial β-receptor agonists. In each case, the effects on blood pressure are similar, although the partial β-receptor agonists are probably acting more as vasodilators than by reducing cardiac output. All β-blockers are contraindicated in asthma due to their potential effects on bronchiolar β_2-receptors. Adverse effects of these drugs include fatigue, negative inotropy, CNS disturbances in some (e.g. nightmares), and worsening and masking of the signs of hypoglycaemia.

α_1-**receptor-selective blockers** are second-line antihypertensives, which cause vasodilatation by inhibiting the ongoing constriction of arteries by the sympathetic neurotransmitter norepinephrine. These drugs are used in preference to non-selective α-antagonists in order to prevent the increased norepinephrine release from sympathetic nerves that would occur if presynaptic α_2-receptors were also blocked. The relatively new drugs **rilmenidine** and **moxonidine** reduce sympathetic outflow by activating central *imidazoline* (I_1) receptors in the rostral ventrolateral medulla (RVLM). This lowers blood pressure with few side effects, but the use of these drugs is limited due to the present lack of evidence from clinical trials that these drugs have beneficial effects on survival.

In cases in which hypertension is secondary to a known condition or factor (e.g. renal stenosis, oral contraceptives), removal of this cause is often sufficient to normalize the blood pressure.

Mechanisms of primary hypertension

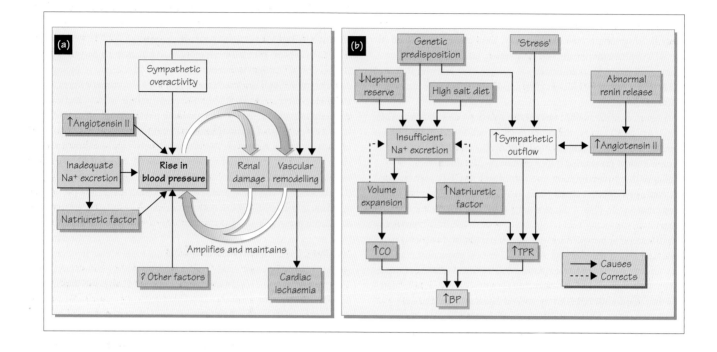

In more than 90% of cases, hypertension has no obvious cause, and is termed **primary** or **essential**. Primary hypertension is a **multifactorial genetic disorder,** in which inheritance of a number of abnormal genes predisposes an individual to high arterial blood pressure (ABP), especially if appropriate *environmental influences* (e.g. high salt diet, psychosocial stress) are also present. The identities of the genes involved are presently unresolved. Attempts to define causative mechanisms have mainly focused on uncovering functional abnormalities associated with hypertension. Many such studies have been carried out in strains of animals which have been selectively bred to develop high ABP, in the hope that the mechanisms causing hypertension are similar across species.

Studies tracking cardiovascular function over many years have shown that early human hypertension is often associated with an increased cardiac output (CO) and heart rate, but a normal total peripheral resistance (TPR). Over a period of years, CO falls to subnormal levels, while TPR becomes permanently increased, thereby maintaining the hypertension (recall that ABP = CO × TPR). One important implication of these observations is that the factors maintaining high ABP may change over time. Therefore the mechanisms which initiate high ABP (e.g. insufficient Na⁺ excretion, sympathetic overactivity) may then be succeeded and/or amplified by additional common secondary mechanisms (e.g. renal damage and vascular structural remodelling) which are caused by, and maintain, the initial rise in pressure. This unifying hypothesis for primary hypertension is shown in Figure 38a.

The kidney and sodium in hypertension

The pressure–natriuresis model The kidneys regulate long-term ABP by controlling the body's Na⁺ content (see Chapter 27). Guyton proposed that hypertension is caused by renal abnormalities which cause *impaired* or *inadequate Na⁺ excretion* (Figure 38b). According to this model, the resulting Na⁺ retention increases blood volume, and therefore CO and ABP. These changes then promote Na⁺ excretion by causing pressure natriuresis (see Chapter 27). Fluid balance is therefore restored, but at the cost of a rise in ABP. Over the long term, the rise in ABP or flow would set in train *autoregulatory* processes resulting in vasoconstriction and/or vascular structural remodelling. This would reduce blood volume to normal levels, but by raising TPR would maintain the high ABP needed for Na⁺ balance.

There is extensive evidence that a renal mechanism of hypertension is important in many people. For example, a high salt diet, which should exacerbate the renal deficiency in Na⁺ excretion, worsens hypertension in many patients and, as shown in the Intersalt study, seems to cause a slow rise in ABP over many years in most people. It has also been shown that ABP falls when the kidneys from normotensives are transplanted into hypertensives. Impairment of renal Na⁺ excretion has been demonstrated directly in the *Liddle syndrome*, a rare form of hypertension in which a mutation of the mineralocorticoid-sensitive Na⁺ channel causes its continual overactivity.

The natriuretic factor hypothesis de Wardener and others have proposed that the body responds to inadequate renal salt excretion by producing one or more **natriuretic factors** (not to be confused with **atrial natriuretic peptide**; see Chapter 27) which promote salt excretion by inhibiting the Na⁺–K⁺-ATPase in the nephron. Na⁺ pumps are also indirectly involved in lowering intracellular Ca²⁺, via regulation of both the membrane potential and Na⁺–Ca²⁺ exchange in smooth muscle cells and neurons. Natriuretic factors would therefore cause additional responses such as vasoconstriction, increased norepinephrine release, and possibly stimulation of brain centres involved in raising ABP. These effects would increase TPR, causing sustained hypertension. In agreement with this hypothesis, several endogenous substances that inhibit the Na$^+$ pump, one being almost identical in structure to ouabain, have been found to be elevated in the plasma from hypertensives.

The reduced nephron number hypothesis Brenner and coworkers have proposed that many hypertensives have a congenital reduction in the number, or filtering ability, of their nephrons which would cause the inadequate Na$^+$ excretion referred to above. Evidence suggests that this may arise from intrauterine growth retardation.

Neurogenic and humoral theories of hypertension

Although renin release should be greatly suppressed by elevated ABP, many hypertensives have normal or even high plasma renin activity. Laragh and coworkers have proposed that many hypertensives have an *abnormality of renin release* which would lead both to increased angiotensin II-mediated vasoconstriction and to Na$^+$ retention via aldosterone, both mechanisms causing hypertension. Angiotensin II is also a potent stimulator of the sympathetic nervous system. Primary hypertension in some individuals has also been linked to a mutation in the **angiotensinogen** gene, which could promote increased angiotensin II production.

The **neurogenic model of hypertension** suggests that ABP elevation is primarily initiated by defective neurohumoral regulation of ABP. Supporters of this concept stress that the central nervous system is ultimately the final determinant of ABP, because it can exert long-term influences on renal function (e.g. renal blood flow), on the production of vasoactive substances, and on vascular and cardiac structure. The neurogenic model is supported by evidence that sympathetic nervous activity is increased in young borderline hypertensives, and also by the fact that drugs which reduce sympathetic outflow effectively lower ABP (see Chapter 37). It may also explain studies in which psychosocial stress has been linked to hypertension.

Insulin resistance is a condition in which the body becomes less responsive to the actions of the hormone *insulin*, leading to a compensatory rise in plasma insulin levels. Both insulin resistance and obesity, with which it is often associated, are very common in hypertensives. There is evidence that excessive insulin can cause multiple effects on the body which could promote hypertension, including activation of the sympathetic nervous system, increased renal Na$^+$ reabsorption, and reduced endothelium-dependent vasodilatation.

Vascular remodelling

Established hypertension is associated with the *structural alteration* of small arteries and larger arterioles. This process, termed **remodelling**, results in the narrowing of these vessels and an increase in the ratio of wall thickness to luminal radius. Remodelling is proposed to be an adaptive mechanism which 'locks in' vascular narrowing and the resulting increase in TPR. This reduces vascular wall stress (see the Laplace/Frank law, Chapter 16) and protects the microcirculation from increased ABP, but at the price of raising the arterial ABP. Remodelling may also be enhanced by the renin–angiotensin–aldosterone and sympathetic nervous systems, the activation of which is known to promote smooth muscle cell growth.

Remodelling will increase basal TPR and also exaggerate any increase in TPR caused by vasoconstriction. In addition, studies in *spontaneously hypertensive rats* indicate that remodelling of renal afferent arterioles may contribute to hypertension by interfering with renal Na$^+$ excretion (see above). This implies that remodelling would accentuate increases in ABP caused by other factors, thereby contributing to the vicious cycle illustrated in Figure 38(a). In addition, remodelling of the coronary arteries as a result of hypertension may increase the risk of myocardial infarction by restricting the ability of these vessels to increase the cardiac blood supply during ischaemia.

Secondary hypertension

In less than 10% of cases, high ABP is secondary to a known condition or factor. Common causes of **secondary hypertension** include:
1 *renal parenchymal* and *renovascular diseases*, which impair volume regulation and/or activate the renin–angiotensin–aldosterone system
2 *endocrine disturbances*, often of the adrenal cortex, and associated with oversecretion of aldosterone, cortisol and/or catecholamines
3 *oral contraceptives*, which may raise ABP via renin–angiotensin–aldosterone activation and hyperinsulinaemia.

Malignant or accelerated hypertension is an uncommon condition that develops quickly, involves large elevations in pressure, is often secondary to other conditions, rapidly damages the kidneys, retina, brain and heart, and if untreated causes death within 1–2 years.

Consequences of hypertension

Chronic hypertension causes changes in the arteries similar to those due to ageing. These include endothelial damage and **arteriosclerosis**, a thickening and increased connective tissue content of the arterial wall that reduces arterial compliance. These effects on vascular structure combine with elevated arterial pressure to promote atherosclerosis, coronary heart disease, left ventricular hypertrophy and renal damage. Hypertension is therefore an important risk factor for *myocardial infarction*, *congestive heart failure*, *stroke* and *renal failure*.

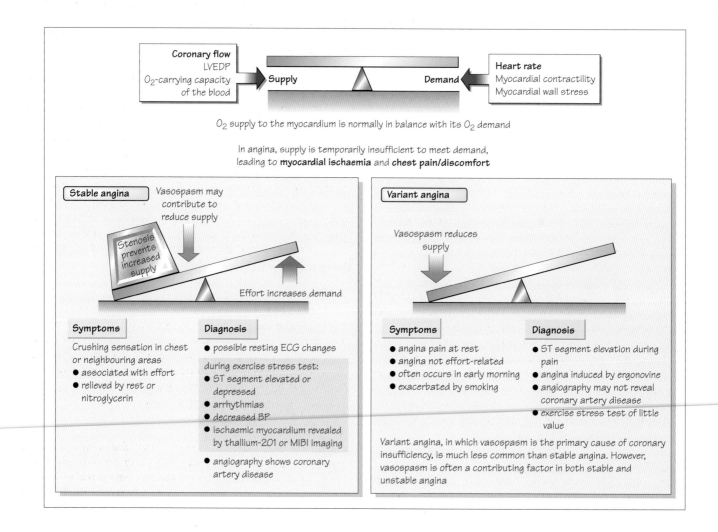

Angina pectoris is an episodic pain or crushing/squeezing sensation in the chest caused by reversible myocardial ischaemia. The discomfort may radiate into the neck, jaw and arms (particularly the left) and, more rarely, into the back. Other common symptoms include shortness of breath, abdominal pain and dizziness. Syncope (unconsciousness) occurs infrequently. Ischaemia may produce classic angina or may be totally *silent* without any symptoms. The clinical outlook from silent ischaemia is similar to symptomatic angina.

Three forms of angina are recognized. **Stable** and **variant** angina are discussed below, and **unstable angina** is described in Chapter 40.

Pathophysiology

The figure shows the factors that determine myocardial O_2 supply and demand. O_2 demand is determined by **heart rate**, **left ventricular contractility** and **systolic wall stress**, and therefore increases with **exercise**, **hypertension** and **left ventricular dilatation** (e.g. during chronic heart failure). Myocardial O_2 supply is primarily determined by coronary blood flow and coronary vascular resistance, which mostly occurs at the level of the intramyocardial arterioles. With exercise the coronary blood flow can increase to four to six times baseline, which is the normal coronary flow reserve (see Chapter 23).

Stable or **exertional/typical** angina arises when the flow reserve of one or more coronary arteries is limited by a significant structural stenosis (> 70%) resulting from atherosclerotic coronary heart disease. Stenoses typically develop in the epicardial region of arteries, within 6 cm of the aorta. Under resting conditions, cardiac O_2 demand is low enough to be satisfied even by a diminished coronary flow. When, however, exertion or emotional stress increases myocardial O_2 demand, dilatation of the non-diseased areas of the artery cannot increase the supply of blood to the heart because the stenosis presents a fixed, non-dilating obstruction. The resulting imbalance between myocardial O_2 demand and supply causes myocardial ischaemia. Ischaemia develops mainly in the **subendocardium**, the inner part of the myocardial wall. This is because the blood flow to the left ventricular wall occurs mainly during diastole as a result of arteriolar compression during systole. The arterioles of the subendocardium are compressed more than those of the mid- or subepicardial layers, so that the subendocardium is most vulnerable to a relative lack of O_2.

In addition to causing pain, ischaemia causes a decline in myocardial cell high-energy phosphates (creatine phosphate and ATP). As a result, both ventricular contractility and diastolic relaxation in the territory of affected arteries are impaired. Consequences of these events may include a fall in cardiac output, symptoms of pulmonary congestion, and activation of the sympathetic nervous system. Stable angina is almost always relieved within 5–10 min by rest or by nitroglycerin, which reduces cardiac O_2 demand.

Some patients with stable angina may have excellent effort tolerance one day, but develop angina with minimal activity on another day. Contributing to this phenomenon of *variable threshold angina* is a dynamic endothelial dysfunction that often occurs in patients with coronary artery disease. The endothelium normally acts via nitric oxide to dilate coronary arteries during exercise. If this endothelium-dependent vasodilatation is periodically impaired, exercise may result in paradoxical vasoconstriction due to the unopposed vasoconstricting effect of the sympathetic nervous system on coronary α-receptors.

Variant angina, also termed **vasospastic** or **Prinzmetal's** angina, is an uncommon condition in which myocardial ischaemia and pain are caused by a severe transient *occlusive spasm* of one or more epicardial coronary arteries. Patients with variant angina may or may not have coronary atherosclerosis, and in the former case, vasospasm often occurs in the vicinity of plaques. Variant angina occurs at rest (typically in the early morning hours) and may be intensely painful. It is exacerbated by smoking, and can be precipitated by cocaine use. About 30% of these patients show no evidence of coronary atherosclerotic lesions. Vasospasm is thought to occur because a segment of artery becomes abnormally over-reactive to vasoconstricting agents (e.g. norepinephrine, serotonin). There is also evidence that flow-mediated vasodilatation, a function of the endothelium, is impaired in the coronary arteries of patients with variant angina, and that this endothelial dysfunction may be due to oxidative stress (see Chapter 22).

Diagnosis

Ischaemic heart disease and stable angina can be distinguished from other conditions causing chest pain (e.g. neuromuscular disorders, gastroesophageal reflux) based on characteristic anginal symptoms and several types of diagnostic investigation. Although *resting ST/T wave changes* indicate severe underlying coronary artery disease, the resting ECG is often normal. In this case, the presence of ischaemic heart disease can be unmasked by an **exercise stress test**, during which patients exercise at progressively increasing levels of effort on a stationary bicycle or treadmill. Development of cardiac ischaemia is revealed by chest pain, ECG changes including *ST segment depression* or *elevation*, arrhythmias, or a fall in blood pressure due to reduced ventricular contractility. The degree of effort at which these signs develop indicates the severity of ischaemia.

The exercise stress test is less useful in uncovering ischaemia-related ECG changes if the baseline ECG is already abnormal due to factors such as left bundle branch block. In such patients, techniques designed to visualize ischaemic myocardium can be combined with the stress test to increase its specificity. **Thallium-201** is an isotope that is taken up by normal but not ischaemic or previously infarcted myocardium. It is given intravenously during the stress test, and a gamma camera is used to image its distribution in the heart both immediately and also after the test, when ischaemia has subsided. A region of exercise-induced ischaemia will cause a 'cold spot' during but not after the stress test, because it will take up thallium-201 only when ischaemia has passed. Technetium-99m (^{99m}Tc)-labelled sestamibi (see Chapter 31) can also be used for this purpose. **Coronary angiography** (see Chapter 31) is used to provide direct radiographic visualization of the extent and severity of coronary artery disease, allowing risk assessment.

The hallmark of variant angina is ST segment elevation on the ECG. Cardiac ischaemia caused by variant angina may cause ventricular arrhythmias, syncope and even myocardial infarction during prolonged attacks. Variant angina can be provoked by intravenous administration of the vasoconstrictor **ergonovine**, forming the basis of a hospital test for this condition.

Prognosis
Stable angina

Uncomplicated stable angina has a good prognosis. Epidemiological studies show that cardiovascular mortality in patients with stable angina is approximately 1% per year. Mortality increases with the number of diseased arteries, especially if there is significant stenosis in the left coronary artery mainstem. Patients who have poor left ventricular function or diabetes are also at particular risk.

Variant angina

Patients without significant coronary artery disease have a benign prognosis; in a recent study only 4% of patients in this group died from a cardiac cause during an average follow-up period of 7 years. However, patients who also have severe coronary artery disease or who develop severe arrhythmias during vasospastic episodes are at greater risk.

Management

The management of angina is designed to control symptoms, reduce underlying risk factors and improve prognosis. **Control of symptoms** involves the use of nitrovasodilators, β-adrenoceptor blockers and Ca^{2+}-channel antagonists (see Chapter 41). Minimization of **risk factors** involves the use of low-dose aspirin, lipid-lowering drugs and lifestyle changes, and is a vital component of treatment. Revascularization (see Chapter 42) can also be used to treat stable angina.

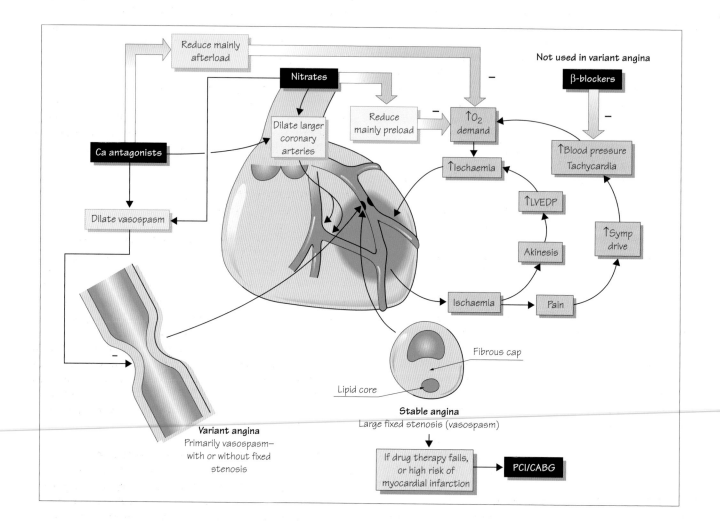

Variant angina
Primarily vasospasm—
with or without fixed
stenosis

Stable angina
Large fixed stenosis (vasospasm)

Treatment of chronic angina aims to control symptoms, and to prevent the progression of coronary heart disease by reducing relevant risk factors. Angina symptoms are controlled by restoring the balance between myocardial O_2 demand and supply. In **stable angina**, the blood flow through stenotic coronary arteries is limited, and therapy is mainly aimed at reducing O_2 demand with **vasodilators** and **β-blockers**. The treatment of **variant angina** is primarily directed at reversing coronary **vasospasm**.

Nitrovasodilators

Nitrovasodilators include **nitroglycerin** (glyceryl trinitrate), **isosorbide mononitrate**, **isosorbide dinitrate**, **erythrityl tetranitrate** and **pentaerythritol tetranitrate**. Rapidly acting nitrovasodilators are used to prevent angina, or to terminate ongoing attacks, while longer-acting preparations are combined with other drugs to provide long-term prophylaxis.

Nitrovasodilators are metabolized to release nitric oxide (NO), thus acting as a 'pharmacological endothelium'. The mechanisms of metabolism are unclear, although nitroglycerin is thought to be metabolized mainly by the enzyme *mitochondrial aldehyde dehydrogenase*. NO stimulates guanylate cyclase to elevate cGMP, thereby causing vasodi-

latation (see Chapter 22). At therapeutic doses, nitrovasodilators act primarily to dilate veins, thus reducing central venous pressure (preload) and as a consequent ventricular end-diastolic volume. This lowers myocardial contraction, wall stress and O_2 demand. Some arterial dilatation also occurs, diminishing total peripheral resistance (afterload). This allows the left ventricle to maintain cardiac output with a smaller stroke volume, again decreasing O_2 demand.

Nitrovasodilators can also increase the perfusion of ischaemic myocardium. They dilate larger coronary arteries (those > 100 microns in diameter). These give rise to **collateral vessels** (see Chapter 3) which can bypass stenotic arteries. Collaterals increase in number and diameter in the presence of a significant stenosis, providing an alternative perfusion of ischaemic tissue which is then enhanced by the nitrovasodilators. Nitrovasodilators also relieve coronary vasospasm, and may diminish plaque-related platelet aggregation and thrombosis by elevating platelet cGMP.

Nitroglycerin and isosorbide dinitrate taken sublingually relieve angina within minutes; this route of administration avoids the extensive first-pass metabolism of these drugs associated with oral dosing. Nitrovasodilators can also be given in slowly absorbed oral, transdermal and buccal forms for sustained effect.

Continuous exposure to nitrovasodilators causes **tolerance**. This is caused in part by increased production within blood vessels of reactive oxygen species, which may inactivate nitric oxide and also interfere with nitrovasodilator bioconversion. Reflex activation of the renin–angiotensin–aldosterone system by nitrovasodilator-induced vasodilatation may also contribute to tolerance. Tolerance is irrelevant with short-acting nitrovasodilators, but long-acting preparations become ineffective within hours. Tolerance can be minimized by 'eccentric' dosing schedules that allow blood concentrations to become low overnight. The most important adverse effect of nitrovasodilators is headache. Reflex tachycardia and orthostatic hypotension may also occur.

Ca^{2+}-channel blockers (CCBs; also Ca^{2+} antagonists)

CCBs act by blocking the L-type voltage-gated Ca^{2+} channels that allow depolarization-mediated influx of Ca^{2+} into smooth muscle cells, and also cardiac myocytes (see Chapters 11, 13, 34). As described in Chapter 34, *dihydropyridine* CCBs such as **amlodipine**, **nifedipine** and **felodipine** act selectively on vascular L-type Ca^{2+} channels, whilst the phenylalkylamine **verapamil** and the benzothiazepine **diltiazem** block these channels in both blood vessels and the heart.

CCBs prevent angina mainly by causing systemic arteriolar vasodilatation and decreasing afterload. They also prevent coronary vasospasm, making them particularly useful in variant angina. Their use is theoretically advantageous in variable threshold angina, in which coronary vasoconstriction contributes to reduced cardiac perfusion (see Chapter 39). The negative inotropic and chronotropic effects of verapamil and diltiazem also contribute to their usefulness by reducing myocardial O$_2$ demand.

The vasodilatation caused by CCBs can cause hypotension, headache and peripheral oedema (mainly dihydropyridines). On the other hand, their cardiac effects can elicit excessive cardiodepression and AV node conduction block (mainly verapamil and diltiazem). CCBs are contraindicated in heart failure, especially if β-blockers are being used.

Beta-adrenergic receptor blockers

As the figure illustrates, myocardial ischaemia creates a vicious cycle by activating the sympathetic system and increasing ventricular end-diastolic pressure; both these effects then worsen ischaemia and anginal pain. **Beta-blockers**, which are used for the prophylaxis of angina, help to block this cycle, thereby decreasing O$_2$ demand. They further reduce O$_2$ demand by decreasing myocardial contractility and wall stress. The resting and exercising heart rate also falls. This increases the fraction of time the heart spends in diastole, thus enhancing perfusion of the left ventricle, which occurs predominantly during diastole. The main therapeutic action of these drugs is on cardiac β$_1$-receptors, but both β$_1$-selective and (β$_1$/β$_2$) non-selective blockers are used.

Potential adverse effects of β-blockers include fatigue, reduced left ventricular function and severe bradycardia. They can precipitate asthma by blocking β$_2$-receptors in the airways, and therefore even β$_1$-selective agents are contraindicated in this condition. Lipid-soluble β-blockers (e.g. propranolol) can enter the central nervous system and cause depression or nightmares. Beta-blockers can also worsen insulin-induced hypoglycaemia in diabetics.

Drugs used less frequently for angina include **nicorandil**, a vasodilator that has nitrate-like effects and also opens potassium channels; **ivabradine**, which reduces cardiac ischaemia by inhibiting the cardiac pacemaker current I_f (see Chapter 10) and slowing the heart; and **ranolazine**, which protects against ischaemia by increasing glucose metabolism compared to that of fatty acids.

Management of angina

Therapy is typically instituted with a short-acting nitrovasodilator taken to prevent and terminate attacks. If control is insufficient, a β-blocker or CCB is added for prophylaxis. The choice between these is influenced by coexisting conditions and contraindications. For example, a CCB is preferable if the patient also has asthma or hypertension, and a β-blocker may be superior if atrial fibrillation is also present. If needed, this regimen can be supplemented with a long-acting nitrovasodilator. Finally, a combination of all of these agents can be employed. CCBs and nitrovasodilators are also used to treat variant angina, but β-blockers are *not*, as they may worsen coronary vasospasm by blocking the β$_2$-mediated (vasodilating), but not α$_1$-mediated (vasoconstricting) effects of sympathetic stimulation. If angina symptoms are refractory to drug treatment, or if the patient is at risk from widespread and serious coronary atherosclerosis, **revascularization** (see Chapter 42) is a preferred option.

Reduction of coronary risk factors

The reduction of risk factors that can contribute to the further progression of coronary heart disease is a key aim of angina management. Angina patients should be treated with daily low-dose aspirin, which suppresses platelet aggregation and greatly reduces the risk of myocardial infarction and death in patients with both stable and unstable angina. Clopidogrel is also sometimes used in angina as an antiplatelet drug. Many are now also treated with 'statins' (see Chapter 35) to reduce their plasma LDL levels to below 100 mg/dL (2.6 mmol/L). The 2001 HOPE trial showed that the angiotensin-converting enzyme inhibitor (ACEI) ramipril reduced the progression of atherosclerosis and enhanced survival over a period of 5 years, in a group with coronary artery disease or diabetes, and ACEI are now recommended for patients with stable angina who also have other conditions (e.g. hypertension or heart failure) for which these drugs are indicated.

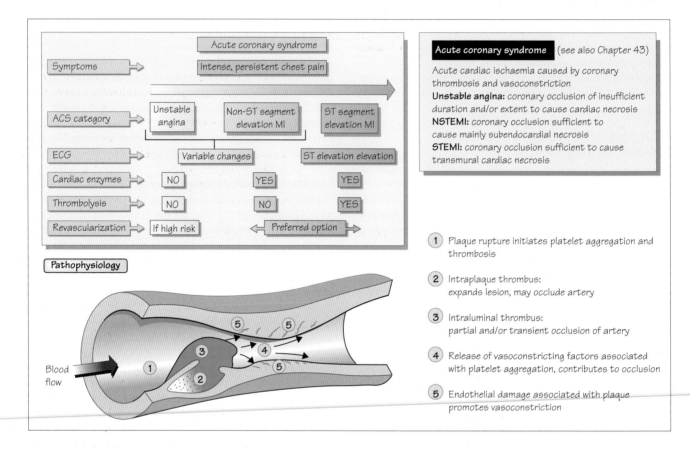

Stable angina is a chronic condition that occurs on a relatively predictable basis when cardiac ischaemia develops due to the inability of a narrowed coronary artery to meet an increased cardiac oxygen demand. Conversely, the **acute coronary syndromes (ACS)**, including in ascending order of severity, **unstable angina**, **non-ST segment elevation myocardial infarction (NSTEMI)** and **ST elevation myocardial infarction (STEMI)**, represent a spectrum of dangerous conditions in which myocardial ischaemia results from *a sudden decrease in the flow of blood through a coronary vessel*. This decrease is almost always initiated by the rupture of an atherosclerotic plaque, resulting in the formation of an intracoronary thrombus which diminishes or abolishes the flow of blood.

When a patient presents with a suspected acute coronary syndrome, an ECG is immediately carried out. The hallmark of **STEMI**, the most serious acute coronary syndrome, is *sustained elevation of the ST segment of the ECG* (see figure, upper left). This indicates that a large area of the myocardium, probably involving the full thickness of a ventricular wall, has suffered *necrosis* (cell death, with subsequent inflammation and scarring) as a result of prolonged ischaemia. Myocardial necrosis causes the release of intracellular proteins, such as **troponins T and I**. These can be detected in the blood, and act as markers of myocardial cell death. STEMI is confirmed when elevated levels of these markers are found. STEMI typically occurs when a thrombus has completely occluded a coronary artery for a significant amount of time, and usually causes more severe symptoms than do unstable angina or NSTEMI.

Incomplete or temporary coronary occlusion, or the existence of collateral coronary arteries which can maintain some supply of blood to the affected region, may result in a smaller degree of myocardial ischaemia and necrosis, usually limited to the subendocardium. This may not result in ST segment elevation, but does cause the release of markers of necrosis. Patients who are found to have elevated levels of these markers, but who do not have ST segment elevation, are deemed to have had **NSTEMI**.

Patients who demonstrate symptoms associated with ACS, but who have neither ST segment elevation nor elevated levels of markers of myocardial necrosis, are deemed to have **unstable angina (UA)**. In this case, it is likely that the coronary obstruction has been of limited extent and/or duration (< 20 min), and is thus sufficient to cause ischaemia but not detectable necrosis.

Both NSTEMI and STEMI are grouped together as **acute myocardial infarctions**, but are managed differently, in that pharmacological reperfusion (thrombolysis) is used to treat STEMI but not NSTEMI (see Chapters 43, 44). On the other hand, the management of unstable angina and NSTEMI utilizes overlapping approaches, and these conditions are often discussed together as 'UA/NSTEMI'. Symptoms of UA/NSTEMI resemble those of stable angina, but they are frequently more painful, intense and persistent, often lasting 30 min. Pain is frequently resistant to nitroglycerin. Typical patient presentations include:
1 crescendo angina, where attacks are progressively more severe, prolonged and frequent
2 angina of recent onset brought on by minimal exertion

3 angina at rest/with minimal exertion or during sleep
4 post-MI angina (ischaemic pain 24 h to 2 weeks after MI).

Pathophysiology of UA/NSTEMI

Studies have shown that episodes of unstable angina are preceded by a fall in coronary blood flow, thought to result from the periodic development of coronary **thrombosis** and **vasoconstriction**, which are triggered by coronary artery disease (see figure).

Thrombosis is promoted by the endothelial damage and turbulent blood flow associated with atherosclerotic plaques. Compared to the lesions of stable angina, plaques found in patients with acute coronary syndromes tend to have a thinner fibrous cap and a larger lipid core, and are generally more widespread and severe. These stenoses are often *eccentric* – the plaque does not surround the entire circumference of the artery. Such lesions are especially vulnerable to being ruptured by haemodynamic stress. This exposes the plaque interior, which powerfully stimulates platelet aggregation and thrombosis. The thrombus propagates out into the coronary lumen, occluding the artery. Rupture may also cause haemorrhage into the lesion itself, expanding it out into the lumen and worsening stenosis.

These events may be exacerbated by impaired coronary vasodilatation, and vasospasm due to plaque-associated endothelial damage, which reduces the local release of endothelium-dependent relaxing factors. Platelet aggregation and thrombosis also cause the local generation of vasoconstrictors such as thromboxane A_2 and serotonin.

Risk stratification

The occurrence of UA and NSTEMI indicates that a patient has a high risk of undergoing subsequent episodes of coronary thrombosis which may cause more significant cardiac damage or death. In the USA, for example, ~4% of the 1.3 million people who enter hospital with UA/NSTEMI die within 30 days, and ~8% experience (re)infarction. Although NSTEMI is by definition a more serious 'event' than UA, these are both heterogeneous conditions, and the risk of (re)infarction is higher in some patients with UA than in others with NSTEMI. Risk assessment is therefore of paramount importance. Risk is scored on the basis of a number of factors, including frequency and severity of angina, elevated markers of cardiac necrosis, ECG changes (ST segment depression and/or T-wave inversion), and prior angiographic evidence of atherosclerotic plaque.

Management

UA/NSTEMI is a medical emergency. Typically, treatment begins with aggressive pharmacological therapy, which focuses on rendering the acute coronary lesion less dangerous, minimizing residual ischaemia and preventing future coronary events. **Urgent revascularization** is considered for patients with high-risk and/or very significant coronary artery disease, or if drug treatment fails to control symptoms (see Chapter 42).

Drug treatment of UA/NSTEMI (see also Chapter 45 for drug mechanisms)

Antiplatelet therapy All patients with UA/NSTEMI are immediately treated with **low-dose aspirin**, which is then continued indefinitely, in order to suppress platelet aggregation, a key initial step in thrombosis. Clinical trials have shown that aspirin, in doses as low as 75 mg/day, reduces mortality or infarction in this group by more than 50%.

The thienopyridine **clopidogrel**, which inhibits ADP-stimulated platelet aggregation, was shown in the 2000 CURE trial to reduce cardiovascular morbidity and mortality by ~20% in patients with UA/NSTEMI. It is recommended that clopidogrel should be added in with aspirin therapy for at least a month, although the optimal duration of its use is not yet defined.

Glycoprotein IIb/IIIa antagonists are the most powerful of the antiplatelet drugs. These drugs are of proven benefit in UA/NSTEMI patients who receive percutaneous coronary intervention (PCI), a type of revascularization procedure in which plaque-stenosed coronary arteries are widened using a balloon catheter (see Chapter 42). PCI usually involves placing a stent (a mesh tube) in the affected coronary to keep it open, and the glycoprotein IIb/IIIa antagonists reduce the tendency of stents to cause thrombosis.

Anticoagulant therapy **Unfractionated heparin (UH)** or **low molecular weight heparins (LMWHs)**, which inhibit the coagulation cascade mainly at factor X and thrombin, are given to all patients with UA/NSTEMI. These drugs are given intravenously (UH) or subcutaneously (LMWH) while patients are hospitalized, but not routinely thereafter. There is evidence that the LMWH enoxaparin may be preferable to UH.

Other drugs **Beta-blockers** have been shown to reduce cardiovascular morbidity and mortality in patients with UA/NSTEMI, and should be given unless contraindicated (e.g. in asthma). **Nitrates** can be given, especially on a temporary basis, to relieve pain, but do not appear to affect mortality. **Ca^{2+}-channel blockers** should *not* be used to treat UA/NSTEMI, although they may be continued if the patient is already receiving them for chronic stable angina. On the other hand, there is increasing evidence that the lipid-lowering '**statins**' and **angiotensin-converting enzyme inhibitors** improve survival in UA/NSTEMI.

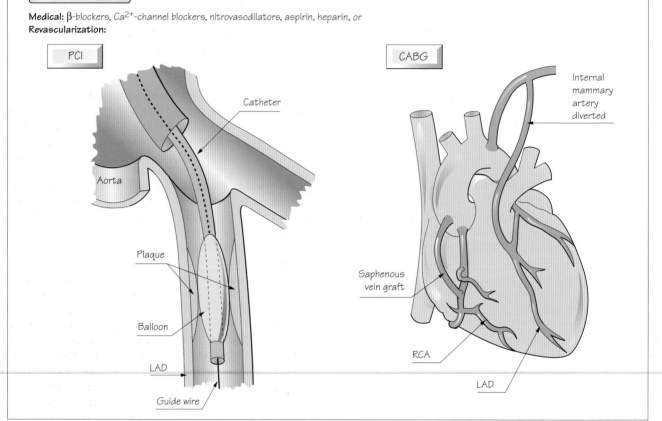

Coronary artery bypass grafting (CABG) and **percutaneous coronary intervention (PCI,** formerly termed percutaneous transcoronary angioplasty) are revascularization techniques that are used to treat patients with both stable angina and acute coronary syndromes. As described below, both procedures are used in higher-risk patients, with the choice of technique determined by several factors including severity of disease and the wishes of the individual. It is estimated that in 2003 CABG and PCI were carried out on approximately 270 000 and 650 000 patients in the USA, respectively.

CABG is a surgical procedure (figure, right) that was introduced in the 1960s. Initially, CABG mainly involved the use of lengths of healthy superfluous blood vessels (conduits) which were removed and then attached (anastamosed) between the aorta and the coronary arteries distal to the stenosis, thus allowing a supply of blood to the heart that bypassed the obstruction. Conduits commonly used for CABG included **saphenous vein** segments harvested from the leg. These, however, have limited long-term patency due to early postoperative thrombosis, intimal hyperplasia with smooth muscle proliferation within the first year, and the development of atherosclerosis after approximately 5–7 years. For this reason, the **left internal thoracic** (also termed **mammary) artery** (LITA) is now used for grafting much more widely than the saphenous vein. In general, the LITA is not disconnected from its

parent (subclavian) artery, but is cut distally and attached to the coronary artery. Unlike the saphenous vein, 90–95% of LITA grafts remain patent after 10 years, and patients with a LITA graft to the crucial left anterior descending coronary artery have improved long-term survival compared to patients receiving saphenous vein grafts. If multivessel disease is present, the use of LITA and saphenous vein grafts can be combined. More recently, the use of both left and right internal thoracic arteries (**bilateral internal thoracic artery**) for grafting has become more common, especially for younger patients. For example, the right internal thoracic artery may be grafted to the left anterior descending coronary artery while the LITA is anastomosed to the circumflex system. The gastroepiploic and radial arteries can also be used for grafting.

CABG is usually perform with the patient on *cardiopulmonary bypass*, with the heart stopped. Blood is typically removed from the right atrium, drained into a reservoir, and then pumped through an oxygenator, then a filter and back into the aorta to perfuse the systemic circulation. The main complications of the procedure are a systemic inflammatory response, atrial fibrillation and persistent neurological abnormalities. These latter are thought to be caused by emboli, either formed in the bypass circuit or produced by disturbance of aortic plaques during cannulation, which lodge in the cerebral vasculature. These complications can be avoided by '*off-pump CABG*', which does not involve stopping the heart. In this case, the region of the cardiac wall encompassing the target coronary segment is immobilized to allow grafting. Randomized trials show that both types of CABG offer similar outcomes. The mortality rate associated with CABG is ~2%.

PCI, first used in 1977, is a much less invasive procedure. A guiding catheter is introduced via the femoral, brachial or radial artery, and is positioned near the target stenosis. A guiding wire is then advanced down the lumen of the coronary artery until it is positioned across the stenosis. A balloon catheter is advanced over this wire, and then inflated at the site of the stenosis to increase the luminal diameter (figure, left). Emergency CABG is required in 1–2% of patients due to acute vessel closure after this procedure. PCI is judged a success if the arterial lumen at the stenosis is increased to more than 50% of the normal coronary artery diameter.

Restenosis at the site of the PCI occurs within 6 months of the procedure in 30% of patients. Restenosis can be caused by elastic recoil of the vessel or by **intimal hyperplasia**, a thickening of the inner layer of the artery which is initiated by endothelial denudation, and which involves proliferation of intimal smooth muscle cells and the production of connective tissue. Restenosis generally causes a return of cardiac ischaemia and angina, in which case PCI is repeated or CABG is performed.

Stents were first introduced in 1986 in an attempt to prevent elastic recoil and restenosis. Stents are cylindrical metal (e.g. stainless steel, platinum) mesh or slotted tubes that are implanted into the artery at the site of balloon expansion following angioplasty. They are mainly used in vessels > 3 mm in diameter and are designed either to be self-expanding, or to be expanded by the catheter balloon, so that they press out against the inner wall of the coronary artery, holding it open. Stenting is currently being used in ~90% of PCI procedures as its introduction has substantially improved acute PCI success, has reduced the rate of restenosis to ~15%, and has correspondingly decreased the need for repeat revascularizations. Various approaches are being tried to reduce this 'in-stent' restenosis still further. Notably, the 2002 RAVEL trial assessed the use of stents that were coated with the proliferation-inhibiting drug **rapamycin** (sirolimus), which gradually eluted from the stent over a month. Rapamycin caused a dramatic decrease in restenosis, and virtually abolished the need for another revascularization over the year following the procedure. Subsequent studies have shown that the use of drug-eluting stents reduces the incidence of major adverse cardiac events during the 9 months following PCI by ~50%, so that drug-eluting stents utilizing rapamycin as well as the alternative agents **paclitaxel** and **everolimus** are now used routinely.

The main potential complication arising from stenting is thrombosis, which can be well controlled with aspirin and clopidogrel. Routine PCI bears a risk of mortality of ≤ 1%.

Revascularization vs medical management: which patients benefit?

In general, revascularization is preferred for patients who are at high risk of developing worsening ischaemic heart disease and/or acute coronary syndromes, or in whom pharmacological ('medical') treatment is either not controlling ischaemic symptoms (e.g. angina) or is causing intolerable side effects. Particularly important indications for revascularization in *stable angina* include the presence of significant plaques in three coronary arteries (particularly when the left anterior descending, which perfuses the largest fraction of the myocardium, is involved) and reduced left ventricular function, which indicates the presence of chronic ongoing ischaemia.

Revascularization is also very frequently used in *UA/NSTEMI* (see Chapter 40), and is recommended for patients who are judged to be at moderate or high risk for death or myocardial infarction, as judged by various indices relating to the seriousness of their signs and symptoms. Revascularization is now also preferred over thrombolysis to produce immediate coronary reperfusion during acute myocardial infarction (STEMI; see Chapters 43, 44). In *heart failure*, revascularization can be used to reperfuse a region of 'hibernating myocardium', in which cells are still alive but are contracting poorly because they are chronically ischaemic.

PCI vs CABG

PCI is preferred when one or two arteries are diseased, as long as the disease is not too diffuse and the plaques are amenable to this approach. CABG is used when all three main coronary arteries are diseased (triple vessel disease), when the left coronary mainstem has a significant stenosis, when the lesion is not amenable to PCI, and when left ventricular function is poor. CABG has been shown to reduce angina symptoms more than does PCI in the first 5 years after the procedure, but symptoms tend to return gradually over the years in either case, and eventually recur similarly after both procedures. Revascularization must be repeated much more often after PCI compared to CABG, although improvements in stenting will probably narrow this difference. The use of PCI is growing rapidly, while that of CABG is diminishing.

Benefits of revascularization

Compared with medical therapy, CABG improves survival in patients with severe atherosclerotic disease in all three major coronary arteries or a more than 50% stenosis of the left main coronary artery, particularly if left ventricular function is impaired. Compared with medical therapy, PCI does not improve survival. However, PCI results in a greater improvement of angina symptoms and exercise tolerance than does medical therapy, and also diminishes the need for drugs.

Pathophysiology of acute myocardial infarction

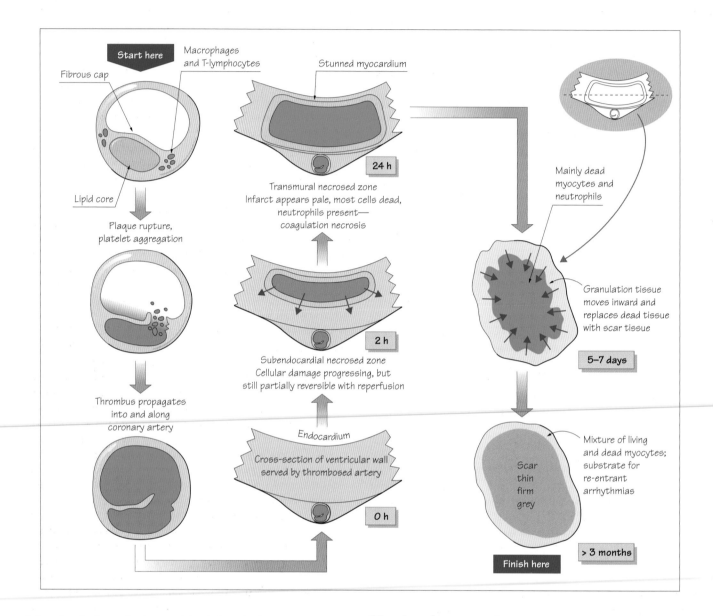

Infarction is tissue death caused by ischaemia. Acute **myocardial infarction** (MI) occurs when localized myocardial ischaemia causes the development of a defined region of **necrosis**. MI is most often caused by rupture of an atherosclerotic lesion in a coronary artery. This causes the formation of a thrombus that plugs the artery, stopping it from supplying blood to the region of the heart that it supplies.

Role of thrombosis in MI
Pivotal studies by DeWood and colleagues showed that *coronary thrombosis* is the critical event resulting in MI. Of patients presenting within 4 h of symptom onset with ECG evidence of transmural MI, coronary angiography showed that 87% had complete thrombotic occlusion of the infarct-related artery. The incidence of total occlusion fell to 65% 12–24 h after symptom onset due to spontaneous fibrinolysis. Fresh thrombi on top of ruptured plaques have also been demonstrated in the infarct-related arteries in patients dying of MI.

Mechanisms and consequences of plaque rupture
Coronary plaques that are prone to rupture are typically small and non-obstructive, with a large lipid-rich core covered by a thin fibrous cap. These 'high-risk' plaques typically contain abundant **macrophages** and **T-lymphocytes** that are thought to release **metalloproteases** and **cytokines** which weaken the fibrous cap, rendering it liable to tear or erode due to the shear stress exerted by the blood flow.

Plaque rupture reveals subendothelial collagen, which serves as a site of platelet adhesion, activation and aggregation. This results in:
1 the release of substances such as *thromboxane A_2 (TXA$_2$)*, *fibrinogen*, *5-hydroxytryptamine (5-HT)*, *platelet activating factor* and *ADP*, which further promote platelet aggregation
2 activation of the clotting cascade, leading to fibrin formation and propagation and stabilization of the occlusive thrombus.

The endothelium is often damaged around areas of coronary artery disease. The resulting deficit of antithrombotic factors such as *thrombomodulin* and *prostacyclin* enhances thrombus formation. In addition, the tendency of several platelet-derived factors (e.g. TXA_2, 5-HT) to cause vasoconstriction is increased in the absence of endothelial-derived relaxing factors. This may promote the development of local vasospasm, which worsens coronary occlusion.

Sudden death and acute coronary syndrome onset show a **circadian variation** (daily cycle), peaking at around 9 a.m. with a trough at around 11 p.m. Levels of catecholamines peak about an hour after awakening in the morning, resulting in maximal levels of platelet aggregability, vascular tone, heart rate and blood pressure, which may trigger plaque rupture and thrombosis. Increased physical and mental stress can also cause MI and sudden death, supporting a role for increases in catecholamines in MI pathophysiology. Furthermore, chronic β-adrenergic receptor blockade abolishes the circadian rhythm of MI.

Autopsies of young subjects killed in road accidents often show small plaque ruptures in susceptible arteries, suggesting that plaque rupture does not always have pathological consequences. The degree of coronary occlusion and myocardial damage caused by plaque rupture probably depends on systemic catecholamine levels, as well as local factors such as plaque location and morphology, the depth of plaque rupture, and the extent to which coronary vasoconstriction occurs.

Severe and prolonged ischaemia produces a region of necrosis spanning the entire thickness of the myocardial wall. Such a *transmural* infarct usually causes ST segment elevation (i.e. STEMI; see Chapter 40). Less severe and protracted ischaemia can arise when:

1 coronary occlusion is followed by spontaneous reperfusion
2 the infarct-related artery is not completely occluded
3 occlusion is complete, but an existing collateral blood supply prevents complete ischaemia
4 the oxygen demand in the affected zone of myocardium is smaller.

Under these conditions, the necrotic zone may be mainly limited to the subendocardium, typically causing non-ST segment elevation MI.

The classification of acute MI according to the presence or absence of ST segment elevation is designed to allow rapid decision-making concerning whether thrombolysis should be initiated (see Chapter 44). This classification replaces the previous one, based on the presence or absence of Q waves on the ECG, which was less useful for guiding immediate therapy.

Evolution of the infarct

Both infarcted and unaffected myocardial regions undergo progressive changes over the hours, days and weeks following coronary thrombosis. This process of postinfarct myocardial evolution leads to the occurrence of characteristic complications at predictable times after the initial event (see Chapter 44).

Ischaemia causes an immediate loss of contractility in the affected myocardium, a condition termed **hypokinesis**. Necrosis starts to develop in the subendocardium (which is most prone to ischaemia; see Chapter 39), about 15–30 min after coronary occlusion. The necrotic region grows outward towards the epicardium over the next 3–6 h, eventually spanning the entire ventricular wall. In some areas (generally at the edges of the infarct) the myocardium is **stunned** (reversibly damaged) and will eventually recover if blood flow is restored. Contractility in the remaining viable myocardium increases, a process termed **hyperkinesis**.

A progression of cellular, histological and gross changes develop within the infarct. Although alterations in the gross appearance of infarcted tissue are not apparent for at least 6 h after the onset of cell death, cell biochemistry and ultrastructure begin to show abnormalities within 20 min. Cell damage is progressive, becomingly increasingly irreversible over about 12 h. This period therefore provides a window of opportunity during which PCI or thrombolysis leading to reperfusion may salvage some of the infarct (see Chapter 45).

Between 4 and 12 h after cell death starts, the infarcted myocardium begins to undergo **coagulation necrosis**, a process characterized by cell swelling, organelle breakdown and protein denaturation. After about 18 h, **neutrophils** (phagocytic lymphocytes) enter the infarct. Their numbers reach a peak after about 5 days, and then decline. After 3–4 days, **granulation tissue** appears at the edges of the infarct zone. This consists of **macrophages**, **fibroblasts**, which lay down scar tissue, and **new capillaries**. The infarcted myocardium is especially soft between 4 and 7 days, and is therefore maximally prone to **rupturing**. This event is usually fatal, may occur at any time during the first 2 weeks, and is responsible for about 10% of MI mortality. As the granulation tissue migrates inward toward the centre of the infarct over several weeks, the necrotic tissue is engulfed and digested by the macrophages. The granulation tissue then progressively matures, with an increase in connective (scar) tissue and loss of capillaries. After 2–3 months, the infarct has healed, leaving a non-contracting region of the ventricular wall that is thinned, firm and pale grey.

Infarct expansion, the stretching and thinning of the infarcted wall, may occur within the first day or so after a MI, especially if the infarction is large or transmural, or has an anterior location. Over the course of several months, there is progressive dilatation, not only of the infarct zone, but also of healthy myocardium. This process of **ventricular remodelling** is caused by an increase in end-diastolic wall stress. Infarct expansion puts patients at a substantial risk for the development of congestive heart failure, ventricular arrhythmias, and free wall rupture.

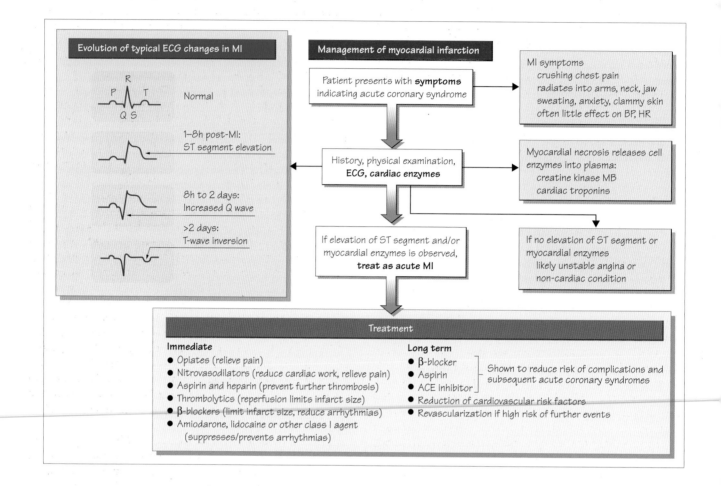

Evolution of typical ECG changes in MI

Normal

1–8h post-MI:
ST segment elevation

8h to 2 days:
Increased Q wave

>2 days:
T-wave inversion

Management of myocardial infarction

Patient presents with **symptoms** indicating acute coronary syndrome

MI symptoms
crushing chest pain
radiates into arms, neck, jaw
sweating, anxiety, clammy skin
often little effect on BP, HR

History, physical examination,
ECG, cardiac enzymes

Myocardial necrosis releases cell enzymes into plasma:
creatine kinase MB
cardiac troponins

If elevation of ST segment and/or myocardial enzymes is observed,
treat as acute MI

If no elevation of ST segment or myocardial enzymes
likely unstable angina or non-cardiac condition

Treatment

Immediate
- Opiates (relieve pain)
- Nitrovasodilators (reduce cardiac work, relieve pain)
- Aspirin and heparin (prevent further thrombosis)
- Thrombolytics (reperfusion limits infarct size)
- β-blockers (limit infarct size, reduce arrhythmias)
- Amiodarone, lidocaine or other class I agent (suppresses/prevents arrhythmias)

Long term
- β-blocker
- Aspirin ⎤ Shown to reduce risk of complications and
- ACE inhibitor ⎦ subsequent acute coronary syndromes
- Reduction of cardiovascular risk factors
- Revascularization if high risk of further events

Symptoms and signs

Patients present with central crushing chest pain, which may radiate into the arms, jaw or neck. The pain lasts longer than 30 min and is not relieved by nitroglycerin. The patient is frequently sweating and may appear cold and clammy. Nausea or vomiting and intense feelings of anxiety are common. Some individuals present atypically, with no symptoms (**silent infarction**, most common in diabetic subjects), unusual locations of the pain, syncope or peripheral embolization. The pulse may demonstrate a tachycardia or bradycardia. The blood pressure is usually normal. However, a systolic pressure of < 90 mmHg and evidence of organ hypoperfusion herald **cardiogenic shock**, where cardiac output is insufficient for adequate tissue perfusion. The rest of the examination of the cardiovascular system may be unremarkable, but there may be a third or fourth sound audible on auscultation as well as a systolic murmur.

Investigations

ECG changes associated with MI indicate the site, extent and thickness of the infarct. ST segment elevation, increased Q waves and inversion of the T wave typically evolve in transmural MI (i.e. STEMI) as shown in the figure. A more than twofold elevation of plasma concentrations of cardiac cellular enzymes indicates that myocardial necrosis has occurred. These include **creatine kinase MB** (CK-MB) and **cardiac**

troponins **T and I**. CK-MB levels begin to rise within 4–8 h, peak at 24 h, and decline to normal at 2–3 days. The cardiac troponins begin to rise within 4–8 h and remain elevated for 4–7 days.

Complications

With large infarctions (> 20–25% of the left ventricle, LV), depression of pump function is sufficient to cause **cardiac failure**. An infarction involving more than 40% of the LV causes cardiogenic shock. **Rupture** of the free LV wall (see Chapter 43) is almost always fatal. Rupture of the ventricular septum may result in leakage of blood between the ventricles. Rupture of the myocardium underlying a papillary muscle, or more rarely of the papillary muscle itself, may cause **mitral regurgitation**. **Arrhythmias** in the acute phase include ventricular ectopic beats, ventricular tachycardia or ventricular fibrillation. Supraventricular arrhythmias include atrial ectopics, flutter and fibrillation. Bradyarrhythmias are also common, including sinus bradycardia, and first-, second- and third-degree AV block. **Infarct expansion** (see Chapter 43) is a dangerous late complication.

Management

Immediate In the ambulance or on first medical contact, individuals with suspected MI are immediately given 300 mg chewable **aspirin** to block further platelet aggregation. The patient is assessed using a

12-lead ECG, and by brief history and examination, and is put on high-flow oxygen. **Morphine** together with an antiemetic is administered to relieve pain. **Nitrovasodilators** may also help to reduce cardiac work and control pain. A **β-blocker** should be given unless there are contraindications (e.g. LV failure). *ST elevation* of more than 0.1 mV in two chest leads or more than 0.2 mV in two limb leads, or *new left bundle branch block*, indicates STEMI. These patients should undergo **thrombolysis** within *30 min* unless contraindications are present (see below), or preferably **percutaneous coronary intervention** (see Chapter 42) of the blocked artery within *90 min* of presentation if appropriate facilities and personnel are available.

Subsequent Long-term treatment with aspirin, β-blockers and **ACE inhibitors** reduces the complications of MI and the risk of reinfarction. Cessation of smoking, treatment of hypertension and diabetes, and reduction of lipids using **statins** (see Chapter 35) are vital. Prior to discharge from hospital, patients are given an exercise stress test. If this indicates that the risk of further events is high, or if they are still experiencing from angina attacks, early revascularization is indicated.

Thrombolytic agents

Thrombolysis is the dissolution of the blood clot plugging the infarct-related coronary artery. As described in Chapter 45, thrombolytic agents induce **fibrinolysis**, the fragmentation of the fibrin strands holding the clot together. This leads to *reperfusion* of the infarct zone. Reperfusion limits infarct size and reduces the risk of complications such as infarct expansion, arrhythmias and cardiac failure. Clinical trials, notably ISIS-2 (1988), have demonstrated that thrombolytic agents reduce mortality by about 25% in STEMI, although patients without ST elevation (indicates NSTEMI) do *not* benefit from thrombolysis. It is critical that thrombolysis is instituted as quickly as possible. Although significant reductions in mortality occur when thrombolytics are given within 12 h of symptom onset, the greatest benefits occur when therapy is instituted within 2 h ('time is muscle').

The two main agents for thrombolysis are **streptokinase (SK)** and **tissue plasminogen activator (tPA)** (see Chapter 45). tPA appears to have a slight survival benefit compared to SK, but the former is much less expensive and so more widely used. Both agents are given by infusion. tPA is very quickly cleared from the plasma, and **reteplase** and **tenecteplase** are newer agents that have been made by modifying the structure of tPA in order to retard plasma clearance. Both can therefore be given by bolus injection, thus facilitating prehospital thrombolysis.

The main risk of thrombolysis is bleeding, particularly intracerebral haemorrhage (stroke), which occurs in ~1% of cases. Contraindications to thrombolytic therapy include prior stroke or substantial risk of intracerebral haemorrhage, and uncontrolled hypertension.

Other drugs used in acute myocardial infarction

Antiplatelet and **anticoagulant** therapy is used after MI to prevent further platelet aggregation and thrombosis in the infarct-related artery. The ISIS-2 trial demonstrated a 23% reduction in 35-day mortality in patients randomized to 160 mg/day of aspirin. Combined aspirin and SK had an additive benefit compared to placebo (42% reduction). Following an initial 300-mg loading dose, 75–150 mg aspirin should be given daily thereafter to all patients to prevent vessel occlusion and infarction. Because tPA, reteplase and tenecteplase are more fibrin specific than SK, intravenous heparin should be given for a duration of 48–72 h to reduce the risk of further thrombosis when these agents are administered, or when the patient is at high risk of developing systemic emboli (e.g. with anterior MI or atrial fibrillation).

Beta-blockers are beneficial in MI for several reasons. They diminish O_2 demand by lowering heart rate and decrease ventricular wall stress by lowering afterload. They therefore reduce ischaemia and infarct size when given acutely. They also decrease recurrent ischaemia and free wall rupture, and suppress arrhythmias (see Chapter 48). Long-term oral β-blockade reduces mortality, recurrent MI and sudden death by about 25%.

ACE inhibitors reduce afterload and ventricular wall stress and improve ejection fraction. Inhibition of ACE raises bradykinin levels, which may improve endothelial function and limit coronary vasospasm. ACE inhibitors also limit ventricular remodelling and infarct expansion (see Chapter 43), thereby reducing mortality and the incidence of congestive heart failure and recurrent MI. Therapy should be instituted within 24 h in patients with STEMI, especially if there is evidence of heart failure or LV dysfunction, and should continue long term if LV dysfunction remains evident.

Severe LV failure as a result of MI is heralded by a large fall in cardiac output, pulmonary congestion and often hypotension. Treatment involves O_2 to prevent hypoxaemia, a diuretic to reduce preload, and nitroglycerin (glyceryl trinitrate) to reduce afterload. Revascularization is crucial. If ventricular failure is severe (cardiogenic shock), **intra-ortic balloon counterpulsation** can be used temporarily to support the circulation. A catheter-mounted balloon is inserted via the common femoral artery and positioned in the descending thoracic aorta. The balloon is inflated during diastole, increasing the pressure in the aortic arch and thereby improving perfusion of the coronary and cerebral arteries. During systole, deflation of the balloon creates a suction effect which reduces ventricular afterload and promotes systemic perfusion.

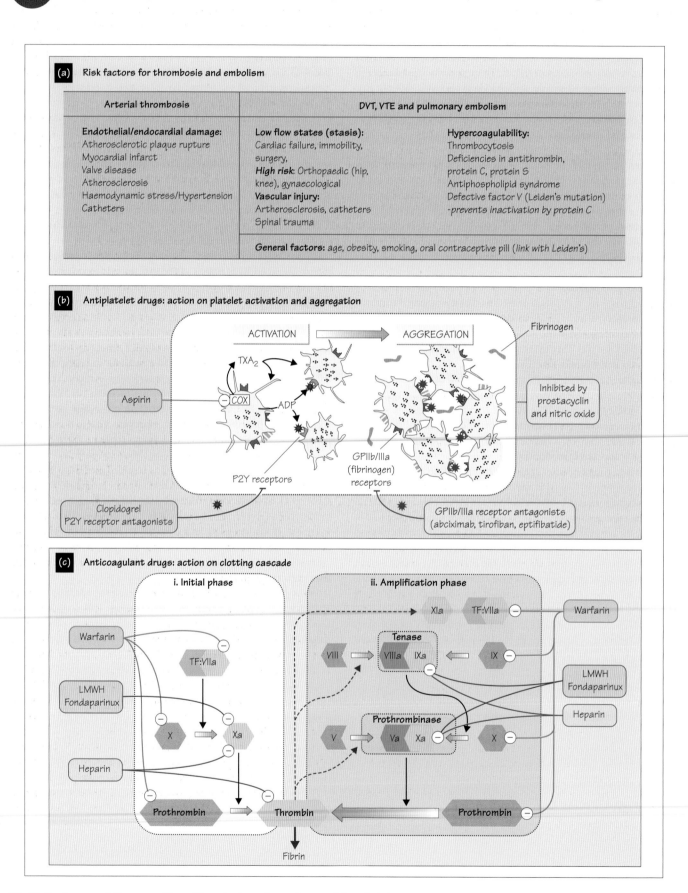

(a) Risk factors for thrombosis and embolism

Arterial thrombosis	DVT, VTE and pulmonary embolism	
Endothelial/endocardial damage: Atherosclerotic plaque rupture Myocardial infarct Valve disease Atherosclerosis Haemodynamic stress/Hypertension Catheters	**Low flow states (stasis):** Cardiac failure, immobility, surgery, **High risk**: Orthopaedic (hip, knee), gynaecological **Vascular injury:** Artherosclerosis, catheters Spinal trauma	**Hypercoagulability:** Thrombocytosis Deficiencies in antithrombin, protein C, protein S Antiphospholipid syndrome Defective factor V (Leiden's mutation) -prevents inactivation by protein C
	General factors: age, obesity, smoking, oral contraceptive pill (link with Leiden's)	

(b) Antiplatelet drugs: action on platelet activation and aggregation

ACTIVATION → AGGREGATION

Fibrinogen

TXA$_2$

Aspirin — COX

ADP

P2Y receptors

GPIIb/IIIa (fibrinogen) receptors

Inhibited by prostacyclin and nitric oxide

Clopidogrel P2Y receptor antagonists

GPIIb/IIIa receptor antagonists (abciximab, tirofiban, eptifibatide)

(c) Anticoagulant drugs: action on clotting cascade

i. Initial phase

ii. Amplification phase

Warfarin

LMWH Fondaparinux

Heparin

TF:VIIa

X → Xa

Prothrombin → Thrombin

Fibrin

XIa   TF:VIIa   Warfarin

Tenase
VIII   VIIIa IXa   IX

LMWH Fondaparinux

Heparin

Prothrombinase
V   Va Xa   X

Prothrombin

Thrombin

Thrombosis

Thrombosis and embolism are ultimately the main cause of death in the Western world. Thrombosis is inappropriate activation of haemostasis, with clots (**thrombi**) forming inside blood vessels. If thrombi fragment they can be carried in the blood as **emboli**, and block downstream blood vessels causing infarction. Most commonly fatalities are due to thrombosis as a result of **atherosclerotic plaque rupture** in acute coronary syndromes, or venous thromboembolism (**VTE**), particular **pulmonary embolism**, following **deep vein thrombosis (DVT)**. **Virchow's triad** of *endothelial damage, blood stasis* and *hypercoagulability* predispose to thrombosis. Endothelial (or endocardial) damage is the most common cause of arterial thrombosis. Stasis (poor flow), which allows platelets to settle, clotting factors to accumulate, and unimpeded formation of thrombi, is the most common cause of DVT and VTE. **Risk factors** are shown in Figure 45a. Once formed, thrombi can undergo **dissolution** by fibrinolysis, **propagation** by accumulation of more fibrin and platelets, or **organization** with invasion of endothelial or smooth muscle cells and fibrosis. In **recanalization** channels form allowing blood to reflow. If not destroyed, thrombi may be incorporated into the vessel wall.

Arterial (white, platelet-rich) thrombi are primarily treated with antiplatelet drugs, whilst venous (red) thrombi are primarily treated with anticoagulants. All such therapies increase risk of bleeding, and may be contraindicated in patients with prior stroke, active ulcers, pregnancy or recent surgery.

Antiplatelet drugs (Figure 45b)

Aspirin (*acetylsalicylic acid*) is the most important antiplatelet drug. It irreversibly inhibits **cyclooxygenase (COX)**, the first enzyme in the sequence leading to formation of **thromboxane A$_2$ (TXA$_2$)** and **prostacyclin (PGI$_2$)**. TXA$_2$ is produced by platelets and is a key platelet activator (see Chapter 7), whereas endothelium-derived prostacyclin inhibits platelet activation and aggregation by increasing cAMP. Because aspirin inhibits COX *irreversibly*, production of prostacyclin and TXA$_2$ only recovers when new COX is produced via gene transcription. This cannot occur in platelets, which lack nuclei (see Chapter 5), so TXA$_2$ production remains depressed until new platelets are formed over several days. Conversely, endothelial cells make new COX within hours. Aspirin therapy therefore produces a sustained increase in the prostacyclin-TXA$_2$ ratio, suppressing platelet activation and aggregation. **Side effects/risks**: gastrointestinal problems and haemorrhage. **Emerging therapy**: nitroaspirin, aspirin with an NO-releasing moiety. NO also inhibits platelet aggregation, and nitroaspirin is better tolerated in terms of gastrointestinal tract problems.

Thienopyridine derivatives such as **clopidogrel** indirectly and irreversibly block purinergic **P2Y receptors**, and thus ADP-induced platelet activation (see Chapter 7); they take > 24 h for maximal effect. They are useful for aspirin-intolerant patients and preventing thrombi on coronary artery stents (see Chapter 40). Long-term treatment with clopidogrel plus aspirin is beneficial in acute coronary syndromes. Novel direct antagonists of P2Y receptors have the advantage of rapidity of action.

The monoclonal antibody **abciximab** and peptides **tirofiban** and **eptifibatide** interfere with fibrinogen binding to **GPIIb/IIIa receptors** on activated platelets, thus inhibiting aggregation (see Chapter 7). In patients with unstable angina or undergoing high-risk angioplasty, GPIIb/IIIa blockade with aspirin and heparin significantly reduces short-term mortality, MI and the need for urgent bypass surgery or revascularization.

Anticoagulant drugs (Figure 45c)

Heparin, a mixture of mucopolysaccharides derived from mast cells, activates **antithrombin**, which inhibits thrombin and factors X, IX and XI (see Chapter 7). Heparin must bind to both thrombin and antithrombin for inhibition of thrombin, but only antithrombin for inhibition of factor X. *Unfractionated* heparin has a large variability of action with dose due to protein binding and inactivation, and causes thrombocytopenia in some patients. **Low molecular weight heparins** (LMWHs; e.g. *enoxaparin*) have largely replaced unfractionated heparin in clinical use, as they exhibit little protein binding or inactivation and so have a longer half-life and predictable dose responses; thrombocytopenia is rare. They are given subcutaneously. LMWHs only bind to antithrombin, and are therefore more effective at inhibiting factor X. They may also have *antithrombin-independent* effects on **tenase** (see Chapter 7). **Fondaparinux** is a synthetic pentasaccharide that inhibits factor Xa in a similar fashion to heparin. It has proved more effective than LMWHs in suppressing VTE and DVT, and could supplant LMWHs for routine thromboprophylaxis.

Warfarin (coumarin) is the most important oral anticoagulant. It inhibits vitamin K reductase, and thus γ-carboxylation of prothrombin and factors VII, IX and X in the liver; this prevents tethering to phospholipids and hence activity (see Chapter 7). Warfarin is only effective *in vivo*. Although slow in onset (~1–2 days), it provides effective support for ~5 days. Numerous factors including disease and drugs affect the sensitivity to warfarin, and the **prothrombin time** is routinely used to monitor dosage (see Chapter 7); this is normally adjusted to give an **INR** of ~3.

Thrombolytics

Thrombolysis is dissolution of the blood clot, and is used in life-threatening coronary artery disease to allows reperfusion of the infarct zone, limiting infarct size and reducing mortality. The greatest benefits occur when it is instituted within 3 h, although short-term mortality is reduced up to 12 h. The risk of gut and intracerebral haemorrhage (stroke) outweighs the benefits of thrombolysis in venous thrombosis, except in life-threatening pulmonary embolism. Thrombolytic agents induce **fibrinolysis** by converting **plasminogen** to the fibrinolytic enzyme **plasmin**; **tissue plasminogen activator (tPA)** is the most important endogenous agent (see Chapter 7). Thrombolysis is gradually being replaced by **angioplasty** in acute MI.

Streptokinase (SK), a *Streptococcus* bacterial protein, is inactive until bound to plasminogen, when it cleaves other plasminogen molecules to produce plasmin. SK has a plasma clearance time of 15–25 min. Unlike tPA, it does not require plasminogen to be bound to fibrin, and so can cause haemorrhage. SK induces antibodies that block its action and may cause severe allergic reactions on second application. **Anistreplase** (APSAC) is a complex of plasminogen and SK rendered inactive by addition of an anisoyl group; the latter is removed slowly in plasma, allowing activation. APSAC has a long plasma clearance time of 50–90 min, but is also allergenic. Aspirin in combination with SK has a *synergistic benefit* on reducing mortality. Recombinant tPA (*alteplase*) binds to fibrin, so has a greater effect on clot-associated plasminogen; it is not antigenic. tPA is cleared from plasma within 4–8 min, and must therefore be given by intravenous infusion; **reteplase**, another recombinant tPA, has a longer clearance time and can be given as a bolus.

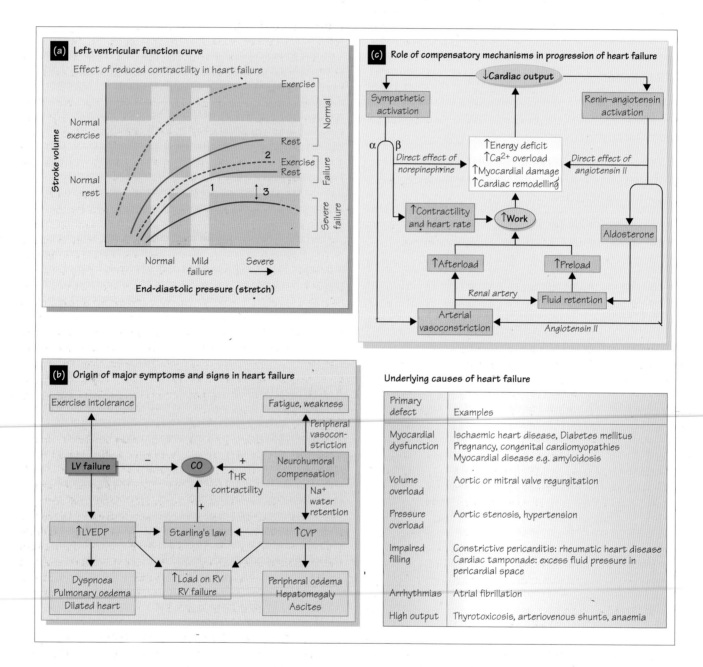

(a) Left ventricular function curve

Effect of reduced contractility in heart failure

(b) Origin of major symptoms and signs in heart failure

(c) Role of compensatory mechanisms in progression of heart failure

Underlying causes of heart failure

Primary defect	Examples
Myocardial dysfunction	Ischaemic heart disease, Diabetes mellitus Pregnancy, congenital cardiomyopathies Myocardial disease e.g. amyloidosis
Volume overload	Aortic or mitral valve regurgitation
Pressure overload	Aortic stenosis, hypertension
Impaired filling	Constrictive pericarditis: rheumatic heart disease Cardiac tamponade: excess fluid pressure in pericardial space
Arrhythmias	Atrial fibrillation
High output	Thyrotoxicosis, arteriovenous shunts, anaemia

In **heart failure**, cardiac output is insufficient to meet the needs of the body, or can do so only with an elevated filling pressure (**preload**). Compensatory mechanisms may be able to maintain cardiac output at rest, but may not be sufficient during exercise. Cardiac function eventually declines, and heart failure becomes severe (**decompensated**). This can be precipitated by other acute diseases, stress and drugs. Nonsteroidal anti-inflammatory drugs (NSAIDs) should be avoided, as they both precipitate and aggravate heart failure through multiple actions. Heart failure is predominantly a disease of old age. It occurs in ~2% of patients under 50, but in more than 10% of patients over 65. Survival is < 50% over 5 years. **Ischaemic heart disease** and **hypertension** are major risk factors. Other causes are shown in the table.

Clinical manifestations

Patients generally present with **dyspnoea** (breathlessness), although initially only during exercise, also weakness, fatigue and **peripheral oedema** (fluid retention in tissues; see Chapter 19), most commonly seen as swollen legs. The heart and liver are enlarged, and a high CVP distends the jugular veins. A **gallop rhythm** may be heard due to high cardiac filling pressure (see Chapter 14). Cardiac output and BP may be normal at rest in moderate heart failure.

Pathophysiology

About 70% of cases are due to **systolic failure**, with impaired ventricular function and an **ejection fraction** (see Chapter 14) of < 50%. Myocardial **contractility** (see Chapter 15) is reduced, and the ventricular function curve is depressed (Figure 46a). In **diastolic failure** ventricular filling is impaired, generally because the ventricular wall is stiff due to fibrosis or hypertrophy (see below and Chapter 15). Contractility may be normal or even increased, and ejection fraction > 50%. Systolic and diastolic failure often coexist. Clinical manifestations are similar because in both output can only be obtained at rest with increased end-diastolic pressure (EDP) (**1** in Figure 46a). In exercise the function curve may never reach the required output (**2**); the increase in contractility is small because sympathetic tone is already high (see below). In severe, decompensated failure, normal resting output cannot be obtained even with substantial increases in EDP (**3**).

Left heart failure Ischaemic heart disease most commonly affects the left ventricle. Decreased output leads to increased left ventricular EDP (preload) and pulmonary venous pressure as blood 'backs up' in the pulmonary circulation (**pulmonary congestion**; Figure 46b). This causes the heart to **dilate**, and the increased pulmonary capillary pressure promotes fluid accumulation in the lung interstitium (see Chapter 19). The increased blood and fluid in the lungs makes them stiff, causing **dyspnoea**. Dyspnoea may only occur when the patient lies down (**orthopnoea**) as fluid redistributes to the lungs. Episodic dyspnoea causing waking at night is called **paroxysmal nocturnal dyspnoea**. When severe, the elevated capillary pressure may force fluid into the alveoli (**pulmonary oedema**), a life-threatening condition causing extreme dyspnoea, reduced gas exchange and hypoxaemia.

Right heart failure Left heart failure increases pulmonary vascular pressure, and can lead to pressure overload and failure of the right heart, a situation called **congestive heart failure** (Figure 46b). Right heart failure alone is associated with chronic lung disease (**cor pulmonale**), pulmonary hypertension or embolism, and valve disease. CVP is greatly increased in right heart failure, seen as **distension of the jugular veins**, and leads to fluid accumulation in peripheral tissues (**peripheral oedema**), peritoneum (**ascites**) and liver, causing tenderness and enlargement (**hepatomegaly**). Ambulatory patients may show **pitting oedema** in the legs (a depression is left following compression with a finger), which is relieved on lying down.

Compensatory mechanisms

Adaptive mechanisms initially compensate for reduced function, but are often deleterious when sustained. They all increase cardiac work and thus oxygen requirement, which is clearly detrimental in ischaemic heart disease.

Starling's law Reduced output and ejection fraction increase preload (see above). Cardiac force therefore increases due to **Starling's law**, partially restoring output (Figure 46a,b; see Chapter 15), but at the expense of an increased filling pressure (EDP).

Neurohumoral system Reduced blood pressure initiates the **baroreceptor reflex**, and stimulates the sympathetic nervous system (Figure 46c; see Chapter 26). This increases heart rate and contractility, and improves cardiac output (see Chapters 11, 15). Venoconstriction increases CVP, and systemic vasoconstriction increases total peripheral resistance (TPR) which helps maintain BP. Afterload is, however, increased, and the redistribution of output from the skeletal muscle and splanchnic circulations leads to muscle weakness and fatigue, and impaired renal function. Vasoconstriction of renal arteries (Figure 46c) reduces filtration and urine production (**oliguria**), and causes the release of **renin**, which activates **angiotensin I**. This is converted to **angiotensin II**, a powerful vasoconstrictor that also potentiates sympathetic activity and stimulates the adrenal glands to produce **aldosterone**. Aldosterone augments Na^+ and hence water reabsorption, thus increasing blood volume and CVP. Sympathetic stimulation also increases **vasopressin** (ADH), leading to further water retention. Sympathetic-mediated effects may be limited in late disease because β-adrenoceptor density falls, and norepinephrine sensitivity decreases.

Myocardial hypertrophy A sustained increase in afterload (hypertension, aortic stenosis) causes the ventricular wall to thicken as the muscle cells grow larger (**myocardial hypertrophy**). It is not usually associated with ischaemic heart disease. Although hypertrophy improves force, the thicker ventricle is less **compliant** (flexible) and EDP must rise further for adequate filling; this can lead to diastolic failure (see above). Hypertrophy also reduces **capillary density**, increasing diffusion distance and reducing **coronary reserve** (difference between maximum and resting coronary flow). Perfusion is therefore reduced in exercise. Changes in contractile protein isoforms (myosin, tropomyosin) also decrease contraction velocity and contractility. Gross hypertrophy may physically impair valve operation.

Exacerbation of cardiac dysfunction

An important component of the transition to full heart failure is a gradual reduction in myocardial function as a direct result of the compensatory mechanisms (Figure 46c). Factors increasing work contribute to any **energy deficit**, and sustained stimulation by norepinephrine and angiotensin II promotes cellular Ca^{2+} **overload**. This causes further cell damage and necrosis, and fosters generation of arrhythmias.

Cardiac dilatation during failure reduces the heart's *efficiency* to develop ventricular pressure because of the **law of Laplace**, which states that pressure in a sphere is proportional to wall tension divided by radius. Large, dilated hearts therefore have to contract harder in order to develop the same pressure as smaller hearts. This becomes a major problem in the grossly dilated, failing heart.

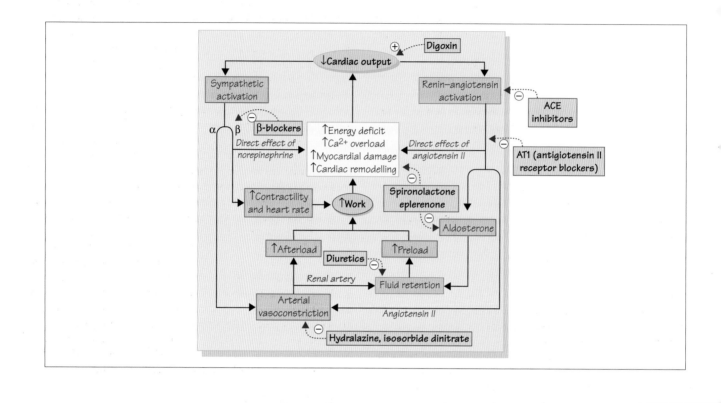

Therapy of chronic heart failure (CHF) is designed to: (i) improve the quality of life by reducing symptoms; (ii) lengthen survival; and (iii) slow the progression of cardiac deterioration. CHF typically has an underlying cause such as ischaemic heart disease, and may be exacerbated by specific **precipitating factors** such as infection or arrhythmias, as well as by myocardial abnormalities which develop as CHF progresses (e.g. valvular dysfunction). As well as the symptoms of CHF *per se*, both underlying and precipitating factors should, if possible, be treated. Restricting activity and reducing dietary sodium help to lessen cardiac workload and fluid retention.

The **sympathetic** and **renin–angiotensin–aldosterone** systems activated in response to reduced pump function initially help to maintain cardiac output, but also drive the progression of cardiac deterioration (see figure; see also Chapter 46). Therapy increasingly involves inhibiting these systems. It is currently recommended that treatment of CHF is initiated with **angiotensin-converting enzyme inhibitors (ACEI)**, which slow CHF progression, lengthen survival time and improve haemodynamic parameters. **Angiotensin receptor blockers (ARBs)** are used as an alternative in patients who cannot tolerate ACEI. A **diuretic** can also be used to control fluid accumulation. Once the patient has stabilized on this treatment, a **β-blocker** can be added in gradually increasing doses. **Digoxin** may be used to support cardiac function and reduce symptoms.

In severe or refractory CHF, or when existing therapy fails to control symptoms adequately, the aldosterone antagonist **spironolactone** can be used, as can vasodilators such as **hydralazine** and **isosorbide dinitrate**. Positive inotropes such as **dobutamine**, **dopamine** or **milrinone** may be used temporarily if decompensation occurs.

ACEI and other vasodilators

As described in Chapter 27, angiotension II causes vasoconstriction and promotes fluid retention via multiple mechanisms. ACEI, which inhibit the conversion of angiotensin I to angiotensin II, therefore dilate arteries and veins, and reduce blood volume and oedema. Arterial vasodilatation decreases afterload and cardiac work, and improves tissue perfusion by increasing stroke volume and cardiac output. Venous dilatation and reduction of fluid retention diminish pulmonary congestion, oedema and central venous pressure (CVP) (preload). Reduction of preload lowers ventricular filling pressure, therefore lowering cardiac wall stress, workload and ischaemia. ACEI also delay abnormal cardiac hypertrophy and fibrosis, which are thought to be promoted by angiotensin II.

Angiotensin (AT1) receptor blockers such as **losartan** are used in patients unable to tolerate the cough or renal dysfunction occasionally caused by ACEI. The combination of the nitrovasodilator isosorbide dinitrate (see Chapter 41) and hydralazine can also prolong survival, although not as effectively as ACEI. Hydralazine causes mainly arterial vasodilatation, possibly via inhibition of Ca^{2+} release from the sarcoplasmic reticulum.

Beta-receptor blockers

The 1993 MDC study reported that the β_1-selective antagonist **metoprolol** reduced mortality when added to conventional therapy for mild to moderate CHF. The benefits of adding metoprolol to standard therapy (ACEI and diuretics) were confirmed in the 1999 MERIT-HF study, which showed that this drug reduced 1-year mortality by 34% in patients with mild to severe CHF. **Bisoprolol**, another

β_1-selective antagonist, was shown by the 1999 CIBIS-II trial to similarly diminish mortality. **Carvedilol** is a non-selective β-blocker which has additional α-antagonist and antioxidant properties, and has also been shown to prolong survival in CHF. The 2003 COMET trial showed that when given to patients being treated with ACEI and diuretics, carvedilol extended survival to a greater extent than did metoprolol.

Long-term treatment with β-blockers has been shown to increase ejection fraction, reduce systolic and diastolic volume, and eventually cause regression of left ventricular hypertrophy. Other beneficial effects of β-blockers in CHF probably include reduced ischaemia and a reduction in heart rate, thus improving myocardial perfusion, and inhibition of the deleterious effects of excess catecholamines on myocardial structure and metabolism. Beta-blockers appear to be particularly effective in reducing sudden death in those with CHF, suggesting that the prevention of *ventricular fibrillation* (see Chapter 51) constitutes an important part of their action.

The negative inotropic effect of β-blockers is potentially hazardous in some patients with CHF, since cardiac function is already compromised. Therapy is therefore initiated with low doses which are carefully elevated over several weeks or months.

Diuretics

Diuretics reduce fluid accumulation by increasing renal salt and water excretion. Preload, pulmonary congestion and systemic oedema are thereby relieved. **Loop diuretics** inhibit the Na^+-K^+-$2Cl^-$ symport in the thick ascending loop of Henle. Na^+ and Cl^- reabsorption is thereby inhibited, and the retention of these ions in the tubule promotes fluid loss in the urine. Diuretics are commonly used in CHF, and include **furosemide, bumetanide, torasemide** and **ethacrynic acid**. Thiazide and thiazide-related diuretics (see Chapter 37) are also used to treat heart failure.

Both loop and thiazide diuretics can cause hypokalaemia and metabolic alkalosis because the increased Na^+ retained in the tubular fluid is partly exchanged for K^+ and H^+ in the distal nephron. This process is stimulated by aldosterone (see Chapter 27), and diuretic-induced hypokalaemia can be controlled by an ACEI or **spironolactone**, an aldosterone antagonist. Hypokalaemia can also be treated with K^+ supplements, or the use of **K$^+$-sparing diuretics** such as **amiloride** or **triamterene**. These inhibit Na^+ reabsorption in the collecting duct. Long-term use of loop diuretics can result in hypovolaemia, reduced plasma Mg^{2+}, Ca^{2+} and Na^+, and hyperuricaemia and hyperglycaemia. This is more common in the elderly, who may require high doses of diuretics to overcome **diuretic resistance**.

Cardiac glycosides

Cardiac glycosides include ouabain, digitoxin and **digoxin**, which is used most widely. Digoxin improves CHF symptoms, but does not prolong life. Cardiac glycosides inhibit the Na^+ pump in cardiac muscle, thereby indirectly inhibiting the Na^+-Ca^{2+} antiport and thus increasing intracellular Ca^{2+} (see Chapter 11). The rise in Ca^{2+} enhances contractility and shortens action potential duration and refractory period in atrial and ventricular cells by stimulating K^+ channels. Digoxin has been shown to increase baroreceptor responsiveness, thereby reducing sympathetic tone.

Digoxin also acts on the nervous system to increase vagal tone. This slows both sinoatrial node activity and atrioventricular node (AVN) conduction, and can be useful in treating atrial arrhythmias (see Chapter 51). It is therefore mainly used in patients with both CHF and atrial fibrillation.

Even a small (two- to threefold) excess of digoxin over the optimal therapeutic concentration can cause arrhythmias. This occurs because an excessive rise in $[Ca^{2+}]_i$ causes oscillations in membrane potential after action potentials. These **delayed afterdepolarizations** can trigger ectopic beats (see Chapter 48), and at higher doses can trigger ventricular tachycardia. Inhibition of the Na^+ pump also decreases intracellular K^+, causing depolarization and facilitating arrhythmias. In addition, excess digoxin can increase vagal tone enough to block conduction at the AVN, and can also raise sympathetic tone, again favouring arrhythmias. Digoxin toxicity is enhanced by **hypokalaemia** (low plasma K^+), because K^+ decreases the affinity of digoxin for the Na^+ pump. Digoxin also causes toxic gastrointestinal effects, including anorexia, nausea and vomiting. Acute toxicity can be treated with intravenous K^+, antiarrhythmics (e.g. lidocaine) and digoxin-specific antibodies.

Spironolactone

Aldosterone levels initially fall during ACEI treatment, but often rise again ('escape') during prolonged treatment. Aldosterone has a number of effects that worsen CHF and its consequences; these include inducing cardiac fibrosis and remodelling, reducing nitric oxide release, and promoting arrhythmias by decreasing plasma K^+ and cardiac norepinephrine release.

The aldosterone antagonist **spironolactone** was shown in the 1999 RALES trial to reduce mortality when added to ACEI in severe CHF. Its use is now recommended in patients with more severe heart failure and good renal function. As it can cause hyperkalaemia, careful monitoring of plasma K^+ levels is important. Spironolactone also causes antiandrogenic side effects such as gynaecomastia, and the more selective aldosterone antagonist **eplerenone** has recently been introduced as an alternative.

Mechanisms of arrhythmia

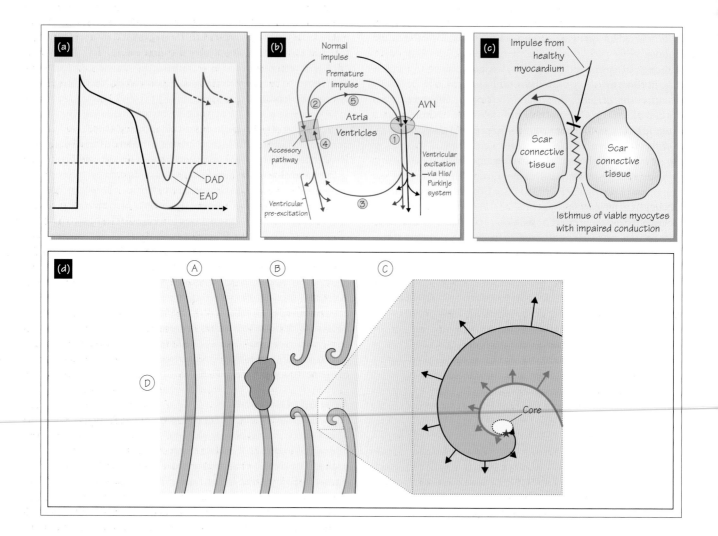

Arrhythmias are abnormalities of the heart rate or rhythm caused by disorders of impulse generation or conduction.

Disorders of impulse conduction: abnormal automaticity

All parts of the cardiac conduction system demonstrate a spontaneous phase 4 depolarization (**automaticity**), and are therefore potential or *latent pacemakers*. Because sinoatrial node (SAN) pacemaking is of the highest frequency (70–80 beats/min), it causes *overdrive suppression* of pacemaking by the atrioventricular node (AVN) (50–60 beats/min) or Purkinje fibres (30–40 beats/min). However, ischaemia, hypokalaemia, fibre stretch or local catecholamine release may increase automaticity in latent pacemakers, which can then 'escape' from SAN dominance to cause arrhythmias.

Cardiac muscle cells are not normally latent pacemakers. However, even these cells can develop repetitive impulse initiation and cause arrhythmias if the membrane potential is sufficiently depolarized. This can result, for example, from ischaemia or high local catecholamine concentrations.

Disorders of impulse conduction: triggered automaticity

Triggered automaticity is caused by **afterdepolarizations**. These are oscillations in the membrane potential that occur during or after repolarization. Oscillations large enough to reach threshold initiate premature action potentials and thus heart beats (Figure 48a). This may occur repeatedly, initiating a sustained arrhythmia either directly or by triggering re-entry (see below). Afterdepolarization magnitude is influenced by changes in heart rate, catecholamines and parasympathetic withdrawal.

Early afterdepolarizations (EADs) occur during the terminal plateau or repolarization phases of the action potential. They develop more readily in Purkinje fibres than in ventricular or atrial myocytes. EADs can be induced by agents that prolong action potential duration and increase the inward current. For example, drugs such as sotalol and *N*-acetyl procainamide (a procainamide metabolite) block K^+ currents, and can cause EADs and triggered activity by delaying repolarization, especially when the heart rate is slow. The abnormal rhythms induced by such drugs resemble **torsade de pointes**, a type of congenital arrhythmia.

Delayed afterdepolarizations (DADs) occur after repolarization is complete, and are due to excessive increases in cellular $[Ca^{2+}]$. This can be caused by catecholamines, which increase Ca^{2+} influx through the L-type Ca^{2+} channel, by digitalis glycosides, which increase $[Ca^{2+}]_i$ (see Chapter 47), and by heart failure, in which myocyte Ca^{2+} regulation is impaired. The **transient inward current** responsible for the oscillation of membrane potential following an increase in $[Ca^{2+}]_i$ appears to involve Na^+ influx. The occurrence and magnitude of DADs and the likelihood that they will cause arrhythmias is increased by conditions that enhance the transient inward current. These include longer action potentials, which cause larger increases in $[Ca^{2+}]_i$. Therefore, drugs prolonging action potential duration may trigger DADs, whereas drugs shortening the action potential have the opposite effect. The magnitude of the transient inward current is also influenced by the resting membrane potential, and is maximal when this is approximately -60 mV.

Abnormal impulse conduction: re-entry

Re-entry occurs when an impulse that is delayed in one region of the myocardium re-excites adjacent areas of the myocardium more than once. One type of re-entry, termed **anatomical**, requires the presence of three conditions.

1 There must exist an anatomical circuit around which the impulse can circulate (a process often termed **circus movement**). This circuit can utilize parallel conduction pathways such as two Purkinje fibre branches, or the AVN and an accessory atrioventricular conduction pathway.

2 Impulse conduction at some point in the circuit should be slow enough to allow the region in front of the impulse to recover from refractoriness. This region is termed the *excitable gap*.

3 The circuit must also include a zone of unidirectional block where conduction is blocked in one direction while remaining possible in the other.

Wolff–Parkinson–White (WPW) syndrome is an uncommon arrhythmia (population incidence 0.1–0.2%) which involves anatomical re-entry (see Chapter 49). In this condition, there is a congenital accessory (extra) conduction pathway (formerly termed the **bundle of Kent**) between an atrium and ventricle, which is often situated on the left free wall of the heart. Thus, as shown in Figure (b), normal atrial depolarization (**black arrows**) is conducted to the ventricles through both the AVN and the accessory pathway (**blue arrows**). The accessory pathway has properties differing from that of the AVN. First, it *conducts more rapidly* than the AVN, so the part of the ventricle to which the pathway connects depolarizes before the rest (**pre-excitation**), resulting in a widened QRS complex. Secondly, the accessory pathway has a *longer refractory period* than the AVN. Thus, if a premature impulse arises in an atrium (**red arrows**), it may be conducted normally to the ventricles via the AVN (**1** in figure), but may not be conducted

forwards through the accessory pathway, which is still refractory from the previous impulse (**2**). However, when the impulse through the AVN is distributed to the ventricles (**3**), it will encounter the distal end of the accessory pathway (**4**) which has now had time to recover its excitability, and will be conducted backwards through this pathway into the atrium (**5**). It can then traverse the AVN again and continue to cycle though the anatomical circuit encompassing the AVN, His–Purkinje system, ventricles, accessory pathway and atrium (**1–3–4–5**). The ventricles are excited with each circuit, which causes a tachycardia because the impulse cycles more quickly than the SAN spontaneously depolarizes.

It is noteworthy that the 'border zone' between healthy myocardium and the scar resulting from the healing of a myocardial infarct (see Chapter 43) typically contains a mixture of living muscle cells and connective tissue. In some cases, a narrow band ('isthmus') of still-viable muscle cells spans an area of non-conducting scar, thereby connecting two regions of healthy myocardium (Figure 48c). Conduction of the impulse by the isthmus may be slowed or even demonstrate effective unidirectional block because this tissue takes so long to recover its excitability between action potentials. This arrangement provides conditions analogous to those that underlie anatomical re-entry, and is thought to cause many ventricular arrhythmias arising in patients following myocardial infarct healing.

Functional re-entry does not require an anatomically defined circuit, and tends to arise when cardiac conduction is impaired, usually as result of ongoing ischaemia or damage from a previous myocardial infarction. Current theories propose that under these conditions, the wave of depolarization (Figure 48d, **A**) originating at the SAN may encounter a scar or non-conducting zone which causes the wave to break up (**B**). In this case, the 'broken' ends of the wave, rather than rejoining and continuing to sweep forward though the myocardium, can curl in on themselves to form spirals (**C**). At the very tip of such spiral waves the leading edge of the action potential (black line and arrows; represents the action potential upstroke) and the trailing edge of the action potential (green line and arrows; represents the end of the refractory period) meet at a 'critical point' (see red star in inset panel). Mathematical models of myocardial conduction indicate that a small zone of myocardium that cannot be excited forms just in front of the critical point, and forms a pivot point (or *core*) around which the spiral continues to rotate. As it does so, it emits waves of depolarization, with a frequency determined by the rotation period of the spiral; these excite the heart and cause tachycardia. The formation of such rotating impulses, or *rotors*, and the further fragmentation of the waves of depolarization they generate, is now thought to underlie the genesis of the chaotic electrical activity which results in the total loss of atrial or ventricular coordinated contraction termed **fibrillation**.

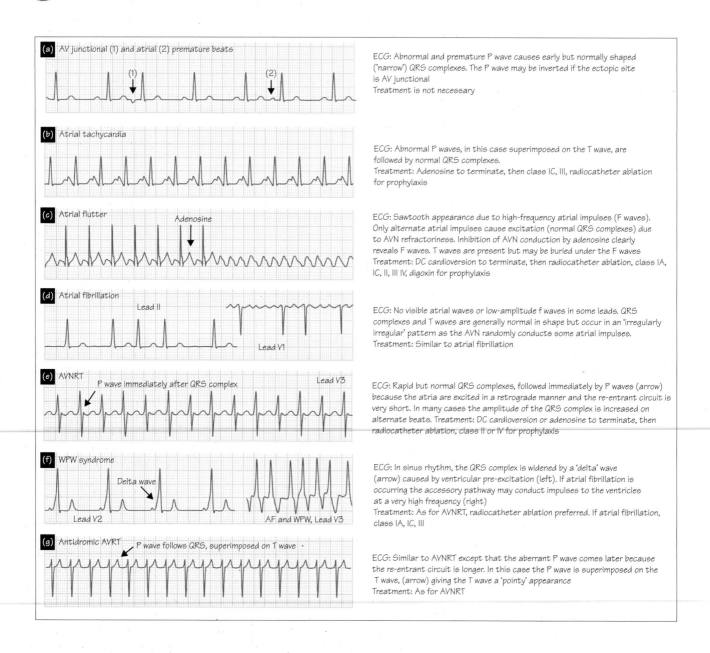

(a) AV junctional (1) and atrial (2) premature beats

ECG: Abnormal and premature P wave causes early but normally shaped ('narrow') QRS complexes. The P wave may be inverted if the ectopic site is AV junctional
Treatment is not necessary

(b) Atrial tachycardia

ECG: Abnormal P waves, in this case superimposed on the T wave, are followed by normal QRS complexes.
Treatment: Adenosine to terminate, then class IC, III, radiocatheter ablation for prophylaxis

(c) Atrial flutter — Adenosine

ECG: Sawtooth appearance due to high-frequency atrial impulses (F waves). Only alternate atrial impulses cause excitation (normal QRS complexes) due to AVN refractoriness. Inhibition of AVN conduction by adenosine clearly reveals F waves. T waves are present but may be buried under the F waves
Treatment: DC cardioversion to terminate, then radiocatheter ablation, class IA, IC, II, III IV, digoxin for prophylaxis

(d) Atrial fibrillation — Lead II — Lead V1

ECG: No visible atrial waves or low-amplitude f waves in some leads. QRS complexes and T waves are generally normal in shape but occur in an 'irregularly irregular' pattern as the AVN randomly conducts some atrial impulses.
Treatment: Similar to atrial fibrillation

(e) AVNRT — P wave immediately after QRS complex — Lead V3

ECG: Rapid but normal QRS complexes, followed immediately by P waves (arrow) because the atria are excited in a retrograde manner and the re-entrant circuit is very short. In many cases the amplitude of the QRS complex is increased on alternate beats. Treatment: DC cardioversion or adenosine to terminate, then radiocatheter ablation, class II or IV for prophylaxis

(f) WPW syndrome — Delta wave — Lead V2 — AF and WPW, Lead V3

ECG: In sinus rhythm, the QRS complex is widened by a 'delta' wave (arrow) caused by ventricular pre-excitation (left). If atrial fibrillation is occurring the accessory pathway may conduct impulses to the ventricles at a very high frequency (right)
Treatment: As for AVNRT, radiocatheter ablation preferred. If atrial fibrillation, class IA, IC, III

(g) Antidromic AVRT — P wave follows QRS, superimposed on T wave

ECG: Similar to AVNRT except that the aberrant P wave comes later because the re-entrant circuit is longer. In this case the P wave is superimposed on the T wave, (arrow) giving the T wave a 'pointy' appearance
Treatment: As for AVNRT

Tachyarrhythmias (tachycardias) and **bradyarrhythmias** (bradycardias) are abnormalities in the origin, timing or sequence of cardiac depolarization which result in a heart rate of > 100 and < 60 beats/min, respectively. The former are much more common and may be **supraventricular**, in which case they arise in either the atria or the AV node (AVN), or are **ventricular** in origin (see Chapter 50). Important bradyarrhythmias are described in Chapter 12. Where appropriate, ECG leads that best illustrate the abnormalities associated with each arrhythmia are shown in this and Chapter 50.

Most **supraventricular tachycardias (SVTs)** are troublesome rather than life-threatening, although rarely sudden death can occur. Common symptoms include lightheadedness, palpitations and shortness of breath.

Supraventricular premature beats (Figure 49a) are caused by **ectopic** (originating from a site other than the SAN) impulses arising in the atria or AVN earlier in the cardiac cycle than would be expected from the normal heart rate. They are typically conducted to the ventricles to cause a premature beat, which is generally followed by a pause as the normal rhythm is reasserted. With an atrial ectopic site the P wave is abnormally shaped because it is not generated in the SAN, and it may be inverted or missing entirely if the ectopic site is in or near the AVN.

Atrial tachycardia heart rate (120–240 beats/min) is frequently caused by an ectopic pacemaker, and can arise in either atrium (e.g. often close to the pulmonary veins in the left atrium). Other atrial tachycardias are re-entrant in nature, frequently following surgery that involves incision into the atrium. The tachycardia may start and stop suddenly or gradually. As with atrial ectopics, the P wave is abnormally shaped (Figure 49b).

Atrial flutter results from re-entry in an atrium (usually the right), often with an area of slowed conduction near the orifice of the inferior vena cava and a circuit involving the whole atrium. The atrial rate is typically ~300 beats/min. However, as shown in Figure 49(c), the AVN is often able to conduct only every other atrial impulse (2:1 AV block) to the ventricles because it is still refractory from the previous impulse, so that the ventricular rate is typically ~150 beats/min. Less commonly, 3:1 or 4:1 block can occur, leading to correspondingly slower rates of ventricular contraction. The ECG has a 'sawtooth' appearance due to presence of rapid regular *F waves* representing atrial depolarization; these become more obvious if AVN conduction and the QRS complex are suppressed by e.g. adenosine (Figure 49c, right). Both atrial flutter and atrial fibrillation (see below) are typically seen in patients with underlying cardiac disease, often associated with atrial dilatation. These conditions are particularly common in older hypertensives, and may also be caused by acute pulmonary thromboembolism or thyrotoxicosis, but can also develop paroxysmally in patients without underlying heart disease. Attempts to **cardiovert** (restore normal sinus rhythm) atrial flutter with class IA drugs may cause severe ventricular tachycardia and sudden death by establishing 1:1 AVN conduction. This occurs because these drugs suppress vagal firing, thereby increasing AVN conduction. This hazard is avoided by preadministering a drug that suppresses AVN conduction (e.g. a β-blocker).

Atrial fibrillation (AF) is a chaotic atrial rhythm resulting in an atrial rate of 350–600 beats/min and a lack of effective atrial contraction. AF is the most common arrhythmia, occurring in ~10% of people over the age of 75. The ventricular rate is described by clinicians as 'irregularly irregular' and is typically less than 200 beats/min because the AVN is unable to conduct most of the atrial impulses impinging upon it (Figure 49d). Studies suggest that this arrhythmia is caused by five to seven unstable re-entrant circuits with very short cycle lengths, which progress across the atrium, temporarily disappearing and then reforming. Palpitations, dyspnoea, dizziness or *syncope* (sudden fainting) may occur due to the increased ventricular rate or the absence of atrial systolic filling. Thrombi may form in the left atrial cavity or appendage because the lack of coordinated atrial contraction leads to stasis of blood. These can then embolize to the systemic circulation, particularly the brain and limbs. For this reason, AF is the most important cause of stroke in the elderly.

AF can occur episodically, or can be permanent, in which case it is more difficult to control. Pharmacological treatment involves restoring normal sinus rhythm, often with amiodarone ('rhythm control'). Alternatively, a class IV or other agent is used to suppress AV conduction, thereby reducing the frequency of impulses which reach and excite the ventricles ('rate control') even though the atria continue to fibrillate.

Atrioventricular nodal re-entrant tachycardia (AVNRT) and **atrioventricular re-entrant tachycardia (AVRT)** result in periodic episodes during which the heart rate abruptly increases to 150–250 beats/min, and they are therefore referred to as **paroxysmal supraventricular tachycardias**. Individuals with AVNRT have an additional or **accessory** conduction pathway between the atrium and the AVN. In most cases, the normal AV pathway (termed α) conducts rapidly and has a long refractory period, while the accessory (β) pathway conducts slowly and has a short refractory period. In these individuals, AVNRT can be initiated by a premature impulse arising in an atrium. This impulse will not be conducted by the α pathway if it is still refractory from the preceding impulse. However, the impulse may travel slowly down the β pathway (which has recovered from the preceding impulse), and then encounter the distal end of the α pathway. Sufficient time has now elapsed for this pathway to be no longer refractory, and the impulse is able to ascend the α pathway in a *retrograde* (backwards) direction, allowing it to return to the atrium. From here it can continue to cycle through the α and β pathways, exciting the ventricles to cause a heart beat with each circuit. An abnormal P wave is also generated each time the impulse cycles through the atrium. This immediately follows the QRS complex because the re-entrant circuit, and thus the cycle time, is very short (Figure 49e).

An accessory pathway allowing impulse conduction between an atrium and ventricle also exists in AVRT, but in this case it is not located within the AVN. Those in whom this pathway can conduct impulses in both directions may suffer from **Wolff–Parkinson–White (WPW)** or **pre-excitation syndrome,** the mechanism of which is described in Chapter 48. When the individual is in normal sinus rhythm, the atrial impulse is conducted in an *anterograde* (forward) direction through both the accessory pathway and the AVN. Since it is conducted more quickly through the accessory pathway, excitation of part of one ventricle occurs more quickly than normal (i.e. pre-excitation occurs), resulting in a shortened PR interval and an initial widening of the QRS complex referred to as a *delta wave* (Figure 49f, left). During the tachycardia, however, the accessory pathway conducts in the *retrograde* direction (see Chapter 48) and so pre-excitation does not occur. Instead, premature P waves (often superimposed on the T wave) caused by rapid excitation of the atria by the retrograde impulse are observed. This type of accessory pathway is particularly dangerous in people with atrial fibrillation, because the it is often better at conducting rapid impulses than the AVN due to its shorter refractory period. Thus, the AVN 'filter' which protects the ventricles from high-frequency atrial activity is bypassed, and the ventricular rate becomes very fast. In this case, the ECG shows rapid and irregular QRS complexes, the majority of which are widened by pre-excitation (Figure 49f, right).

Less common forms of AVRT also exist. In *antidromic* AVRT, the accessory pathway conducts in an anterograde direction during the tachycardia (Figure 49g). In other cases, the accessory pathway is capable of conducting only in the retrograde direction. Thus, pre-excitation does not occur, and the bypass pathway is said to be *concealed*.

50 Ventricular tachyarrhythmias and non-pharmacological treatment of arrhythmias

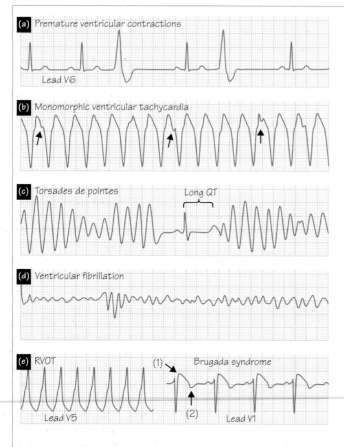

(a) Premature ventricular contractions

Lead V6

ECG: QRS complexes (3rd and 5th) occur prematurely compared with the normal rhythm and are broad and bizarrely shaped.
Treatment: Not necessary, although in cardiac disease VPCs may be harbingers of more serious arrhythmias requiring treatment

(b) Monomorphic ventricular tachycardia

ECG: Wide bizarre QRS complexes of similar shape occur with high frequency. In this case, P waves can be seen (arrows) superimposed on the ventricular complexes, indicative of continuing SA nodal activity
Treatment: Terminate with DC cardioversion or class 1A, 1C, then Class II or III for prophylasis.

(c) Torsades de pointes   Long QT

ECG: A type of polymorphic VT characterized by an abnormally long QT interval apparent during sinus rhythm. Can be congenital or caused by many drugs or other conditions that delay AP repolarization.
Treatment: Remove precipitating factor if possible, if congenital, use β-blockers and an implantable defibrillator.

(d) Ventricular fibrillation

ECG: Chaotic ventricular rhythm characterized by irregular wavelets of electrical activity and no coordinated contraction
Treatment: Immediate DC cardioversion, followed by class II, II and implantable defibrillator in high risk patients

(e) RVOT   (1)   Brugada syndrome

Lead V5   (2)   Lead V1

ECG: For RVOT, the pattern resembles that caused by left bundle branch block (see Chapter 15) because left ventricular depolarization is slowed since the impulse reaches it from the right ventricle rather than via the normal conduction pathway. For Brugada syndrome, the ST segment is elevated (1) and T wave is negative (2).
Treatment: For AVOT, adenosine to terminate, class II, IV. For Brugada, implantable defibrillator in high-risk patients

---

Tachyarrhythmias originating in the ventricles are most often associated with ischaemic heart disease. They are common during and up to 24 h after acute MI, when increases in sympathetic activity and extracellular [K$^+$] as well as slowed conduction favour their initiation. Such *peri-infarction* arrhythmias may be immediately life-threatening, and indeed the vast majority of deaths associated with MI are due to ventricular **fibrillation** occurring before the individual reaches the hospital. If survived, these arrhythmias generally do not recur and are not associated with a subsequent increased risk over and above that conferred by the MI itself. Subsequently, however, the border zone of the healed infarct scar may serve as a substrate for the development of dangerous reentrant ventricular tachyarrhythmias which can recur or become incessant weeks to years after the MI. Their seriousness and prognostic significance are related to the extent of cardiac damage and impairment of ventricular function that has been sustained. These late arrhythmias themselves confer an additional risk of death, and must be treated either with drugs or with an **implantable defibrillator** (see below). Ventri-cular tachyarrhythmias can also be associated with cardiomyopathy, and valvular and congenital heart disease, and specific *idiopathic* varieties may occur in structurally normal hearts.

Specific ventricular tachyarrhythmias

Premature ventricular contractions (PVCs) are caused by a ventricular ectopic focus and may occur randomly or following every (*bigeminy*, see Figure 50a) or every second (*trigeminy*) normal beat. Because depolarization is initiated at a site within ventricular muscle, it spreads throughout the ventricles more slowly than normal impulses which are distributed rapidly by the specialized His–Purkinje conduction system. Thus, the QRS complex is broad and abnormally shaped. PVCs may be of no prognostic consequence, but can predispose to more serious arrhythmias if they develop during or after MI, and/or occur during the T wave of the preceding beat.

Ventricular tachycardia (VT) originates in the ventricles, and is defined as a run of successive ventricular ectopic beats occurring at a rate of > 100 beats/min (usually 120–200 beats/min). VT is classified as *non-sustained* or *sustained* based on whether it lasts for > 30 s. Depending on the heart rate, VT can cause symptoms such as syncope, angina and shortness of breath, and if sustained can compromise cardiac pumping, leading to heart failure and death. VT can also deteriorate into ventricular fibrillation (see below), particularly with a heart rate of > 200 beats/min.

The ECG in VT demonstrates high-frequency, bizarrely shaped QRS complexes which are abnormally broadened (> 120 ms in duration). Normal atrial activation may continue to be driven by the SAN (Figure 50b), or the abnormal ventricular pacemaker may cause atrial tachycardia via retrograde impulses traversing the AVN. The configuration of the QRS complex can be used to classify VT into two broad categories. In *monomorphic* VT (Figure 50b), the QRS complexes all have a similar configuration and the heart rate is generally constant, whereas in *polymorphic* VT both the QRS configuration and the heart rate vary continually. Monomorphic VT generally indicates the presence of a stable re-entrant pathway, the substrate for which is typically an MI-related scar (see Chapter 48). Polymorphic VT is thought to be caused by multiple ectopic foci or re-entry in which the circuit pathway is continually varying, and most often occurs during or soon after an MI.

Torsade de pointes ('twisting of the points') is a type of polymorphic VT in which episodes of tachycardia, which may give rise to fibrillation and sudden death, are superimposed upon intervals of bradycardia, during which the QT interval (indicative of the ventricular action potential duration) is prolonged (Figure 50c). During the tachycardia, the ECG has a distinctive appearance in which the amplitude of the QRS complexes alternately waxes and wanes. Torsade de pointes may be caused by drugs or conditions that delay ventricular repolarization (e.g. class IA and III antiarrhythmics, hypokalaemia, hypomagnesaemia). It is also associated with **congenital long QT (LQT) syndrome**, which can be caused by mutations in *KvLQT1* or *HERG*, genes coding for cardiac K^+ channels mediating repolarization, or *SCN5A*, the gene coding for the cardiac Na^+ channel. In congenital LQT syndrome, torsades de pointes is often triggered by sympathetic activity (e.g. caused by stress), which may give rise to early or delayed afterdepolarizations, and may also involve functional re-entry mediated by spiral waves of depolarization (see Chapter 48).

Ventricular fibrillation (VF) is a chaotic ventricular rhythm (Figure 50d) causing an immediate loss of cardiac output and death unless the patient is resuscitated. VF may follow episodes of VT or acute ischaemia, and frequently occurs during MI. It is the main cause of sudden death, which is responsible for ~10% of all mortality. VF is generally associated with severe underlying heart disease, including ischaemic heart disease and cardiomyopathy.

Right ventricular outflow tract tachycardia (RVOT) and **fascicular tachycardia** are two forms of VT that can occur in structurally normal hearts (i.e. idiopathically). RVOT (Figure 50e, left) is associated with increases in sympathetic activity, and is thought to be caused by delayed afterdepolarizations, whereas fascicular tachycardia may in some cases be caused by a re-entrant circuit involving the Purkinje system. These have a good prognosis, and can usually be successfully eliminated with radiofrequency catheter ablation. Occasionally, VF can also occur idiopathically, for example in people with LQT syndrome or **Brugada syndrome** (Figure 50e, right). This latter condition is associated with ion channel mutations (e.g. in *SCN5A*) which shorten the action potential in epicardial but not endocardial cells of the right ventricle, a situation favouring the development of re-entry.

Non-pharmacological treatment for arrhythmias

Direct current (DC) cardioversion allows rapid cardioversion (reversion to sinus rhythm) of VF and haemodynamically unstable SVT and VT. Shocks of 50–360 J are delivered to the anaesthetized patient via paddles placed over the sternum and the right ventricular apex.

In **radiofrequency catheter ablation** the accessory pathways or focally automatic myocardium causing certain tachyarrhythmias are ablated by focal heating delivered via a catheter. The catheter is placed transvenously (through a vein) and the tip is located at the surface of the endocardium at the site of the abnormality. Radiofrequency energy is delivered to the catheter tip, and dissipated to a large indifferent plate, usually over the back. The tip temperature is set to 60–65°C, resulting in a lesion 8–10 mm in diameter and of a similar depth. This technique, which seldom causes complications, is curative in > 90% of certain supraventricular arrhythmias and may also be effective in some scar-related ventricular arrhythmias.

Implantable defibrillators consist of a generator connected to electrodes placed transvenously in the heart and superior vena cava. A sensing circuit detects arrhythmias, which are classified as tachycardia or fibrillation on the basis of rate. The treatment algorithm is either as burst pacing, which can terminate VT with a high degree of success, or by the delivery of a shock at up to 40 J, which can cardiovert VT and VF. Shock delivery is between an electrode in the right ventricle and another in the superior vena cava or to the body of the generator (active can). Refinements in detection allow the distinction of supraventricular and ventricular arrhythmias, so that several tiers of progressively more aggressive therapy can be set up. The AVID study reported in 1997 that in patients with malignant ventricular arrhythmia, this approach improved survival by 31% over 3 years compared to antiarrhythmic drug therapy (mainly amiodarone).

Electronic pacemakers can be used either temporarily or permanently to initiate the heart beat by imposing repeated cardiac depolarizations. Temporary pacing is generally accomplished using a catheter-tipped electrode introduced transvenously and provides for the rapid treatment of bradycardias. A temporary pacemaker can also be used to terminate a persistent arrhythmia by pacing the heart at a rate somewhat faster than that of the arrhythmia; sinus rhythm is often restored when this *overdrive pacing* is stopped. Permanent pacemakers are usually implanted to treat bradycardias, for example due to AV block or sick sinus syndrome (see Chapter 12). The pacemaker is implanted under the skin on the chest, and stimulates the heart through leads introduced into the heart transvenously, usually through the subclavian vein. Contemporary pacemakers are able to pace both the atria and ventricles to maintain atrioventricular synchronization, and to adjust the pacemaking frequency to respond to changes in physical activity by sensing parameters such as respiration and the interval between the stimulated depolarization and the T wave, a measure of sympathetic nervous system activity.

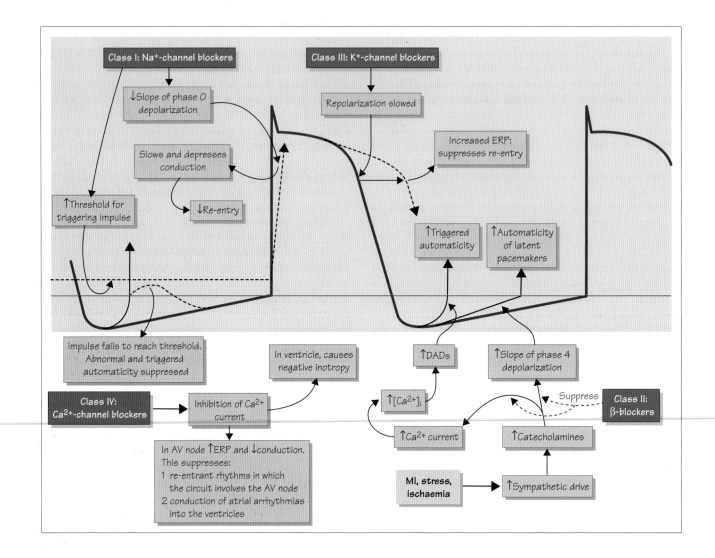

Most antiarrhythmic drugs, whatever their specific mechanisms, have two actions that allow them to reduce abnormal electrical activity, while having tolerably small effects on normal myocardium.

1 They suppress abnormal (ectopic) pacemakers more than they do the sinoatrial node.

2 They increase the ratio of the effective refractory period to action potential duration: ERP/APD.

Antiarrhythmic drugs have been divided into four classes, based on their cellular mechanisms (see figure). However, most antiarrhythmic drugs have properties of more than one of these classes, often because drug metabolites have their own separate antiarrhythmic effects, or because the drugs exist as 50/50 mixtures of two stereoisomers with different actions. This classification system, introduced by Vaughan Williams and Singh, also excludes several drugs, and is of limited use in matching specific drugs to particular arrhythmias. A more clinically relevant classification scheme is presented in Table 51.1.

Clinical trials have shown that class I agents do not enhance survival, and in fact are deleterious if used for some purposes (e.g. prevention of

Table 51.1 Site-based classification of antiarrhythmic drugs.

Atria	Classes IC, III
Ventricles	Classes IA, IB, II
AV node	Adenosine, digoxin, classes II, IV
Atria and ventricles, AV accessory pathways	Amiodarone, sotalol, classes IA, IC

ventricular ectopic beats). Conversely, the class III agent amiodarone modestly increases survival, and class II agents (β-blockers) are increasingly seen to be beneficial for a wide spectrum of arrhythmias. There is therefore a trend away from the use of class I drugs towards the use of class II and III drugs. Moreover, the success of radiofrequency catheter ablation in curing many supraventricular tachyarrhythmias and the effectiveness of implantable defibrillators in controlling some lethal ventricular arrhythmias is shifting the emphasis of arrhythmia management towards device-based therapy.

Class I drugs

Class I drugs act primarily by blocking Na^+ channels, thereby slowing and depressing impulse conduction. This effect can suppress re-entrant circuits which depend on an area of impaired conduction, as further Na^+ channel blockade here may block conduction, and therefore the arrhythmia, entirely. Class I drugs can also suppress automaticity (figure, upper left).

Because they have a higher affinity for Na^+ channels when they are open and/or inactivated, these drugs bind to Na^+ channels during each action potential and then progressively dissociate following repolarization. Dissociation is slowed in cells in which the resting potential is decreased, and this deepens channel blockade in tissue that is depolarized due to ischaemia.

Three subclasses of class I drugs were originally designated based on studies of their effects on the action potential (AP) in canine Purkinje fibres, which showed that each class of drug dissociates from the Na^+ channel at different rates. Class IB drugs (**lidocaine**, **mexiletine**) dissociate from the channel very rapidly and almost completely between APs. They therefore have little effect in normal myocardium because the steady-state level of drug bound to the channel remains minimal. However, in tissue that is depolarized, or firing at a high frequency, dissociation between impulses is decreased, promoting channel blockade and depression of conduction. These drugs are therefore useful in treating ventricular tachyarrhythmias associated with MI, which mainly originate in myocardium depolarized by ischaemia. Conversely, class IC drugs (**flecainide**, **propafenone**) dissociate so slowly that they remain bound to channels between APs, even at low frequencies of stimulation. This strongly depresses conduction in both normal and depolarized myocardium, thereby reducing cardiac contractility. The intermediate dissociation rate of class IA drugs (**procainamide**, **disopyramide**) causes a lengthening of the ERP. These drugs also have class III activity, which prolongs the AP.

Class I drugs cause many side effects, not the least of which are several types of arrhythmia. This **proarrhythmic** effect is not surprising, given that depression of conduction and prolongation of the AP are important causes of arrhythmia development (see Chapter 48).

Class II drugs

Beta-blockers such as **propranolol** and **atenolol** form the second class of antiarrhythmics. The rationale for their use is that sympathetic activation and resulting catecholamine elevation associated with MI stimulates cardiac β-receptors, and this is thought to cause arrhythmias through multiple mechanisms (figure, lower right). Stress-related sympathetic activation can also initiate ventricular tachycardia in patients with MI scarring, cardiomyopathy and heart failure.

Class III drugs

Class III drugs increase APD and therefore prolong ERP. Re-entry occurs when an impulse is locally delayed, and then re-enters and re-excites adjacent myocardium (see Chapter 48). Drugs that prolong ERP can prevent this re-excitation because the adjacent myocardium is still refractory (inexcitable) at the time when the delayed impulse reaches it. The class III agents **amiodarone** and **sotalol** increase APD by inhibiting K^+ channels and slowing repolarization. However, each drug has additional actions, which may be useful.

Amiodarone is effective against many supraventricular and ventricular arrhythmias, probably because it also has class IA, II and IV actions (it also blocks α-receptors!). Clinical trials show that amiodarone modestly reduces mortality after MI and in congestive heart failure. However, its long-term use is recommended only if other antiarrhythmic drugs fail, because it has many cumulative adverse effects and must be discontinued in about one-third of patients. Hazards include pulmonary fibrosis, hypo- and hyperthyroidism, liver dysfunction, photosensitivity and peripheral neuropathy. Amiodarone also has a very unpredictable and long (4–15 weeks) plasma half-life, which complicates its oral administration. Sotalol is a mixed class II and III drug used for ventricular and supraventricular arrhythmias. Although it causes far fewer side effects than amiodarone, it is more likely to cause torsades de pointes (see Chapter 50). **Dofetilide**, **ibutilide** and **azimilide** are newer drugs that are considered to be 'pure' class III agents in that they are relatively selective for the voltage-gated K^+ channels involved in repolarization. These drugs are used to terminate atrial flutter and fibrillation. They can also cause torsades de pointes in some patients, although azimilide is less apt to do so.

Class IV drugs, adenosine, and digoxin

Class IV drugs (**verapamil**, **diltiazem**) exert their antiarrhythmic effects on the atrioventricular node (AVN) by blocking L-type Ca^{2+} channels. These channels mediate the AVN action potential, and their blockade therefore slows AVN depolarization and conduction, and also increases its refractory period. Ca^{2+}-channel blockade is use dependent, and AV block is enhanced by cell depolarization and high-frequency firing. These drugs are used to treat supraventricular tachycardias. They suppress AVN re-entrant rhythms by depressing conduction, and can slow the ventricular rate in atrial flutter and fibrillation by preventing a proportion of atrial impulses from being conducted through the AVN. Negative inotropy can occur due to L-type channel inhibition, especially if left ventricular function is impaired. Negative inotropic and chronotropic effects are exacerbated by coadministration of β-blockers.

Adenosine, an endogenous nucleoside (see Chapter 21), acts on myocardial A_1-receptors, suppressing the Ca^{2+} current and enhancing K^+ currents. These effects depress AVN conduction. Adenosine, given by injection, is the drug of choice for rapid termination of many supraventricular tachycardias. It commonly causes transient flushing and breathlessness. **Digoxin** slows AV conduction by stimulating the vagus and is used to treat atrial fibrillation and other supraventricular tachycardias, especially in patients with heart failure (see Chapter 47).

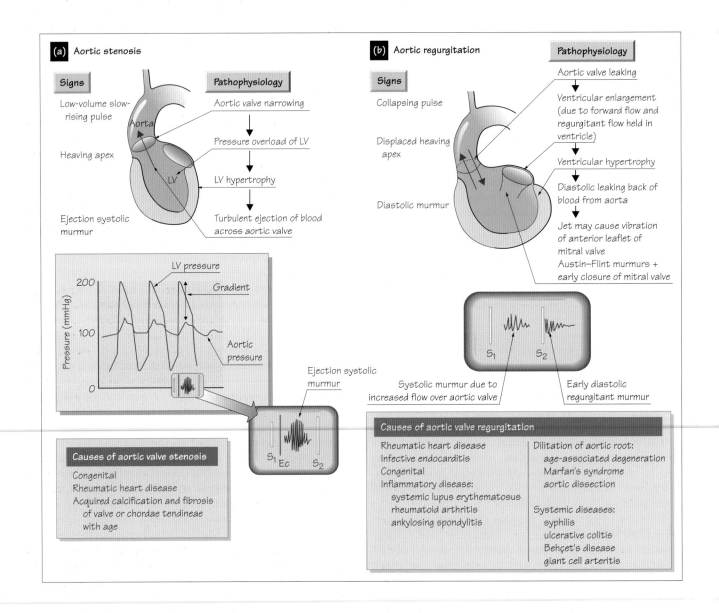

The **aortic valve** is normally tricuspid and separates the left ventricle (LV) from the aorta. Impaired aortic valve opening (**aortic stenosis**, AS) impedes outflow of blood and imposes a pressure load on the LV. Deficient valve closure (**aortic regurgitation**, AR, *incompetence*) allows blood to flow back from the aorta, and imposes a volume load on the LV.

Aortic stenosis
Causes
Acquired calcific aortic stenosis is the most common cause. Calcium deposits occur at the base of the cusp, without involvement of the commissures. This is most likely related to prolonged mechanical stress, and is more common in people with congenital bicuspid valves. About 50% of patients under 70 years old with significant AS have bicuspid valves, whereas most old patients with AS have tricuspid valves.

Rheumatic AS as a result of rheumatic heart disease is unusual without coexisting mitral valve disease. Male sex, diabetes and hypercholesterolaemia are also risk factors for AS.

Congenital A **unicuspid aortic valve** is usually fatal within 1 year of birth. **Bicuspid** aortic valves develop progressive fusion of the commissures, and symptoms usually present after 40 years. Infants with atherosclerosis due to lipid disorders may develop AS in conjunction with **coronary artery disease** (CAD).

Pathophysiology
A slow reduction of aortic valve area causes **left ventricular hypertrophy** and eventual myocardial dysfunction, arrhythmias and **left heart failure** (see Chapter 46). 'Critical' AS occurs with > 75% reduction of valve area to < 0.5 cm^2/m^2 body surface area, and a > 50-mmHg

gradient between peak systolic LV and aortic pressure at a normal cardiac output. With worsening AS, cardiac output cannot increase adequately during exercise and eventually becomes insufficient at rest. At this point the LV dilates, and left ventricular end-diastolic pressure (EDP) increases to the point where overt LV failure ensues.

Clinical features

Patients present usually between the ages of 50 and 70 years, most commonly with **angina** (50% have concurrent CAD). Angina is due to the increased oxygen needs of the hypertrophied LV and inadequate cardiac output during exercise. Exercise tolerance is decreased, and if brain blood flow is insufficient patients may develop **exercise-associated syncope**. Once patients with AS develop angina, syncope or LV failure, their median survival is less than 3 years.

Patients with mild AS have a normal blood pressure and pulse. In moderate to severe AS there is a slow-rising, low-volume pulse that may demonstrate a **thrill** (vibration) and decreased pulse pressure. Auscultation reveals a normal S_1, a single S_2 because of an absent aortic component, an S_4, and a harsh late **systolic murmur**, preceded by an ejection click (Ec) (see Figure 52a and Chapter 30), heard best in the right second intercostal space and transmitted to the carotids and apex. It is louder with squatting and softer with standing or during the **Valsalva manoeuvre** (forced expiration against a closed glottis). With worsening AS and a fall in cardiac output, the murmur may become softer (**silent AS**).

Investigations

The ECG shows LV hypertrophy with strain (depressed ST, inverted T), and left atrial delay. Atrial fibrillation and ventricular arrhythmias are often seen when LV function has deteriorated. Echocardiography shows reduced valve opening and calcification of cusps, and allows calculation of valve area. Doppler imaging allows calculation of the pressure gradient between the LV and aorta.

Management

It is important that systemic hypotension and arterial vasodilatation are avoided, so β-adrenergic blockers and other negative inotropic agents should not be used. Once symptoms develop, cardiac catheterization with **coronary angiography** must be performed prior to valve replacement, and coronary artery bypass performed if significant CAD is present. Several types of mechanical valve are available, including those of a 'ball and cage' variety or tilting disc. These will always require **anticoagulant therapy** (see Chapter 45). Valves can also be obtained from pigs or human cadavers and these have the advantage that anticoagulants are not generally required. **Balloon valvuloplasty** can be performed in children with non-calcified valves, but is of little value in adults.

Aortic regurgitation
Causes

Causes of aortic regurgitation (AR) include **rheumatic disease**, where fibrous retraction of the valve cusps prevents apposition, **infective endocarditis** causing valve damage, and **congenital malformations** (e.g. bicuspid valve) (see Figure 52b).

Pathophysiology

AR imposes a volume load on the LV because of flow back into the ventricle. **Acute AR** (trauma, infective endocarditis, aortic dissection) is usually catastrophic. Here the LV cannot accommodate the acute increase in volume and LV EDP rises. The early increase in LV EDP causes premature closure of the mitral valve and inadequate forward LV filling, resulting in cardiovascular collapse and acute respiratory failure.

In **chronic AR**, volume load and LV EDP increase gradually, and **LV hypertrophy** allows adequate output to be maintained. As the aortic valve never completely closes, there is no LV isovolumetric relaxation phase (see Chapter 14) and the pulse pressure is wide.

Clinical features

Patients usually do not present with symptoms until LV failure develops. Signs include a wide pulse pressure (caused by reduction in diastolic pressure) and a **collapsing pulse** (see Chapter 14). This may occasionally cause visible nail bed pulsation and pulsatile head bobbing. The LV apex is displaced laterally and is hyperdynamic. Auscultation reveals a high-pitched **early diastolic murmur** at the left sternal border, and a **systolic flow murmur** across the aortic valve. A low-frequency **rumbling late diastolic murmur** at the apex (**Austin–Flint murmur**) may be caused by premature closing of the mitral valve.

Investigations

Echocardiography can determine the aetiology and severity of AR by imaging the valve leaflets and LV dimensions, aortic root diameter, and diastolic closure or fluttering of the mitral valve. Doppler imaging quantifies the amount of regurgitation.

Management

Acute severe AR requires urgent valve replacement. Chronic AR has a generally good prognosis until symptoms develop. Patients with moderate AR should be followed with serial echocardiography. Valve replacement should be considered in patients with symptoms, or in asymptomatic patients with worsening LV dimensions, LV function or aortic root diameter. Valve replacement is similar to that for aortic stenosis, except that replacement of the aortic root may also be required in patients with a severely dilated ascending aorta.

53 Diseases of the mitral valve

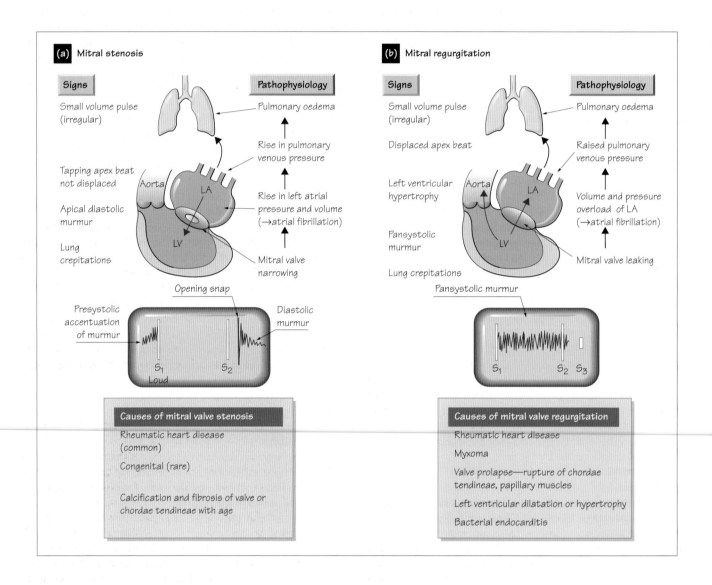

(a) Mitral stenosis

Signs

- Small volume pulse (irregular)
- Tapping apex beat not displaced
- Apical diastolic murmur
- Lung crepitations

Aorta • LA • LV

Pathophysiology

- Pulmonary oedema
- Rise in pulmonary venous pressure
- Rise in left atrial pressure and volume (→atrial fibrillation)
- Mitral valve narrowing

Opening snap

Presystolic accentuation of murmur

Diastolic murmur

S_1 Loud S_2

Causes of mitral valve stenosis

- Rheumatic heart disease (common)
- Congenital (rare)
- Calcification and fibrosis of valve or chordae tendineae with age

(b) Mitral regurgitation

Signs

- Small volume pulse (irregular)
- Displaced apex beat
- Left ventricular hypertrophy
- Pansystolic murmur
- Lung crepitations

Aorta • LA • LV

Pathophysiology

- Pulmonary oedema
- Raised pulmonary venous pressure
- Volume and pressure overload of LA (→atrial fibrillation)
- Mitral valve leaking

Pansystolic murmur

S_1 S_2 S_3

Causes of mitral valve regurgitation

- Rheumatic heart disease
- Myxoma
- Valve prolapse—rupture of chordae tendineae, papillary muscles
- Left ventricular dilatation or hypertrophy
- Bacterial endocarditis

The **mitral valve** is normally bicuspid and separates the left atrium (LA) and left ventricle (LV). The valve may narrow (**mitral stenosis**) or leak (**mitral regurgitation**).

Mitral stenosis

Causes

Mitral stenosis (MS) is usually due to prior episodes of acute **rheumatic fever**. This causes thickening and fusion of the mitral **commissures**, **cusps** or **chordae tendineae**, making the cusps less flexible and narrowing the orifice. Symptoms from MS usually develop more than 10 years after the acute attack, which patients may not recall. The normal area of a mitral valve is 6 cm^2; critical MS occurs when this area falls to 1 cm^2.

Pathophysiology

Mitral stenosis prevents the free flow of blood from the LA to the LV, and slows ventricular filling during diastole. The left atrial pressure rises to maintain cardiac output, and there is **atrial hypertrophy** and **dilatation**. The elevated left atrial pressure causes pulmonary congestion and can result in **pulmonary hypertension** and **oedema**, and **right heart failure** (see Chapter 46). Patients with MS rely on atrial systole for ventricular filling, and **atrial fibrillation** (caused by atrial enlargement) significantly reduces cardiac output. The fibrillating atrium is liable to develop **thrombi** that may be **embolized** (dislodge and move freely in the blood) causing stroke (see Chapter 45). The LV is usually normal in MS, but may be abnormal due to either chronic underfeeding of the LV or rheumatic scarring.

Clinical features

Patients present in their 20–30s with **dyspnoea** on exertion or conditions that raise cardiac output (e.g. fever, pregnancy). This is a result of **pulmonary congestion**, which causes the lungs to become stiffer. Patients may present with **haemoptysis** (coughing up of blood), **palpitations** or **stroke** (via embolization of thrombi). Symptoms may be precipitated by arrhythmias such as atrial fibrillation. Auscultation reveals an **opening snap** (OS) soon after S_2 that is heard best at the apex, and by a **rumbling diastolic murmur** leading to a loud S_1. The duration of the murmur is related to the severity of the MS. It is brief in mild MS and **holodiastolic** (*pandiastolic*, i.e. over the whole diastolic period) in severe MS. Patients in sinus rhythm may have **presystolic accentuation** of the murmur due to atrial contraction, and a large venous 'a' wave (see Chapter 14). If the mitral valve is completely immobile there may be no OS or a loud S_1. As MS becomes more severe, there will be a less prominent arterial pulse, **lung crackles** (*crepitations*; audible crackles because of fluid in the lungs), and elevation of the **jugular venous pressure**.

The ECG may show only LA enlargement, although many patients are in atrial fibrillation. The chest radiograph may show left atrial enlargement with normal left ventricular size, but with increasing severity of MS there may be pulmonary vascular congestion, enlarged pulmonary arteries, and right ventricular enlargement.

Management

Mild MS may require little treatment, although management should include avoidance of **anaemia** and **tachyarrhythmias** as these may precipitate decompensation and cardiac failure (see Chapter 46). Prophylactic antibiotics for **endocarditis** should be administered before invasive procedures, and patients in atrial fibrillation should receive **anticoagulation** to decrease the occurrence of stroke. Patients with MS can remain minimally symptomatic for many years, but deteriorate quickly once symptoms begin to worsen. Therefore, **valve replacement** with a mechanical valve, **valvotomy** (surgical separation of commissures) or **balloon valvuloplasty** (use of a balloon catheter to force open cusps) should be performed in moderately symptomatic patients with a mitral valve area < 1.7 cm².

Mitral regurgitation
Causes

Acute mitral regurgitation (MR) is usually a result of **bacterial endocarditis, ruptured chordae tendineae** or ischaemic **papillary muscle rupture**. Chronic MR is now most likely to arise from **myxomatous degeneration** of the mitral leaflets or **valve prolapse** (reversal into atrium). Chronic MR may also develop in any disease causing LV dilatation, so preventing apposition (coming together) of the mitral leaflets, or because of ischaemic dysfunction of the papillary muscles.

Pathophysiology

In **acute MR** the LV ejects blood back into the LA, imposing a sudden volume load on the LA during ventricular systole. Left atrial pressure rises suddenly and this is rapidly followed by a rise in pulmonary venous pressure and capillary pressure. This leads to fluid entering the lung interstitium, causing stiffness and dyspnoea, or alveoli causing **pulmonary oedema**.

Chronic MR is sufficiently slow to allow compensatory LV dilatation and hypertrophy, and dilatation of the LA. The latter protects the pulmonary circulation from the effects of the regurgitant volume. MR imposes a diastolic volume load on the LV that causes dilatation, because each systolic stroke volume is composed of a portion that enters the aorta (LV output) and an ineffective portion that re-enters the LA (LV regurgitant volume) and adds to the venous return. The regurgitant volume increases when LV emptying is impaired, such as with aortic stenosis or hypertension.

Clinical features

Patients with mild chronic MR are usually asymptomatic. As MR worsens, patients develop **fatigue, dyspnoea on exertion, orthopnoea** and **pulmonary oedema** as a result of progressive LV failure and elevation of pulmonary capillary pressure (see Chapter 46). The development of atrial fibrillation is common because of dilatation of the LA. Chronic MR is associated with a **holosystolic** murmur which is heard best at the apex, with transmission to the axilla and the left infrascapular region. S_1 is soft and S_2 is split widely because of an early aortic component. Echocardiography can detect a prolapsing or rheumatic valve, and determine LV size and function. Doppler imaging of the regurgitant jet can assess the severity of MR.

Management

Management is focused on promoting LV emptying into the aorta. Reduction of afterload with **ACE inhibitors** is beneficial (see Chapter 47). Patients with atrial fibrillation receive **anticoagulants** to prevent stroke. A prolapsing valve may sometimes be repaired. Dilatation of the mitral valve ring may be corrected by implantation of an artificial ring. Rheumatic valves and those damaged by endocarditis often need replacement with an artificial valve. Valve replacement is best performed prior to the development of LV dysfunction or chronic pulmonary hypertension, and should always be performed in patients with symptomatic MR despite medical therapy. The risks of surgery are higher in acute MR; however, valve replacement should be performed in patients with uncontrollable heart failure or end-organ failure, even in cases of acute infective endocarditis.

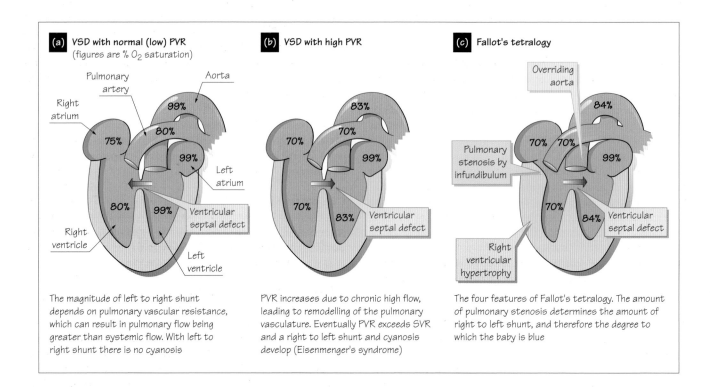

(a) VSD with normal (low) PVR
(figures are % O$_2$ saturation)

Pulmonary artery
Aorta
Right atrium
99%
80%
75%
99%
Left atrium
80%
99%
Ventricular septal defect
Right ventricle
Left ventricle

The magnitude of left to right shunt depends on pulmonary vascular resistance, which can result in pulmonary flow being greater than systemic flow. With left to right shunt there is no cyanosis

(b) VSD with high PVR

83%
70%
70%
99%
70%
83%
Ventricular septal defect

PVR increases due to chronic high flow, leading to remodelling of the pulmonary vasculature. Eventually PVR exceeds SVR and a right to left shunt and cyanosis develop (Eisenmenger's syndrome)

(c) Fallot's tetralogy

Overriding aorta
84%
Pulmonary stenosis by infundibulum
70%
70%
99%
70%
84%
Ventricular septal defect
Right ventricular hypertrophy

The four features of Fallot's tetralogy. The amount of pulmonary stenosis determines the amount of right to left shunt, and therefore the degree to which the baby is blue

Definition

Congenital heart diseases (CHDs) are abnormalities of cardiac structure that are present from birth. They result from abnormalities in cardiac development occurring between 3 and 8 weeks' gestation.

Incidence

The incidence of CHD is ~1% of live births, not including congenital valve disorders such as mitral prolapse or bicuspid aortic valve. Many spontaneously aborted fetuses or stillborns have cardiac malformations, or chromosomal abnormalities associated with structural heart defects. Maternal factors such as **rubella infection**, alcohol abuse and some medications are associated with CHD.

Physiology

In the normal fetal circulation (see Chapter 24) blood crosses the **foramen ovale** from the right to the left atrium. Most of the blood ejected by the right ventricle enters the aorta via the **ductus arteriosus**, because pulmonary vascular resistance (PVR) is higher than systemic vascular resistance (SVR). After birth, PVR falls to one-tenth of SVR, allowing blood flow from the right ventricle through the lungs. Closure of the foramen ovale and ductus arteriosus establishes the adult circulations in series.

Clinical features

CHDs normally present in infancy with either **congestive heart failure** or **central cyanosis**. Congestive heart failure in an infant is usually due to a left to right shunt, such as a **ventricular septal defect** or a **patent ductus arteriosus** (PDA), or as a result of aortic coarctation or stenosis. Infants with congestive heart failure fail to thrive, and demonstrate

symptoms similar to those in adults (see Chapter 46). **Central cyanosis**, blueness of the trunk and mucous membranes, is due to > 3–5 g/dL of deoxygenated haemoglobin in the arterial circulation. Central cyanosis may result from severe pulmonary disease, and intrapulmonary right to left shunt (arteriovenous malformation, AVM) or extrapulmonary right to left shunting. It is characteristic of **transposition of the great vessels** and **tetralogy of Fallot**.

Ventricular septal defect

This is the most common CHD (0.2% of births), and may occur in isolation or with other abnormalities. Flow across the defect is determined by the relationship between the resistances of the pulmonary and systemic circulations. *In utero*, when PVR > SVR, most blood exits the left ventricle via the aorta. However, after birth PVR < SVR, and blood is shunted from the left to the right ventricle, and into the pulmonary artery (Figure 54a). The magnitude of the shunt is related to the size of the defect as well as the relative sizes of PVR and SVR.

Clinical features

A ventricular septal defect (VSD) should be suspected in an infant who fails to gain weight, and has frequent respiratory difficulties or infections. The VSD is diagnosed by a harsh systolic murmur at the left sternal border. In young children a moderate VSD may cause exercise limitation or fatigue, an enlarged heart and biventricular hypertrophy. Echocardiography with Doppler imaging allows estimation of the size and location of the VSD. Shunting of blood from the left ventricle into the pulmonary circulation leads to pulmonary hypertension, which if persistent causes irreversible **pulmonary vascular remodelling**. Once PVR exceeds SVR the direction of the shunt reverses and cyanosis develops (Figure 54b; **Eisenmenger's syndrome**). At this point surgical correction is not possible, and therefore infants with a significant VSD benefit from early surgery. In the case of smaller VSDs, 50% close spontaneously within 3–4 years. Children with VSDs have an increased risk of endocarditis and should receive prophylactic antibiotics before dental procedures.

Patent (or persistent) ductus arteriosus

PDA may arise because the duct does not close properly due to malformations, and is more common in females. The malformation may be caused by maternal rubella. The duct may not close in premature babies due to immaturity.

Clinical features

Frequently PDA is not diagnosed immediately after birth, and then only after development of heart failure or infective endocarditis. A loud murmur is characteristically heard in both systole and diastole. The left atrium and ventricle are enlarged. Treatment should be initiated as soon as possible to prevent development of full heart failure. Ligation of the ductus arteriosus is a safe procedure, but must be performed within 5 years of birth. In some cases treatment with indometacin, a cyclooxygenase inhibitor, to reduce PGE_1 is sufficient to promote closure on its own.

Transposition of the great arteries

Transposition of the great arteries occurs when the left ventricle empties into the pulmonary artery and the right ventricle empties into the aorta. This may be associated with VSD, atrial septal defect (ASD) or PDA. The transposition results in two parallel circulations, where deoxygenated systemic venous blood is returned to the body and oxygenated pulmonary venous blood returns to the lungs. This causes severe central cyanosis. Unless corrected, this defect is fatal in one-third of cases within 2 weeks and in 90% of cases within a year. Surgical correction involves an arterial switch where the great vessels are transected and connected to their appropriate ventricles. Prior to surgery infants can be stabilized by the creation of an ASD with a catheter, which allows mixing of blood in the atria and oxygenation of systemic blood. Administration of PGE_1 delays closure of the ductus arteriosus and allows further access of oxygenated blood to the systemic circulation.

Fallot's tetralogy

This is the most common cyanotic CHD found in children surviving to 1 year (Figure 54c). It consists of a VSD, pulmonary stenosis, an overriding aorta (positioning of the aorta over the VSD) and right ventricular hypertrophy. These lead to a high right ventricular pressure and right to left shunt. The degree of cyanosis depends on the pulmonary stenosis, which is usually a combination of infundibular stenosis and obstruction of the pulmonary valve. The subvalvular stenosis is caused by misalignment of the infundibular septum; when the latter contracts it may exacerbate the stenosis.

Clinical features

Infants with Fallot's tetralogy are slow to develop, and may present with dyspnoea, fatigue and hypoxic episodes (**Fallot's or tetralogy spells**), characterized by rapidly worsening cyanosis, progressing to limpness, stroke and loss of consciousness. There is usually a palpable RV impulse and a thrill at the left sternal border. There is no pulmonary component to the second heart sound, and a systolic ejection murmur which is inversely proportional to the degree of pulmonary stenosis. Surgical correction of the VSD and ventricular obstruction is performed in infancy and has less than 5% mortality.

Atrial septal defects

These defects usually go unrecognized until adulthood. They generally involve the midseptum in the ostium secundum and are distinct from a patent foramen ovale. The left to right shunt increases pulmonary blood flow, which if sustained into adulthood leads to pulmonary vascular remodelling and fixed pulmonary hypertension. Adults with ASDs may also present with atrial arrhythmias or left ventricular failure. Once severe pulmonary hypertension develops, there may be reversal of the left to right shunt, and cyanosis due to a right to left shunt.

Clinical features

There is normally a pulmonary ejection murmur, a wide fixed split S_2 and elevated jugular venous pressure. As pulmonary hypertension worsens, the murmur becomes softer and the S_2 becomes louder. If discovered early, ASDs with significant left to right shunts should be repaired to prevent the development of irreversible pulmonary hypertension. Once a right to left shunt has developed, surgical repair of an ASD is not performed.

Case studies and questions

Case 1: Heart failure

A 62-year-old man is transferred to your hospital because of recurrent chest pain and dyspnoea 5 days after suffering a large myocardial infarction. On the day of arrival he is free of chest pain but is still breathing with moderate difficulty. You obtain a chest radiograph, which confirms increased distended pulmonary vasculature, septal lines and an enlarged heart. An echocardiogram shows an enlarged heart and an ejection fraction of 30% with minimal systolic motion of the anterior and apical portions of the heart. The patient is in normal sinus rhythm, with a heart rate of 110. Arterial blood pressure is 96/68, mean 82, respiratory rate 25/min. On cardiac auscultation you hear an S_3 gallop, an S_4 gallop, a normal S_1 and S_2, and a soft murmur that encompasses systole (holosystolic), and has uniform intensity that is heard at the apex and radiates to the left axilla. There are fine late inspiratory crackles (crepitations) heard about a third of the way up both lung fields. Arterial blood gases reveal a Pao_2 of 60 mmHg, $Paco_2$ of 30 mmHg and pH of 7.37.

1 *What is the left ventricular end-diastolic pressure likely to be in this patient and why?*
2 *What is the significance of the S_3 and S_4 gallop sounds?*
3 *Why is heart rate likely to be increased?*
4 *The arterial pressures are low. What is the peripheral vascular resistance likely to be in this case? What is the preload volume likely to be? How would similar arterial and venous loads probably affect arterial pressure in a normal heart?*
5 *You place a right heart catheter to assess the haemodynamics better, and find that the cardiac output is 3.0 L/min, and the right atrial pressure has a mean value of 10 mmHg. What is systemic vascular resistance? Is this normal?*

6 *How do abnormalities in contractile function, preload and afterload resistance play a role in this patient's current problem?*
7 *What might happen to cardiac output and arterial blood pressure if an arterial vasodilator was administered to this patient?*
8 *Would it be useful to alter contractility? In what direction? What might be a potential disadvantage of increasing contractility in this particular patient?*
9 *Suppose the arterial perfusion pressure during diastole could be increased while at the same time lowering it during systole. Would this intervention be useful? Why?*

Case 2: Valvular heart disease

You are asked to supervise an exercise stress test on a 65-year-old man. He saw his doctor last week for exertional chest pain and mild dyspnoea. He has had chest discomfort for about a year, but the increased frequency of angina prompted him to see his doctor. He has chest pain when he walks more than one block, and if he continues he becomes breathless. He never has chest pain or dyspnoea at rest. He has no ankle swelling, orthopnoea or paroxysmal nocturnal dyspnoea. When you examine him before the stress test, his blood pressure is 120/86 mmHg heart rate 82 and regular, jugular venous pressure 5 cmH$_2$O, and lungs are clear. His apex beat is slightly lateral to the midclavicular line and mildly sustained. He has a normal S_1 and a single S_2. An S_4 gallop is noted. He has a soft crescendo–decrescendo systolic murmur, best heard at the upper right sternal border, radiating to the carotids and the apex. The carotid pulses are delayed and diminished.

You call the referring doctor to discuss the signs and symptoms, cancel the stress test and perform an echocardiogram instead.

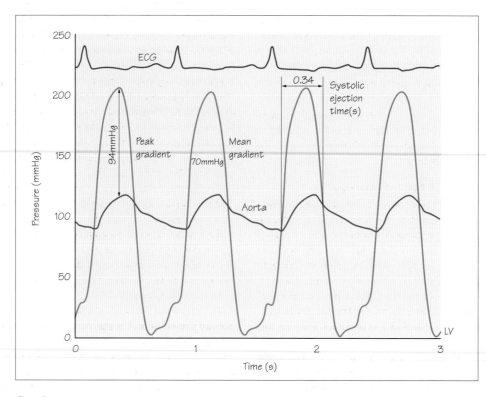

Case 2

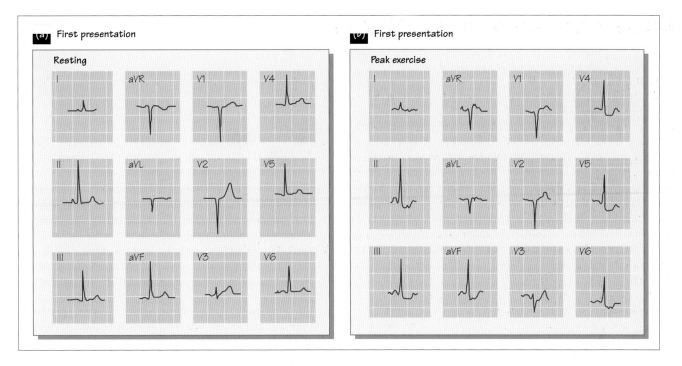

(a) **First presentation**

Resting

I aVR V1 V4
II aVL V2 V5
III aVF V3 V6

(b) **First presentation**

Peak exercise

I aVR V1 V4
II aVL V2 V5
III aVF V3 V6

Case 3

1 *What is the likely diagnosis based on the physical examination? What are the pathophysiological mechanisms underlying these findings?*

2 *He only had a soft systolic murmur. If you knew that his murmur last year was louder and harsher in intensity, would this have reassured you? What could go wrong if he did do the stress test?*

3 *What was likely to be observed on the echocardiogram and why?*

Catheterization data The patient is formally referred to you, and you recommend valve replacement. He undergoes cardiac catheterization, and the haemodynamic data are shown in Fig. Case 2 Cardiac output is 5.2 L/min and heart rate is 77. There is no significant coronary artery disease.

4 *The aortic valve area can be estimated by the simplified formula:*

Valve area = cardiac output/$\sqrt{pressure\ gradient}$

Based on the data given, what is his estimated valve area?

5 *When admitted for surgery, he complains of chest pain. The intern orders sublingual nitroglycerin for him. Why is this a bad idea? What is the chest pain due to? What therapeutic options are available for protracted chest pain in this case?*

Case 3: Ischaemic heart disease

A 53-year-old woman presents with a prolonged episode of chest discomfort. The discomfort is under her sternum, and is a squeezing feeling that extends to her left arm and jaws. She has had this on and off for 3 months. It usually occurs when she goes up two flights of stairs, but never when resting. Tonight, the discomfort began while walking to buy cigarettes, and lasted for 40 min. She has no known medical problems and has not seen a doctor in more than 20 years. Her last menstrual period was 4 years ago. She takes no medications. Her family history is only significant in that her father died of a heart attack when he was 74 years old.

On examination, she appears well and in no acute distress. Her height is 5 feet 6 inches (1.68 m) and weight 120 pounds (55 kg). Her blood pressure is 132/84 mmHg and heart rate 74. There is no jugular venous distension, and her lungs are clear to percussion and auscultation. Cardiac

examination is normal. Her abdomen is benign, and there is no oedema. Pulses are full and equal bilaterally without thrills. An ECG shows normal sinus rhythm without abnormalities.

1 *Is this angina pectoris?*

2 *What predisposing factors does she have for coronary artery disease (CAD)? What other risk factors might she have? Could this have been a myocardial infarction (MI)?*

She is admitted for monitoring. Serial serum enzyme tests are negative, and ECG remains normal after 18 h. Fasting serum glucose is 92, and fasting lipid profile is: total cholesterol 198, HDL 36, LDL 137, and triglycerides 126. She undergoes a graded exercise test for 12 min, and has chest discomfort with the ECG abnormalities shown in Fig. Case 3 (b). Her blood pressure rose from 124/78 to 180/76 mmHg at peak exercise. Her heart rate rose from 78 to 143. The chest discomfort resolved within 5 min of stopping exercise, and the ECG returned to normal. Coronary angiography showed a focal 70% narrowing in the right coronary artery and a focal 30% narrowing in the left anterior descending artery (LAD). She is treated with anti-ischaemic medicines, advised on low-cholesterol diets and aerobic exercise, instructed on the use of sublingual nitroglycerin, started on aspirin and atenolol, and discharged. She agrees to stop smoking. She will return for follow-up in 7 days for another exercise test.

3 *What serum enzymes are useful in diagnosing myocardial damage?*

4 *Why not perform angioplasty on the coronary lesions?*

5 *Her cholesterol is not high. Why a low-cholesterol diet? Would lowering blood cholesterol help her existing CAD? What other risk factors can she modify?*

6 *Why perform a follow-up exercise test?*

Second presentation The patient does well on the medicines and stops smoking. She has no chest discomfort, even during vigorous exercise. However, within the week she is awakened from sleep by the same chest discomfort. As nitroglycerin is ineffective, she is brought to hospital. Her ECG is shown in Fig. Case 3 (c). She is given oxygen, aspirin, intravenous nitroglycerin and heparin, and her chest discomfort then

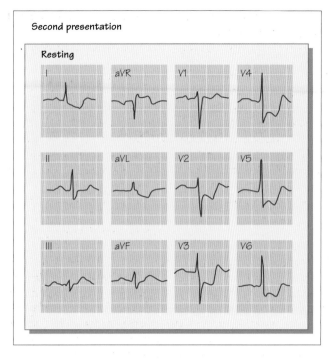

Second presentation

Resting

Case 3 (continued)

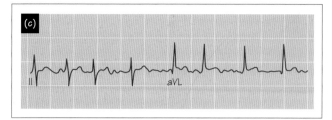

Case 4 (continued)

recedes. It lasted for 35 min. Because of recurrent chest discomfort in hospital, she has another coronary angiogram. This shows the same 70% narrowing in the right coronary artery, but the 30% LAD narrowing has now grown to 99%. Cardiac enzymes are still negative.

7 *What does the new ECG show? What is your diagnosis? How is the pathophysiology of the current chest discomfort different from her previous effort-related angina?*

8 *Do the ECG abnormalities correlate with the coronary angiogram? What is the 'culprit' lesion? How could the LAD lesion progress so fast? Why use aspirin and heparin? How about thrombolytic agents?*

Case 4: Arrhythmias (1)

Initial presentation: A 64-year-old man with a history of longstanding hypertension and diabetes presents complaining of shortness of breath and weakness. He has orthopnoea but no chest pain. His physical examination is notable for a heart rate of 150 beats/min, a blood pressure of 100/70 mmHg, and a respiratory rate of 24. There are bilateral crackles a third of the way up the lung fields, the first heart sound is soft, and there is a summation gallop. His ECG is shown in Fig. Case 4 (a).

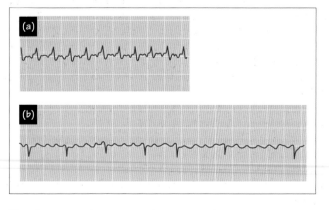

Case 4

Carotid sinus massage then changes the rhythm to the one shown in Fig. Case 4 (b).

1 *What is the ventricular rate in Fig. Case 4 (a)? Is this a ventricular or supraventricular arrhythmia?*

2 *Based on the effect of carotid sinus massage, what is the diagnosis? How does carotid sinus massage affect the ventricular response?*

3 *What pharmacological agents can be used to slow the ventricular response?*

Results of treatment The patient is admitted to hospital and begun on digitalis and amiodarone. The next morning he feels better, but his pulse is irregularly irregular with an apical pulse of 110 and a radial pulse of 70. An ECG is shown in Fig. Case 4 (c).

4 *What is the rhythm now? Is the change from the day before common?*

5 *Is the current antiarrhythmic regimen appropriate?*

6 *What other therapy may be indicated? Why?*

Case 5: Arrhythmias (2)

Initial presentation: A 55-year-old man presents with a 24-h history of shortness of breath and palpitations. He has mild dizziness and diaphoresis. There is no prior record of MI, but he has a longstanding history of hypertension and cigarette smoking. His blood pressure is 80/52 mmHg, his heart rate is 186 beats/min and regular, and his respiratory rate is 26. There are crackles bilaterally, jugular venous pressure (JVP) is raised, and a grade III/IV holosystolic murmur (see Chapter 30) at the apex radiates to the axilla but not the neck. His ECG is shown in Fig. Case 5 (a).

1 *What does the III/IV holosystolic murmur indicate?*

2 *Is this tachycardia more likely supraventricular or ventricular? Why? What is the axis and the QRS morphology?*

3 *Why is he short of breath and hypotensive? Why is his JVP elevated?*

4 *What would be appropriate treatment?*

Results of treatment The patient receives lidocaine. This fails to convert him to sinus rhythm and he is therefore electrically cardioverted. The resulting ECG is shown in Fig. Case 5 (b) and (c).

5 *What is the rhythm now?*

6 *What is the likely cause of his acute presentation?*

7 *What would be the appropriate evaluation with this information?*

Case 6: Haemorrhage and shock

You are a casualty officer in a busy department in the late evening. A young man comes in supporting his friend; he gives his name as John, and that of his friend as Bill. He is very worried about Bill, who he says was hurt when they were involved in a traffic accident. Bill's legs are covered in blood from a wound in his thigh, which has been inexpertly bandaged. He also has a livid bruise on his forehead. John appears very pale, nervous and uncomfortable, and is evasive about the accident; it is not clear how long ago this occurred, although he implies that it was within the last half hour. Both John and Bill smell

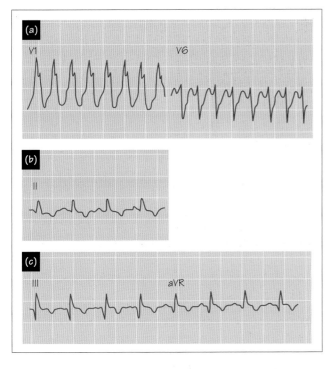

Case 5

tocrit is 0.44. You are unsure of the diagnosis, so he is admitted overnight for observation.

6 *Why was John so thirsty? Why might security have thought he was drunk?*

7 *Why might John's blood pressure fall so much on standing?*

The next morning Bill has recovered well. John, on the other hand, still has a raised heart rate, and his haematocrit has fallen to 0.35. He has not passed any urine. A CT scan reveals an accumulation of more than 2 litres of blood in the peritoneum, and subsequent surgery a torn peritoneum and renal artery. On the recovery ward John's blood pressure is shown to be 120/80 mmHg, but you remain concerned, and place him under ongoing observation.

8 *Why did John's haematocrit fall, and why was he not passing any urine?*

9 *Why are you concerned about John, considering his blood pressure has recovered and his urine output is improved?*

John's urine output, which partially recovered after the operation, gradually decreases and after 8 hours ceases. He shows some signs of oedema. Acute renal failure is diagnosed, and he is put on a regime of low fluid, salt and protein intake to reduce accumulation of toxins. Whilst Bill is discharged the following day, John's renal function takes 3 days to recover, and he remains in hospital for more than a week. It is several months before he is well enough to return to work.

10 *What might have caused the acute renal failure?*

11 *Why might he develop oedema, and why would it take a few days to recover?*

12 *How long will it take for John's haematocrit to return to normal?*

Case 7: Hypertension

A 52-year-old overweight Caucasian male is referred to your clinic by his optician, who noted retinopathy, specifically 'dot' and 'blot' haemorrhages, on a routine eye examination. The patient complains of blurred vision, increased thirst and lethargy. You elicit the following history:

PC – blurred vision; polydipsia.
HPC – both eyes, for 2 months; becoming increasingly lethargic.
PMH – unremarkable.
DH – nil; no known drug allergies.
SH – 30 pack-years; 25 units EtOH per week.
FH – father had hypertension; mother RIP aged 72, stroke.

PC, presenting complaint; HPC, history of PC; PMH, previous medical history; DH, drug history; SH, smoking history; FH, family history; EtOH, alcohol.

On examination he is comfortable at rest, there are no peripheral stigmata of cardiovascular disease, his radial pulse is 86, BP 150/95 mmHg, the JVP is not raised, nor is the apex beat displaced. On auscultation heart sounds S_1 and S_2 are normal. Dorsalis pedis and posterior tibialis pulses are palpable. Ophthalmoscopy reveals dot and blot haemorrhages on the retinae. The patient is 1.76 m tall and weighs 102 kg.

A lipid profile reveals HDL cholesterol to be 0.98 mM (38 mg/dL) and triglyceride 1.80 mM (164 mg/dL).

A random glucose tolerance test reveals a plasma glucose concentration of 14.0 mM (255 mg/dL).

1 *What is your diagnosis and what do you do?*

2 *What is the target blood pressure in non-diabetic and diabetic patients?*

3 *Why do as many as 75% of type 2 diabetics have hypertension?*

of alcohol, and although John says they are 18 years old, they both look a couple of years younger. You suspect they may have been joy-riding. Whilst you are uncovering Bill's wound, John says he feels dizzy and nauseous; you suggest he goes out and sits in the waiting room.

Bill is conscious, but unable to stand unsupported and is only partly coherent. When you get him lying on the trolley you find his skin is pale and clammy, his pulse rate 110 bpm, and his blood pressure 110/70 mmHg. He has a raised respiratory rate. On investigation, you find that the wound is not as serious as it appeared, though there has clearly been significant blood loss. You decide that blood transfusion is required, and take a blood sample for cross-matching and measurement of haematocrit. The blood tests reveals a haematocrit of 0.43, which does not reassure you, and an AB blood group. Within an hour of transfusion Bill becomes coherent, his pulse falls to 95 bpm, and his blood pressure is 115/80 mmHg.

1 *In Bill's case, what symptoms and signs should alert you to hypovolumic shock?*

2 *What are they caused by?*

3 *Why are you not reassured by Bill's haematocrit? Why might you suspect that the accident happened rather longer ago than John said?*

4 *What blood group could be used for Bill's transfusion, and why?*

5 *What did you omit to do concerning John?*

Bill asks for John so he can call his family. However, when the nurse goes to the waiting room she finds that John had kept asking for water and then became abusive; security, believing him to be drunk, had escorted him outside and told him to go home. An hour later a young man is brought in having been found looking very ill on a bench by the bus stop. It is John. He is very disorientated, his skin is cold and clammy, and he has abdominal discomfort. His heart rate on the trolley is 115 bpm, and his blood pressure 100/70 mmHg. When helped to stand his blood pressure falls to 85/40 mmHg and he faints. His haema-

4 *Which antihypertensive drug do you prescribe as first-line therapy and why is this class of drug preferred?*

5 *Which is the most important prognostic indicator of a cardiovascular event: systolic, diastolic or the pulse pressure?*

6 *What additional risk of cardiovascular mortality is conferred by type 2 diabetes?*

The patient begins taking the medication you prescribed, but on follow-up his blood pressure remains above the appropriate target.

7 *Why should this patient now receive a diuretic, in addition to the other antihypertensive agent? And from which class?*

Your patient's blood pressure is proving refractory to the two types of drug you have prescribed. But he does not have proteinuria.

8 *Which adjunct therapy should be given?*

His BP is still not at target but his pulse has lowered to 82.

9 *What action do you take now?*

10 *Which glucose-lowering drug do you prescribe?*

The patient's blood pressure and blood glucose levels remain well controlled on this treatment regimen.

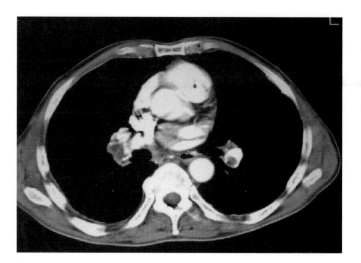

Case 8 CT scan

Case 8: Pulmonary embolism

You are the medical SHO looking after a 69-year-old man, who was admitted to hospital with an acute exacerbation of his chronic obstructive airways disease a week ago and has fallen during routine physiotherapy. He has osteoporosis following multiple courses of steroids for his chronic obstructive pulmonany disease (COPD) and he has fractured his right lower leg. A plaster splint has been fitted and he must not weight-bear on his right leg for at least 2 weeks. As he lives alone in a second floor flat without lifts he is now awaiting social services support before discharge. Late on a Friday evening, 3 days after the fracture, he becomes confused and hypotensive. He is reviewed by the on-call SHO. Examination demonstrates a temperature of 37.5°C, normal pulse and blood pressure, widespread wheeze and occasional crepitations at the right base on chest auscultation. Blood tests, ECG and CXR are all normal. The on-call doctor diagnoses an acute confusional state secondary to chest infection with a further exacerbation of the COPD. Antibiotics, nebulized bronchodilators and a further course of steroids are started. He is also treated with haloperidol for the confusion. Overnight the confusion resolves and the patient appears to recover. However, he has several similar short-lived episodes over the next 48 h that resolve spontaneously. The nurses remain concerned about the patient and you are asked to review him on Monday morning.

1 *What is the most likely diagnosis and what is your differential diagnosis?*

2 *Which investigations will you perform, and in what order, to confirm your diagnosis and why?*

3 *In what other ways can this condition present?*

4 *What immediate treatment would you recommend?*

Later the same day, following return from further investigations in the radiology department, the patient reports a sudden onset of severe breathlessness. He rapidly becomes cyanosed with a saturation of 65%. You are on the ward and have been able to briefly assess the patient. He is cold, clammy, cyanosed and confused, with a thready pulse, low blood pressure and raised jugular venous pressure. The CT scan images are available but have not been reported (Fig. Case 8). The oxygen flow has been increased to maximum and you have inserted a venous catheter when the patient suddenly arrests.

5 *What is the likely cause of the arrest and what immediate management would you institute whilst awaiting the arrest team?*

6 *Would you consider thrombolytic therapy in this patient?*

Answers

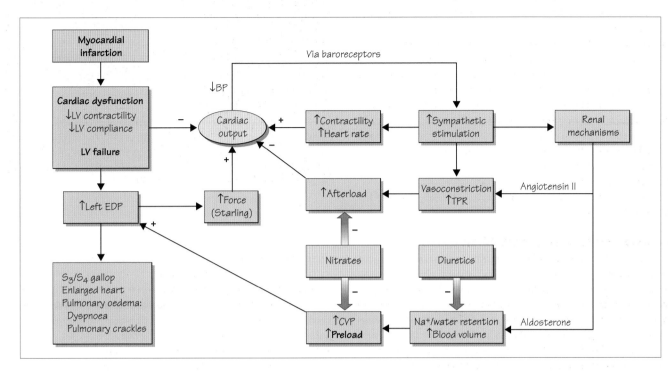

Case 1 Mechanisms of heart failure

Case 1: Heart failure (refer to above figure)

1 The left ventricular diastolic pressure is likely to be elevated. The recent myocardial infarction has diminished the pumping capacity of the ventricle, and to compensate the heart has filled to a larger diastolic volume to partially restore cardiac output and arterial pressures. The elevated cardiac filling pressures are reflected in the pulmonary venous pressures, and this has contributed to the pulmonary oedema. Cardiac enlargement is evident on the chest X-ray as an increase in heart size. The crackles are consistent with increased pulmonary interstitial and alveolar oedema.

2 The S_3 gallop is associated with early diastolic filling and is an indication of increased chamber stiffness. The S_4 gallop is associated with atrial contraction – late diastolic filling – and is associated with elevation of the end-diastolic pressures. Both sounds are analogous to tapping a drumhead that is pulled taut. Normally, diastolic compliance is high and the chamber compliance declines if filling is increased. When end-diastolic pressures are elevated, the distensibility declines and one hears a low-pitch sound associated with filling.

3 Heart rate is likely to be increased as a compensation for reduced pump function due to the infarction. This is driven by sympathetic stimulation and vagal withdrawal.

4 Peripheral resistance is likely to be high even though arterial pressures are low. Remember that arterial pressure results from the interaction of the heart with the vascular system, and is not itself a reflection of arterial tone. In this case, reduced cardiac output would have resulted in a much lower arterial pressure had the systemic arteries not constricted. Preload volume is increased, as discussed in answer **1**. If preload volume were increased and peripheral resistance increased in a normal

heart, the arterial pressure would be very elevated. This can be illustrated using pressure–volume loops (see Chapter 14).

5 Systemic vascular resistance (SVR) = (mean arterial pressure, MAP – right atrial pressure, RAP)/CO. From the data given, MAP is 82, RAP is 10 and CO is 3.0. Therefore, SVR = (82 − 10)/3 = 24. The units here are mmHg/L/min which are clinical units, but not those typically used to express resistance. The units that are more often used are dynes/s/cm^{-5}. To convert, you multiply 24 by 80 = 1920. Normal resistance is closer to 1200.

6 Net contractile function is reduced because of the recent heart injury (infarction). The heart after a MI is heterogeneous, with a necrotic non-contractile zone surrounded by compensating regions that are functionally closer to normal. The net effect, however, is still a decline in overall contractile function. Preload is elevated as noted, and afterload resistance increased. To improve cardiac output further and to reduce pulmonary oedema, you need to reduce preload with venodilators and diuretics, and lower afterload resistance with arterial vasodilators. Nitrates are an excellent class of drug for this purpose.

7 Cardiac output would very likely increase, and arterial pressures may not change much. If too much vasodilatation is induced, pressures will decline. However, with careful titration, one can often obtain an improvement in pump performance and coronary perfusion, and actually see a slight increase in pressure as the heart is better perfused.

8 Increasing contractile function is the last resort. One is particularly cautious in using inotropic therapy in a heart attack patient, because it is quite possible to make matters worse by increasing cardiac work and extending the territory of damage. Such patients often have coronary disease in places other than that directly responsible for the heart attack.

9 Blood flow to the left ventricle occurs primarily during diastole, when myocardial pressure surrounding the arterioles is low and arterial perfusion pressure remains elevated (thanks to systemic vascular compliance and wave reflections). During systole, flow through the myocardium is inhibited by ventricular muscle contraction. So, if one had a method to enhance diastolic arterial pressures while simultaneously reducing systolic pressures, you are likely to improve cardiac perfusion while reducing ventricular load during ejection. Such a device exists and is called an **aortic counterpulsation balloon pump**. By inflating a balloon placed in the proximal descending aorta rapidly during diastole and deflating it during systole, you can augment the diastolic perfusion to the heart while improving forward output. In patients with ischaemic heart disease and reduced arterial pressures, this device is very useful indeed.

Concluding remarks

The overall objectives in heart failure are to improve quality of life, lengthen survival and slow progression of the disease. Any underlying causes or precipitating factors should of course be treated as a matter of priority. The main aims of drug treatment are to reduce oedema, increase exercise tolerance, and reduce cardiac work and stimuli leading to myocardial remodelling and hypertrophy. This improves both symptoms and survival in heart failure. In practice, the drug regime should initially involve diuretics and an ACE inhibitor (or AT1 receptor blocker), and gradually increasing doses of β-blockers. Increasingly commonly, an aldosterone antagonist (e.g. spironolactone) (see Chapter 47).

Case 2: Valvular heart disease

1 He is likely to have severe aortic stenosis. The crescendo–decrescendo systolic murmur usually arises from stenosis of either the aortic or pulmonary valve. The stenotic valve creates turbulence during ejection that causes a murmur. The murmur gets louder as flow increases during ejection, then diminishes as flow decreases. This murmur is transmitted to the carotid arteries because of the high velocity of the ejected blood. The apical murmur is probably caused by high-frequency vibration of the aortic valve during ejection and can sometimes be louder than that at the sternal border.

Aortic stenosis causes left ventricular hypertrophy, which displaces the apex beat laterally. The apex beat can be sustained because the ventricle takes longer to empty. The carotid pulse contour reflects flow across the aortic valve. Because peak ejection flow is delayed and decreased in aortic stenosis, the carotid pulses are delayed and diminished.

2 The loudness of murmur depends on *flow* across the valve; therefore it may not reflect the severity of valve stenosis. In the case of aortic stenosis, other physical examination parameters are more indicative of the severity of valve stenosis. As valve area becomes smaller, the peak loudness of the murmur occurs later in systole. This is presumably due to the difficulty in opening the valve. In severe aortic stenosis left ventricular stroke volume is decreased. This manifests as low-amplitude carotid pulsation with a delayed peak (***pulsus parvus et tardus***).

Normally, the aortic valve closes before the pulmonary valve, causing splitting of S_2. During inspiration more blood volume is returned to the right heart and the pulmonary valve closes even later. The increased splitting of S_2 during inspiration is termed physiological splitting. In severe aortic stenosis, the ejection time becomes longer, and the aortic valve closes later. This may eliminate splitting of S_2 (single S_2), or create paradoxical splitting.

If this murmur was previously louder, it would suggest that flow across the valve has decreased as the stenosis worsened. Decrease in flow (lower cardiac output) is an ominous sign of a failing left ventricle or a decrease in valve size. This is not reassuring.

During exercise, blood vessels dilate and peripheral resistance decreases. When the peripheral resistance falls, the blood pressure tends to fall. Normal individuals compensate by increasing stroke volume and heart rate. However, this patient cannot increase his stroke volume because of the tight aortic valve. When blood pressure falls, coronary perfusion decreases and the subendocardial area of the hypertrophied ventricle is not perfused adequately. As heart rate and oxygen demand increase, the supply and demand mismatch may worsen and cause ischaemia. If a significant portion of the myocardium is affected, cardiac output can fall, causing a further drop in coronary perfusion and further worsening ischaemia. This vicious cycle can continue until the patient drops dead, an event that may not look particularly good on your record.

3 The echocardiogram showed uniform left ventricular hypertrophy. His left ventricular ejection fraction was estimated at 45%, and the aortic valve appeared calcified with impaired cusp mobility. Doppler studies showed the peak instantaneous gradient across the aortic valve was 98 mmHg with a mean gradient of 68 mmHg. Estimated aortic valve area was 0.6 cm^2.

The most common cause of aortic stenosis in this age group is calcific degeneration of the aortic cusps. The valvular pathology leads to left ventricular hypertrophy, a pressure gradient and impaired emptying of the chamber, which were all demonstrated on the echocardiogram.

4 Using the formula the estimated valve area is 0.62 cm^2. This formula is a simplified version of the Gorlin formula, which states that the valve area is related to cardiac output, and inversely related to mean pressure gradient, systolic ejection period and the gravitational acceleration constant. In most cases, the systolic ejection period multiplied by the acceleration constant is close to 1, so that term is not used in the estimate formula.

5 This patient's left ventricle (LV) needs all the help it can get to eject an adequate supply of blood through the pinhole-sized aortic valve. Nitroglycerin is primarily a venodilator, and it will pool his blood in the veins. This will reduce blood returning to the heart and decrease preload. Even though the ejection fraction is only 45%, his thick LV still has high contractility and a steep end-systolic pressure–volume relation. This means that he is very sensitive to preload changes, and a slight drop in preload volume can drop blood pressure significantly, which will decrease coronary perfusion, worsen subendocardial ischaemia, decrease systolic dysfunction, lower blood pressure, and so on. Thus, nitrates are a bad idea. Beta-adrenergic blockers or calcium-channel blockers are also not good because they can reduce contractility. Calcium-channel blockers can also dilate peripheral arterioles and reduce blood pressure further.

What *can* you do? You may actually give some fluid to increase preload and increase cardiac output. The other mode of therapy, if the valve cannot be replaced promptly, is intra-aortic balloon counterpulsation. This can improve coronary perfusion in some cases and relieve subendocardial ischaemia.

Concluding remarks

Valve replacement is best performed before development of ventricular dysfunction or pulmonary hypertension. Either tissue (xenografts, commonly from pig) or mechanical valves can be used. Although the latter are harder wearing, they can promote thrombosis, so anticoagulant therapy will be required.

Case 3: Ischaemic heart disease

1 This sounds like angina. The location, radiation and type of discomfort are consistent with cardiac ischaemic pain. However, the traditional dividing line between 'angina' and possible MI is 30 min of discomfort. Because her discomfort lasted more than 30 min, it is possible she suffered an MI, even with a normal ECG. To determine whether an MI occurred, look for evidence of myocardial damage such as cardiac-specific serum enzymes.

2 Her risk factors for CAD are smoking and being postmenopausal. Her family history is *not* positive for premature CAD, because her father was 74 when he had his MI. She does not have hypertension. We do not yet know her cholesterol levels, or whether she is diabetic.

3 Increased serum levels of the cardiac (MB) isoform of creatine kinase and of the cardiac troponins T and I are indicative of myocardial damage. Unlike CK-MB, troponins are selective for cardiac injury, and are therefore now the preferred markers.

4 She does not have unstable angina at this point, and her effort tolerance is reasonable. Such patients have a good prognosis whether they take medicines or have single-vessel angioplasty. A recent study showed that angioplasty was no better than medicines for single-vessel CAD.

5 Her cholesterol was not high, but studies indicate that lowering LDL cholesterol below ~110 mg/dL may stabilize coronary lesions and possibly cause regression of CAD. However, greater effects were seen on reduced incidence of unstable angina or MI. These may be due to reducing the lipid-rich area of plaques and making them less susceptible to rupture.

The most important thing was to stop smoking. Reducing cholesterol is a secondary prevention. Another risk factor is lack of oestrogen. Postmenopausal women with CAD may benefit from hormone replacement therapy.

6 Reasons for exercise testing are diagnosis, prognosis, and to test effectiveness of treatment. Here, we want to know if her anti-anginal regimen is adequate.

7 The ECG shows marked ST segment depression in the precordial (V1–V6) and lateral (I and aVL) leads. She has cardiac ischaemia, due to either unstable angina or an MI. The chest discomfort occurred during sleep, indicating that it is unstable rather then stable angina. She is unlikely to have had an MI, as her cardiac enzymes are not elevated.

Cardiac ischaemia occurs when myocardial oxygen demand exceeds supply. This typically happens with exertion in CAD patients, because blood flow through the stenosis is usually adequate during rest. Rest ischaemia is caused when the oxygen supply falls below that required for even basal myocardial metabolic needs. This implies an occlusion more serious than that caused simply by a structural stenosis. It is believed that unstable angina is initiated by plaque rupture, causing aggregation of platelets and fibrin deposition. This can cause direct occlusion of the artery, and also trigger vasospasm.

8 The angiogram suggests the 'culprit' is the LAD lesion. It is serious enough to cause rest angina. The ECG abnormalities are consistent with the ischaemic area being that served by the LAD. Unstable angina involves platelets and the clotting cascade. Thus it makes sense to use inhibitors of platelet aggregation such as aspirin and clopidogrel. Clot formation and dissolution are dynamic processes, and although antiplatelet drugs cannot directly disperse clots, they can promote resolution. Thrombolytics make theoretical sense, but are not used because in trials no improvement in outcome of unstable angina patients was seen, and morbidity was *higher*.

Case 4: Arrhythmias (1)

1 The ventricular rate is 150 beats/min. The narrow QRS complex implies that the tachycardia is supraventricular. The differential diagnosis for this tachycardia includes AV nodal re-entrant tachycardia, atrial flutter or sinus tachycardia. Atrial fibrillation is unlikely because the rhythm is regular.

2 Carotid sinus massage demonstrates the sawtooth pattern of flutter waves, particularly in the inferior leads (II, III, aVF). This proves that the initial rhythm was atrial flutter with 2 : 1 conduction (i.e. only one of every two atrial waves is conducted through the AVN to the ventricle). Because the flutter waves have a rate of nearly 300 beats/min, the ventricular rate is 150 beats/min. Carotid sinus massage increases vagal tone, slowing conduction through the AVN and increasing AV block.

3 Beta-blockers, digoxin, Ca^{2+}-channel blockers and adenosine slow conduction through the AVN. This slows the ventricular rate, allowing adequate time for left ventricular filling, and relieving the symptoms of left heart failure (shortness of breath, weakness, orthopnoea).

4 This is atrial fibrillation; note the irregularly irregular ventricular rate. Atrial flutter is an unstable rhythm, and commonly degenerates into atrial fibrillation.

5 Yes. Amiodarone and digoxin are commonly used to treat atrial arrhythmias. Digoxin helps to slow the ventricular rate by increasing vagal tone at the AVN. Amiodarone similarly helps to slow the ventricular response. Amiodarone is also used to cardiovert patients with atrial arrhythmias back into sinus rhythm and/or help maintain sinus rhythm once they have been electrically cardioverted.

6 Patients with intermittent or persistent atrial fibrillation should receive anticoagulation because of the risk of embolic stroke. In this patient, who seems to be having his first episode of atrial fibrillation, electrical cardioversion should be attempted if amiodarone does not convert the rhythm to sinus.

Case 5: Arrhythmias (2)

1 This indicates a moderate murmur of mitral regurgitation (see Chapters 30, 53).

2 This rhythm is most likely ventricular in origin. When a patient has a wide-complex tachycardia, the differential diagnosis is ventricular tachycardia (VT) vs supraventricular tachycardia with aberrant conduction (i.e. the tachycardia is conducted with a bundle branch block). A wide variety of clinical and ECG criteria aid in distinguishing between these possibilities. The most important clinical criterion is whether the patient has a history of heart disease (see below). If this is the case, and in particular if there is a history of MI, the most likely origin of the tachycardia is ventricular, because an infarct creates a substrate for re-entry. ECG criteria which suggest a ventricular origin include: (i) a very wide QRS complex; (ii) an extreme axis; (iii) evidence of atrial–ventricular dissociation; (iv) certain specific QRS morphologies. This patient's QRS morphology is that of a right bundle. Note the terminal S waves in V6, and the R in V1. The extreme axis, the very wide QRS duration and the morphology (R/S < 1 in V6 and the large primary R in V1) suggest the rhythm is VT.

3 He is short of breath and hypotensive because the tachycardia does not allow enough time for ventricular filling. Therefore, cardiac output is low, causing hypotension, and left atrial pressure is high. The high left atrial pressure has backed up into his pulmonary capillaries, causing pulmonary oedema and breathlessness. His increased JVP is caused by raised central venous pressure, indicative of inadequate right ventricular function. His arrhythmia is therefore causing congestive heart failure.

4 Treatment requires cardioversion to sinus rhythm with either appropriate drugs (lidocaine, procainamide or amiodarone) or electrical cardioversion. Because this patient's symptoms indicate that his arrhythmia is causing his heart to fail, immediate conversion to sinus rhythm is mandatory. Therefore in this case electrical cardioversion is preferable.

5 The rhythm is now sinus, with the rate of 95 beats/min.

6 He has evidence on his ECG of an inferior wall MI (note the Q waves in leads II, III, aVF with slight ST elevation). The aetiology of his ventricular tachycardia is likely to be re-entry into left ventricular (LV) scar caused by an undetected recent acute MI.

7 Following stabilization, appropriate treatment includes evaluation of LV function and of coronary anatomy.

Concluding remarks

In this case, the patient had severe inoperable coronary artery disease and poor LV function. Because a poor ejection fraction identifies high risk for recurrent VT and sudden death, the patient underwent electrophysiology testing and was readily inducible into hypotensive VT. This indicated: (i) that he was at a high risk of spontaneously developing VT again; and (ii) that his tachycardia was fast enough to lower his cardiac output dangerously. His already poor LV function meant that he would not be able to tolerate tachycardia. He therefore subsequently underwent successful placement of an internal cardioverter-defibrillator and has since been stable.

Case 6: Haemorrhage and shock

Note: Refer to Chapter 29 for all answers.

1 and 2 The loss of blood is obvious, but the cold, clammy skin, high heart rate and confusion are strongly suggestive of cardiovascular shock. Reduced blood volume will lead to activation of the baroreceptor reflex which may allow blood pressure to be maintained by vasoconstriction and diversion of blood from the periphery and splanchnic circulations. Sympathetic activation of the skin also causes sweating, and thus the clamminess. If the fall in blood pressure is sufficient, reduced blood flow through the carotid bodies would cause chemoreceptor activation and an increase in rate of breathing, although in this case it may be just anxiety. Reduced blood flow also causes acidosis which will similarly activate the chemoreceptors. The disorientation, especially initially when standing, could be due to reduced cerebral perfusion and consequent hypoxia, but the bruising to the forehead might indicate some concussion.

3 Bill's haematocrit is towards the bottom of the normal range for males (0.43 compared to the normal value of ~0.47). He could be normally slightly anaemic, but this might reflect haemodilution due to movement of fluid from the tissues into the blood (internal transfusion). As the latter takes place over a few hours, this would suggest that the accident occurred at least a couple of hours ago. He may also have drunk a lot of fluids. It is likely that Bill and John delayed coming to the hospital because they were afraid of being caught for joy-riding and drunk-driving.

4 Bill's blood group is AB, and as his red blood cells therefore have both A and B antigens (agglutinogens), he has no antibodies (agglutinins) to either. He can therefore receive blood of any group. People of group AB are often called universal recipients, and those of group O universal donors. However, in massive transfusions agglutinins in the donor blood could reach a level to cause problems, and close matching is required unless these have been previously removed.

5 John was also involved in the accident. You initially noted he was pale and obviously uncomfortable, and soon after he said he felt dizzy and nauseous. As a minimum, you should have asked whether he had suffered any injury himself. It later transpires of course that he has also lost a significant amount of blood to internal bleeding; early correction might well have prevented the later complications.

6 (See Chapter 27) Activation of the baroreceptor reflex leads to increased activity of renal sympathetic nerves, and therefore release of renin and consequently increased production of angiotensin II. The fall in blood volume and reduction in atrial stretch receptor activation may also have been sufficient to cause increased production of ADH. Both ADH and angiotensin II are strong stimulators of thirst.

It is clear that John's cardiac output and blood pressure must have been low, leading to insufficient cerebral perfusion and consequent hypoxia. This would impair cognitive function, leading to behavioural differences, slurred speech and unsteadiness – not dissimilar to the effects of alcohol. Moreover, it is clear that he had been drinking as he smelt of alcohol.

7 (See Chapter 25) John's blood pressure and central venous pressure when lying down are being maintained by the baroreceptor reflex, peripheral vasoconstriction and venoconstriction. On standing, blood pools to the legs and because the baroreceptor reflex is now unable to provide any further support for central venous pressure, cardiac output falls due to Starling's law of the heart, and consequently so does blood pressure. He faints because this is insufficient to maintain adequate cerebral perfusion.

8 (See Chapters 18, 27) A fall in capillary pressure due to a generalized arterial vasoconstriction will reduce the hydrostatic pressure, so that the plasma oncotic pressure due to proteins now predominates, with the result that fluid moves from the interstitial space into the tissues (internal transfusion). This will, however, cause haemodilution, and so reduce the haematocrit. Urine production is severely reduced because vasoconstriction of the renal afferent arterioles, activation of the renin–angiotensin axis and increased production of ADH reduce renal filtration and increase reabsorption of Na^+ and water.

9 In view of the volume of blood loss and the delayed treatment, John would need ongoing observation to exclude underlying ischaemia in other organs. Typically, the gut is most affected by this type of ischaemia, which then allows translocation of bacteria from the bowel to the blood, causing sepsis that can then cause multiorgan failure (MOF) and irreversible shock. However, it would be unusual for a young man to go into MOF this quickly (although less so in a 75-year-old man). MOF usually occurs after some time in intensive care.

10 Prolonged activation of the sympathetic system with vasoconstriction of the renal circulation can lead to renal ischaemia, and 'acute renal necrosis'. The renal medulla is particularly sensitive to ischaemia and hypoxia, as the counter-current system of the vasa recta means that the Po_2 of the deep medulla is relatively hypoxic even under normal conditions. In acute renal necrosis function normally returns in 3–21 days; renal replacement therapy (dialysis or haemofiltration) might be necessary if function was still impaired after 4–5 days.

11 (See Chapter 19) Prolonged vasoconstriction can lead to peripheral ischaemia and raised metabolites, damaging the vascular endothelium and causing it to become leaky to plasma proteins. Movement of these proteins into the interstitium would reduce the net oncotic pressure across the capillary wall, leading to fluid loss to the tissues. If he received saline instead of blood or plasma during the operation, the resulting haemodilution and thus decreased plasma protein concentration would also reduce oncotic pressure and thus lead to fluid loss to the tissues. Plasma proteins are synthesized in the liver, and it takes around a week for normal levels to be restored.

12 (See Chapter 6) About 3 weeks, due to increased erythropoietin and thus erythropoiesis.

Concluding remarks

This case emphasizes the need for suspicion of internal injury and blood loss following trauma. Both the amount and rate of blood loss are important. A very rapid loss of ~30% can be fatal, where 50% over 24 h may be survived. The risk of developing irreversible shock is drastically increased if treatment is not initiated within the 'golden hour' after major haemorrhage.

Case 7: Hypertension

1 You diagnose hypertension associated with type 2 diabetes (DM2). These conditions, in addition to his low HDL, high triglycerides and obesity (BMI = 31), are consistent with a diagnosis of the **metabolic syndrome**. You advise him to stop smoking, reduce his alcohol intake (21 units per week is the maximum recommended intake for men; 14 units per week for women) and follow a diabetic diet, in which daily sodium intake does not exceed 6 g. You also prescribe him a statin and an antihypertensive agent.

2 Although antihypertensive drug therapy in non-diabetics is appropriate if the systolic reading is sustained at > 160 mmHg, or the diastolic reading is > 100 mmHg, in DM2 patients therapy should be commenced at lower pressures (> 140 mmHg systolic and/or > 90 mmHg diastolic), with the aim of reducing BP to < 130/80 mmHg.

3 There are a number of mechanisms by which the hyperinsulinaemia and insulin resistance characteristic of DM2 may cause hypertension. For example, glycosylation of proteins caused by hyperglycaemia is thought to lead to cross-linking of collagen and loss of elasticity of major arteries, which can result in systolic hypertension. Moreover, insulin resistance and hyperinsulinaemia are associated with hypertension because high insulin levels suppress renal Na^+ excretion and stimulate the sympathetic nervous system (see Chapter 38).

4 You prescribe an ACEI. A meta-analysis (Pahor *et al.* (2000) *Diabetes Care* 23: 888–92) of four clinical trials comparing the efficacy of ACEI in DM2 versus other antihypertensives revealed ACEI to be superior. However, the long-held belief that ACEI are especially beneficial in diabetics, due to their *renoprotective* benefit, in addition to their blood pressure-lowering effect, is being challenged. A meta-analysis (Casas *et al.* (2005) *The Lancet* 366: 2026–33) suggests ACEI do not confer renoprotection.

5 The pulse pressure is the most accurate predictor of a cardiovascular event. A wide pulse pressure largely reflects a high systolic level. At all ages systolic pressure is more predictive of risk than is diastolic, and this is especially important in the elderly.

6 Diabetics have a 2–5 times higher chance of dying from coronary heart disease than do non-diabetics, depending on whether other risk factors are also present. About two in every three people with diabetes will die of cardiovascular disease.

In the Joint British Societies' guidelines, diabetes is judged to confer the risk equivalent to established CHD.

7 Since his blood pressure is inadequately controlled on one antihypertensive, he needs additional therapy. He should receive a thiazide diuretic, such as bendroflumethiazide (2.5 mg/day), because thiazides are associated with reduced stroke mortality, and this benefit offsets the concerns that thiazides, at least in large doses, may reduce glucose tolerance. The combination of an ACEI with a thiazide is particularly attractive, as the ACEI will inhibit the diuretic-stimulated activation of the renin–angiotensin-system and the K^+-sparing activity of the ACEI may protect against cardiac mortality.

8 You prescribe a long-acting calcium-channel blocker (CCB). The HOT and Syst-Eur trials found that treatment of hypertension in diabetics with a CCB reduced cardiovascular mortality, and the ASCOT trial reported that the combination of the CCB amlodipine with the ACEI perindopril was more effective in reducing mortality than the combination of a β-blocker and a thiazide diuretic.

Since he does not have proteinuria (an indicator of renal disease), you select a CCB from the dihydropyridine class: amlodipine. (If he did have > 300 mg per day proteinuria, you would select a non-dihydropyridine, such as verapamil, as some dihydropyridines worsen proteinuria.)

9 You add in a low-dose β-blocker, such as bisoprolol (2.5 mg/day).

10 You prescribe metformin, and if this fails to reduce blood glucose, then you add in rosiglitazone.

Concluding remarks

There has long been a recognized relationship between diabetes and hypertension and the **metabolic syndrome** encompasses these distinct conditions, along with hyperinsulinaemia, reduced HDL cholesterol, hypertriglyceridaemia and central obesity. The metabolic syndrome is defined as more than three of the following: hypertension; diabetes mellitus; BMI > 30; triglycerides > 1.69 mM; HDL cholesterol < 1.04 mM.

Hypertension is extremely common in DM2, affecting up to 75%. Aggressive hypertension control reduces macro- and microvascular risks, such as decreased visual acuity and end-stage renal disease. The risk reduction seen in diabetics with hypertension is substantially greater than in the general population with similar levels of blood pressure.

In the HOT study, a reduction in diastolic blood pressure of 4 mmHg resulted in a 50% decrease in cardiovascular events in patients with diabetes. Non-diabetics participating in the same trial received much less benefit after the same drop in diastolic pressure.

The priority of diabetes treatment in terms of *macrovascular* disease lies not in the control of blood glucose but in the control of hypertension. Glycaemic control is much more effective in reducing *microvascular* complications (retinopathy, nephropathy and neuropathy).

Case 8: Pulmonary embolism

1 The most likely diagnosis is recurrent small pulmonary emboli as this patient is at high risk due to immobility and the need for a plaster cast, lower limb trauma with potential vascular damage and the clinical history of recurrent short-lived episodes of hypotension. Although less likely, chest infection, arrhythmias and ischaemic heart disease are other possibilities that should be considered.

2 Arterial blood gas abnormalities are common following a pulmonary embolus, including hypoxaemia with a widening of the alveolar–arterial (A–a) gradient, hypoxaemia and hypocapnia (despite increased dead space). In the majority of patients the ECG is not helpful and shows non-specific ST segment changes. However, about one-third of patients with large pulmonary emboli develop a right ventricular strain pattern with the classical changes of an S wave in lead I and a Q wave and T wave inversion in lead III ($S_1Q_3T_3$ pattern), right axis deviation and right bundle branch block. Most patients have non-specific abnormalities on chest X-ray including atelectasis due to reduced surfactant production in areas of poorly perfused lung. The presence of a lower limb deep venous thrombosis (DVT) should be sought with a Doppler ultrasound scan (or impedance plethysmography). Echocardiography may show right ventricular dysfunction and pulmonary hypertension. A transoesophageal echocardiograph may detect emboli in the main pulmonary arteries but not in lobar or segmental arteries.

A V/Q scan is usually the initial diagnostic investigation. A negative perfusion scan rules out a pulmonary embolus, whereas a 'high-probability' scan (i.e. multiple segmental perfusion defects and associated normal ventilation) has a > 85% probability of a pulmonary embolus. With a high clinical suspicion, a high-probability V/Q scan has a positive predictive value > 95%. Unfortunately, most V/Q scans are not diagnostic or are indeterminate with a 15–50% likelihood of pulmonary embolism, necessitating further imaging. Absence of a DVT combined with a low-probability V/Q scan permits withholding treatment, whereas a negative Doppler ultrasound scan with an intermediate-probability V/Q scan (or underlying cardiac or pulmonary disease) necessitates further imaging. Spiral CT scans have a sensitivity for pulmonary embolus of 70–95% (higher for more proximal emboli) and a specificity > 90%. CT also allows visualization of parenchymal abnormalities and is useful in patients with COPD or extensive chest X-ray abnormalities where V/Q scanning is indeterminate. MRI scans are more specific and sensitive but not widely available. Pulmonary angiography remains the diagnostic standard but is invasive.

3 Patients with pulmonary embolism present with pleuritic pain and haemoptysis in about 65% of cases, isolated dyspnoea occurs in about 25% and circulatory collapse in about 10% of cases. Dyspnoea is not present in about 30% of patients with confirmed pulmonary embolism. Other non-specific features include apprehension, tachypnoea, tachycardia, cough, sweating and syncope. Following a large pulmonary embolus features of right ventricular failure (e.g. hypotension, jugular venous distension) may occur.

4 Anticoagulation stops propagation of existing lower limb thrombus and allows organization of the remaining clot, which reduces the risk of further emboli. Immediate therapy in patients with a high suspicion of a pulmonary embolus may prevent further life-threatening emboli. Unfractionated heparin (UH) or low molecular weight heparin (LMWH) for 5–7 days, is followed by warfarin for 4–6 weeks when temporary risk factors (as in this case) are the cause and for 3–6 months in idiopathic cases. UH and warfarin must be monitored, as subtherapeutic levels increase the risk of recurrent thromboembolism. LMWH is more bioavailable and does not require monitoring. About 20% of patients with thromboembolic disease have inherited or acquired hypercoagulation problems (e.g. antithrombin III deficiency, protein C deficiency, lupus anticoagulant) and may require lifelong therapy. If contraindications prevent anticoagulation (e.g. recent surgery, haemorrhagic stroke, CNS metastases, active bleeding) or emboli occur whilst on therapeutic anticoagulation, an inferior vena cava filter may prevent further pulmonary embolism.

5 The CT scan in Figure Case 8 confirms the presence of pulmonary emboli in both pulmonary arteries. A single, sudden, large embolus with marked obstruction of pulmonary blood flow is the likely cause of the cardiac arrest. In general, circulatory collapse occurs with > 50% obstruction of the pulmonary arterial bed. Smaller emboli may be fatal when pre-existing lung or heart disease coexist. Cardiopulmonary resuscitation must be started immediately. The cardiac massage may help break up a large clot into smaller segments which travel distally and reduce the degree of pulmonary bed occlusion. Following intubation high-dose oxygen must be administered. Immediate plasma expanders and inotropic support are often given in an attempt to increase right ventricular pressure and to displace clot distally, but risks of right ventricular distension and subsequent myocardial damage are severe.

6 Thrombolytic therapy is recommended in severe life-threatening massive pulmonary embolism with cardiovascular collapse. Thrombolytics hasten resolution of perfusion defects and correct right ventricular dysfunction, but there is limited evidence of survival benefit. Nevertheless, they would have been appropriate in this patient with life-threatening cardiovascular collapse. In patients without massive pulmonary embolism there is no survival benefit with thrombolysis and there is a substantial increase in bleeding complications, including a 0.3–1.5% risk of intracerebral haemorrhage. Consequently thrombolysis is not recommended in these patients.

Index

Page numbers in *italics* represent figures, those in **bold** represent tables

abciximab 99
abdominal examination 69
ABO system 24
absolute refractory period 2
acetylcholine 61
actin 13, 17, 30
action potential 28–9
  Na$^+$-Ca^{2+} exchange 29
  upstroke velocity 33
activated partial thromboplastin time 23
active transport 27
acute coronary syndromes 90
acute respiratory distress syndrome 67
adenosine 51, 55, 111
adenosine deaminase 51
ADMA 53, 75
ADP 23
adrenal medulla 61
adrenaline *see epinephrine*
adrenergic receptors 61
afterload 39
agglutination 24
Akt 52
albumin 19
aldosterone 63, 67, 101
alpha$_1$-receptor blockers 83
amiloride 103
amiodarone 111
amlodipine 77, 83, 89
anaemia *20*, 21, 115
  see also different types
anaphylactic shock 67
anatomy
  heart *12*, 13
  vascular system 14–15, *14*
aneurysm 41, 80
angina 69, 113
  drug treatment 88–9, *88*
  Prinzmetal's 87, 90–1, *90*
  stable/exertional 81, 86–7, *86*
  variant 86–7, *86*
angiography 71, 87, 113
angiotensin I 63, 101
angiotensin II 35, 63, 67, 101
angiotensin receptor blockers 76–7, *76*, 83, 102
angiotensin-converting enzyme 53, 63
angiotensin-converting enzyme inhibitors 76–7, *76*, 83, 91, 97, 102, 115
angiotensinogen 63
anistreplase 99
annulus fibrosus *12*, 13, 33, 73
anti-D agglutinin 25
anticoagulants 97, 98–9, *98*, 113, 115
antidiuretic hormone 59, 62, 63
antiphospholipid syndrome 23
α$_2$-antiplasmin 23
antiplatelet therapy 97, 99
antithrombin 23
aortic arch 15, 58
aortic regurgitation 113
aortic stenosis 112–13, *112*
aortic valve 37

aplastic anaemia 21
apo A1 78
apo(a) 74
apolipoproteins 78
apoproteins 78
arrhythmias 104–5, *104*, 120, *120*, 125–6
  atrial fibrillation 107
  atrial flutter 107
  atrial tachycardia 106
  atrioventricular nodal re-entrant tachycardia 107
  atrioventricular re-entrant tachycardia 107
  fascicular tachycardia 109
  non-pharmacological treatment 109
  paroxysmal supraventricular tachycardia 107
  pharmacological treatment 110–11, *110*, **110**
  right ventricular outflow tract tachycardia 109
  supraventricular tachycardia 106–7, *106*
  triggered 104
  ventricular fibrillation 108, 109
  ventricular tachycardia 108
arterial anastomoses 15
arterial blood pressure 42
arteries *10*, 11, *14*, 15, 42–3, *42*
  see also individual arteries
arterioles 11, 15, 42–3, *42*, **43**, 44
arteriosinusoidal vessels *12*, 13
arteriovenous anastomoses 55
ascites 101
aspirin 91, 96
atenolol 76, 111
atherosclerosis 53, 80–1, *80*
  fatty streaks 80
atherosclerotic plaques 80
atorvastatin 79
atrial conduction 33
atrial fibrillation 107, 114
atrial flutter 107
atrial hypertrophy 114
atrial natriuretic peptide 63, 67
atrial septal defects 117
atrial systole 37
atrial tachycardia 106
atrioventricular nodal re-entrant tachycardia 107
atrioventricular node *12*, 13, 29, 33, 61
atrioventricular re-entrant tachycardia 107
atrium 11
auscultation 69
Austin-Flint murmur 113
autocoids 51
automaticity, abnormal 104
autonomic nervous system *38*, 39, 60–1, *60*
  parasympathetic system *60*, 61
  sympathetic system *60*, 61, 102
autonomic reflexes 58, 65
autoregulation 50–1
azimilide 111

Bachman tract 33
Bainbridge reflex 59
balloon valvuloplasty 113
baroreceptors 58, 67

baroreceptor reflex 58, 101
basal lamina 17
basilar and carotid arteries 55
basophils 19
beta-blockers 76–7, *76*, 83, 89, 91, 97, 102, 111
bezafibrate 79
Bezold-Jarisch effect 59
bile acid sequestrants 79
bilirubin 21
biliverdin 21
bipolar leads 73
bisoprolol 76, 102–3
bleeding time 23
blood 11
  constituents of *18*, 19
  ionic composition 19
  proteins 19
  storage 25
blood cells 19
blood flow, local control 50–1, *50*
blood groups 24–5, *24*
  ABO system 24
  Rh system 24–5
blood pressure *68*, 69
  arterial 42
  arteries 42–3
blood transfusion 24–5, *24*
  haemolytic transfusion reaction 25
blood vessels 11
blood viscosity 41
blood volume 11, *18*, 62–3, *62*
blood-brain barrier 17, 45
bone marrow 19
Bowditch effect 31
brachiocephalic artery 15
bradyarrhythmias 106
bradycardia 33
bradykinin 51, 55, 77
breathlessness 68–9, 101, 114
bronchial circulation 56
Brugada syndrome 109
bruits 69
bumetanine 103
bundle branch block 33
bundle of His 33
bundle of Kent 105

c wave 37
C-reactive protein 75
calcium channels, voltage-sensitive 29, 30
calcium channel blockers 76–7, *76*, 89, 91
calcium extrusion 35
calcium influx 35
calcium overload 31
calcium sensitization 35
calcium sequestration 35
calcium-activated chloride channels 35
calcium-activated potassium channels 35
calcium-ATPase 31
calcium-channel blockers 83
calcium-induced calcium release 30
calmodulin 34
calsequestrin 30
candesartan 77
capacitance vessels 49

capillaries *10*, 11, 17, 44
  continuous 17
  discontinuous 17, 45
  fenestrated 17, 45
  solute exchange 44–5, 47
capillary recruitment 64
captopril 77, 83
cardiac cycle 36–7, *36*
cardiac dilatation 101
cardiac failure 96
cardiac glycosides 31, 103
  see also digoxin
cardiac muscle
  action potential 28–9, *28*
  excitation-contraction coupling 30–1, *30*
cardiac myocytes 13
cardiac output 38–9, *38*
cardiogenic shock 67, 96
cardiopulmonary reflex 58
cardiothoracic ratio 71
cardiovascular reflexes 58–9, *58*
cardioversion 107, 109
carotid sinuses 58
carvedilol 76, 103
catecholamines 61
catheterization 71
cell membrane 27
central command *64*, 65
central cyanosis 116
central venous pressure 39, 49
cerebral arteries 55
cerebral circulation 54–5, *54*
cerebral ischaemia 51
cerebrospinal fluid 55
charge separation 27
chemoreceptors 65, 67
chemoreceptor reflex 58
chemotaxis 19
chest examination 69
chest pain 69
chest radiography 71
cholera 67
cholesterol 78
cholesteryl esters 78
cholestipol 79
cholestyramine 79
cholinergic sympathetic fibres 55
chordae tendineae *12*, 13, 114
Christmas disease 23
chronotropic agents 29, 39
chylomicrons 78
chylomicron remnants 78
chymase 77
ciprofibrate 79
circadian variation 95
circle of Willis 55
circumflex artery *12*, 13
circumventricular organs 45
circus movement 105
claudication 69
clofibrate 79
clopidogrel 91, 99
clotting *22*, 23
coagulation cascade 23
coagulation necrosis 95
collagen 17
collapsing pulse 113
collateral circulation 15
collateral vessels 88
colloid osmotic pressure 18, 47
common carotid artery 15

common iliac artery 15
compliance 37, 49
conduction pathways *32*, 33
congenital heart disease 116–17, *116*
congestive heart failure 101
connexons 13, 17, 33
continuous capillaries 17
contractility 37, 39
cor pulmonale 101
coronary arteries *12*, 13, 54
coronary artery bypass grafting 92, 93
coronary chemoreflex 59
coronary circulation *10*, *12*, 13, 54–5, *54*
coronary heart disease 74
coronary reserve 101
coronary sinus *12*, 13, 54
coronary veins *12*, 13
cortisol 59
creatine kinase 96
crossbridging 30–1
crystalloid osmotic pressure 18
Cushing reflex 55, 59
cutaneous circulation 54–5, *54*
cyclic AMP 35
cyclic AMP-dependent protein kinase 35
cyclic GMP-dependent protein kinase 35
cyclooxygenase 23, 99
cytokines 81, 94
cytoskeleton 17

D-dimers 23
Darcy's law 40
decompensation 101
delayed afterdepolarizations 105
dense bands 17
dense bodies 17
dense granules 19, 23
desmin 17
desmosomes 13
diabetes mellitus 53, 75
diacylglycerol 35
diads 13
diastole 37
diastolic failure 101
diastolic pressure *10*, 11
diastolic run-off 43
dicrotic notch 37
diffusion 44
digoxin 27, 31, 102, 103, 111
dihydropyridines 30
diltiazem 77, 83, 111
dimethylarginine dimethylaminohydrolase 53
discontinuous capillaries 17, 45
disopyramide 111
disseminated intravascular coagulation 23, 67
diuretics 103
dobutamine 102
dofetilide 111
dominance 29
dopamine 102
Doppler ultrasound 71
dorsal motor nucleus 59, 61
ductus arteriosus 57, 116
ductus venosus 57
dyslipidaemias 74
dyspnoea 68–9, 101, 114

early afterdepolarizations 104
echocardiography 71

Einthoven's triangle 73
Eisenmenger's syndrome 117
ejection 37
ejection fraction 37, 39, 101
elastin 17
electrical axis 73
electrical conduction 32–3, *32*
electrocardiogram 72–3, *72*
electrochemical gradient 27
electronic pacemakers 109
electrophysiology *28*, 29
emboli 99
enalopril 77, 83
end-diastolic pressure 37, 39
end-diastolic volume 37, 39
end-systolic volume 37
endocardium *12*, 13
endothelial cells 17
endothelin 35
endothelin-1 52, 53
endothelium 13, 17, 52–3, *52*
endothelium-derived hyperpolarizing factor 52
endothelium-derived relaxing factor *see* nitric oxide
eosinophils 19
epicardium *12*, 13
epinephrine 31, 61, 67
eplerenone 83, 103
eptifibatide 99
erythrityl tetranitrate 88
erythroblastosis fetalis 21, 25
erythroblasts 20
erythrocyte sedimentation rate 19
erythrocytes 11, 19
  hypochromic 21
  microcytic 21
erythropoiesis 20–1, *20*, 21, 67
erythropoietin 20
ethacrynic acid 103
everolimus 93
exchange vessels 17, 44
excitation-contraction coupling
  cardiac muscle 30–1, *30*
  vascular smooth muscle 34–5, *34*
exercise 64–5, *64*, **64**
  training 65
exercise stress test 87
exercise tolerance test 73

face and neck, examination 69
factor IX 23
factor X 23
factor XIIIa 23
Fåhraeus-Lindqvist effect 41
Fanconi's anaemia 21
fascicular tachycardia 109
felodipine 77, 89
fenestrae 17, 45
fenestrated capillaries 17, 45
fenofibrate 79
ferritin 21
fetal circulation 56–7, *56*
fibrates 79
fibrin *22*, 23
fibrin monomers 23
fibrinogen 19, 23
fibrinolysis *22*, 23, 97, 99
fibroblasts 95
fibrous cap 80
filling pressure 39

fixed risk factors 75
flecainide 111
flow 40–1
fluid filtration 46–7, *46*
fluvastatin 79
foam cells 81
folate 21
folate deficiency 21
fondaparinux 99
foramen ovale 57, 116
Frank-Starling relationship 39
functional re-entry 105
functional syncytium 13
furosemide 103

G-protein-mediated pathways 35
gallop rhythm 69, 101
gap junctions 13, 17, 28, 33
    myoendothelial 53
gated acquisition 71
gating 27
gemfibrazole 79
Gibbs-Donnan equilibrium 27
globulin 19
glycocalyx 17
glycoprotein IIb/IIIa antagonists 91
glycoprotein receptors 23
golden hour 67
Goldman equation 27
granulation tissue 95
granulocytes 19

haemoconcentration 67
haemodynamics 40–1, *40, 41*
haemoglobin *20*, 21
haemoglobinopathies 21
haemolysis 24, 25
haemolytic anaemia 21
haemolytic disease of newborn 21, 25
haemolytic jaundice 25
haemolytic transfusion reaction 25
haemophilia A 23
haemoptysis 114
haemorrhage 66–7, *66*, 120–1, 126–7
haemorrhagic shock 67
haemostasis *22, 23*
    anti-haemostatic therapy 98–99
    defects in 23
    inhibitors 23
    suppression of 25
hands, examination 69
heart *10*, 11
    anatomy *12*, 13
    catecholamine effects 61
    electrical conduction 32–3, *32*
heart beat *28*, 29
heart block 29, 33
    second-degree 33
    third-degree 33
heart failure 100–1, *100*, 118, 123–4
    treatment 102–3, *102*
heart murmurs *see* murmurs
heart rate 31, 86
    exercise 64
heart sounds 37, 69
heart valves 37
    defects 69
    see also valvular heart disease; and
        individual valves
heparin 23, 91, 99
hepatic failure 67

hepatomegaly 69, 101
hereditary haemolytic anaemia 21
high-density lipoprotein 75, 78
histamine 51
history and examination 68–9, *68*
HMG-CoA reductase inhibitors 75, 79
Holter test 73
homocysteine 75
hydralazine 102
hydrophilic 44
hydrops fetalis 21, 25
hydrostatic force 47
hydrostatic pressure 47
hydroxy-methylglutaryl coenzyme A
    reductase 78
hypercapnia 51
hypercholesterolaemia 79
hyperkalaemia 29
hyperkinesis 95
hyperlipidaemias 78–9, *78*
    Frederickson/WHO classification 79
hyperosmolarity 51, 55
hypertension 121–2, 127
    consequences of 85
    isolated systolic 82
    mechanisms 84–5, *84*
    secondary 85
    treatment 82–3, *82*, **83**
hypertriglyceridaemia 79
hypocapnia 51, 55, 57, 59
hypokalaemia 29, 103
hypokinesis 95
hypothalamic osmoreceptors 62
hypovolumic shock 67
hypoxia 51, 55, 57, 59
hypoxic pulmonary vasoconstriction 57

ibutilide 111
iliac arteries 15
imaging 71
implantable defibrillators 108, 109
infarction 94
    see also myocardial infarction
infective endocarditis 113, 115
inferior vena cava 15
injury currents 73
inorganic phosphate 51
inositol triphosphate 35
inotropic agents 31, 39
insulin resistance 75, 85
integrins 17, 51
intercalated discs *12*, 13, 33
intercostal arteries *14*, 15
intermediate-density lipoprotein 75, 78
intermediolateral columns of spinal cord 61
internal carotid arteries 55
international normalized ratio 23, 99
intimal hyperplasia 93
intraortic balloon counterpulsation 97
intrinsic factor 21
investigations 70–1, *70*
    see also electrocardiogram
ion channels *26*, 27
ion exchangers 27
ion pumps *26*, 27
ionic current 27
iron deficiency 21
ischaemic heart disease 101, 119–20,
    120, 125
isosorbide dinitrate 88, 102
isosorbide mononitrate 88

isovolumetric contraction 37
isovolumetric relaxation 37
ivabradine 89

jaundice 21, 25
    haemolytic 25
jugular venous pressure 69, 115
jugular venous pulse 37

kininase II 63

lactic acid 51
lamellae 17
laminar flow 41
Laplace/Frank law 41, 101
latent pacemakers 104
left axis deviation 73
left heart failure 101
left ventricular contractility 86
left ventricular hypertrophy 75
leucocytes *see* white blood cells
lidocaine 111
light chains 34
lipids 78
lipophilic 44
lipoproteins 74, 78, 81
lipoprotein (a) 74
lipoprotein lipase 78
lisinopril 77, 83
long QT syndrome 109
losartan 77, 83, 102
lovastatin 79
low molecular weight heparin 91, 99
low-density lipoprotein 74, 78
    oxidized 81
low-resistance shock 67
lung crackles 115
lymph nodes 45
lymphatic system *14*, 15, 44–5, *44*
lymphocytes 19

macrophages 19, *20*, 81, 94
magnetic resonance imaging 71
mean arterial blood pressure 11
mean cell haemoglobin 19
mean cell haemoglobin concentration 19, 21
mean cell volume 19, 21
mechanoreceptors 58, 65
megakaryocytes 19
megaloblasts 21
megaloblastic anaemia 21
membrane depolarization 35
membrane potential *26*, 27
metabolic hyperaemia 51, 55, 65
metabolic syndrome 75, 79
metabolic vasodilatation 50
metalloproteases 94
metarterioles 44
metoprolol 76, 102
mevastatin 79
mexilitine 111
microcirculation 15, 44–5, *44*
    fluid filtration in 46–7, *46*
    organization of 44
microcytic hypochromic anaemia 21
milrenone 102
mitochondrial aldehyde dehydrogenase 88
mitral regurgitation 96, 115
mitral stenosis 114–15, *114*
mitral valve 37
modifiable risk factors 74–5, **74**

monocytes 19, 81
morphine 97
moxonidine 83
multiorgan failure 67
murmurs 37, 69, 113, 115
myocardial hypertrophy 101
myocardial infarction 73
  clinical aspects 96–7, *96*
  non-ST elevation 90–1
  pathophysiology 94–5, *94*
  silent 96
  ST elevation 90
myocardial stunning 95
myocardium *12, 13*
  structure 13
myoendothelial gap junctions 53
myogenic response 51
myosin 13, 17, 30
myosin light-chain kinase 34
myosin light-chain phosphatase 34

natriuresis 63
natriuretic factor 84–5
necrosis 94
Nernst equation 27
neurogenic model of hypertension 85
neurohumoral system 101
neutrophils 19, 95
niacin 79
nicorandil 89
nicotinic acid 79
nicotinic receptors 61
nifedipine 30, 77, 83, 89
nitrates 91
nitric oxide 51, 52–3
nitric oxide synthase 52
  inducible 53
nitroglycerin 88
nitrovasodilators 88–9
non-selective cation channels 27
noradrenaline *see norepinephrine*
norepinephrine 31, 35, 61
normoblasts 20
normocytic normochromic anaemia 21
nuclear imaging 71
5′-nucleotidase 51
nucleus ambiguus 59, 61
nucleus tractus solitarius 59

obesity 75
oedema 47, 101
oliguria 67, 101
oncotic pressure 18
opening snap 69, 115
organization 81
orthopnoea 69, 101, 115
osmolality 18
osmolarity 18
osmoregulation 62–3
osmotic pressure 47
overdrive suppression 29

P wave 37, 73
pacemaker potential 29
packed cell volume 18
paclitaxel 93
palpation apex beat 69
palpitations 69
pancytopenia 21
parasympathetic system *60*, 61
paroxysmal nocturnal dyspnoea 69, 101

paroxysmal supraventricular tachycardia 107
patent ductus arteriosus 116, 117
pentaerythritol tetranitrate 88
percutaneous coronary intervention 92, 93, 97
pericardial space *12, 13*
pericarditis 69
pericardium *12, 13*
pericytes 17
pernicious anaemia 21
peroxynitrite 52
phagocytosis 19
phosphatidylinositol 3-kinase 52
phospholamban 31
phospholipid 23
phospholipids 78
physical inactivity 75
pindolol 76
piretanide 103
pitting oedema 101
placenta 57
plasma 11, 18–19
plasma membrane calcium-ATPase 35
plasma volume 62–3
  exercise 65
  renal control 63
plasmin 23, 99
plasminogen 23, 99
plasminogen activator inhibitor-1 23
plateau phase 29, 30
platelets 11, 19
platelet activating factor 51
platelet adhesion 23
platelet plug *22*, 23
Poiseuille's law 40
polycythaemia 20, 41
portal circulation *14, 15*
portal vein *14, 15*
positive feedback 28
postcapillary venules 44
postural effects 49
postural hypotension 69
potassium channels 35
potassium ions 51, 55
PR interval 33, 73
PR segment 73
pravastatin 79
pre-eclampsia 53
pre-excitation 105
pre-excitation syndrome 105, 107
precapillary sphincters 44
preload 101
premature ventricular contractions 108
pressor reflex 65
pressure 40–1
pressure natriuresis 63, 84
pressure–volume loop 37
Prinzmetal's angina 87, 89
procainamide 111
propafenone 111
propranolol 76, 111
prostacyclin 23, 51, 52, 99
prostaglandin E$_2$ 51
prostaglandin H$_2$ 52
prostaglandin I$_2$ 51 (*see prostacyclin*)
prostanoids 53
protein arginine methyltransferases 53
protein C 23
protein kinase C 35
protein S 23
prothrombin 23
prothrombin time 23, 99

pulmonary arteries *14*, 15
pulmonary circulation *10*, 11, *14*, 15,
  56–7, *56*
pulmonary congestion 101
pulmonary embolism 99, 122, *122*, 127–8
pulmonary hypertension 114
pulmonary oedema 47, 57, 101, 115
pulmonary valve 37
pulmonary vascular remodelling 116
pulmonary veins *14*, 15
pulmonary wedge pressure 71
pulse 37, 69
pulse pressure 11
pulsus alternans 69
pulsus bigeminus 69
pulsus paradoxus 69
Purkinje fibres 29
Purkinje system 33
purpura 23

QRS complex 37, 73
Quincke's sign 69
quinidine 111

radiofrequency catheter ablation 109
ramopril 77
ranolazine 89
rapamycin 93
rapid ejection phase 37
rapid ventricular filling 37
re-entry 105
reactive hyperaemia 51
recanalization 99
receptor-gated channels 27, 35
red blood cells *see* erythrocytes
reduced ejection phase 37
reduced refilling 37
refilling 37
reflection coefficient 47
relative refractory period 2
relaxation 31
renal failure 67
renin 59, 63, 101
renin-angiotensin system 67
renin-angiotensin-aldosterone system 63, 102
renin-producing granular cells 76
renovascular hypertension 81
repolarization 29
resistance 40–1
respiratory pump 49
restenosis 93
resting membrane potential 27, 28
reteplase 97, 99
reticuloendothelial system 19
revascularization 90–1, *90*, 92–3, *92*
Rhesus blood groups 24–5
  inheritance of 25
rheumatic fever 113, 114
rhoA kinase 35
right axis deviation 73
right heart failure 101
right ventricular outflow tract tachycardia
  109
rilmenidine 83
risk factors 74–5, *74*, **74**
rosuvastatin 79
rouleaux 19
rubella 116

saphenous vein 92
sarcolemma 13, 30

sarcoplasmic reticulum 13, 17, 30
Scandinavian Simvastatin Survival Study 79
scavenger receptors 81
septic shock 67
serotonin 19, 23, 51
serum 18
shock 66–7, *66*, 120–1, 126–7
  haemorrhagic 67
  irreversible 67
  low-resistance 67
  traumatic/surgical 67
sick sinus syndrome 33
sickle cell anaemia 21
sickle cell trait 21
simvastatin 79
single photon emission computed tomography (SPECT) 71
sinoatrial block 33
sinoatrial node 29, 33, 37, 61
sinus arrhythmia 69
sinus node *12*, 13
sinus tachycardia 33
sinusoids 17
skeletal muscle circulation 54–5, *54*
skeletal muscle pump 49
sliding filament theory 39
slow inward current 29
smoking 69, 75
smooth endoplasmic reticulum calcium-ATPase 35
smooth muscle cells *16*, 17
SOCRATES 69
sodium
  in hypertension 84–5
  renal control 63
sodium pump 27, 31
sodium-calcium exchange 29, 31, 35
sotalol 111
spironolactone 102, 103
splanchnic circulation *14*, 15
ST segment 73
staircase effect 31
Starling curve 39
Starling equation 47
Starling's law 38–9, *38*, 101
statins 75, 79, 91, 97
stem cells 19
stenosis 81
stents 93
Stokes-Adams attacks 69
store-operated calcium channels 35
streptokinase 97, 99
stretch-activated channels 51
stroke 81
stroke volume 37, 39
  exercise 64
stroke work 37
subclavian artery 15
subendocardium 86
superior vena cava 15
superoxide 52
supraventricular premature beats 106, *106*
supraventricular tachycardia 106–7, *106*
Swan-Ganz catheters 71

sympathetic system *60*, 61, 102
syncope 69
syncytium 17, 33
systemic circulation 11, *14*, 15
systemic oedema 47
systolic failure 101
systolic pressure *10*, 11
systolic wall stress 86

T tubules 30
T wave 37, 73
T-lymphocytes 94
tachyarrhythmias 106
tenase 23, 99
tenecteplase 97
terminal cisternae 13
tetralogy of Fallot 116, 117
thalassaemia 21, 25
thallium-201 87
thebesian veins *12*, 13, 54
thermoregulation 55
thiazide diuretics 82–3
thienopyridine 99
thoracic duct 45
Thorel tract 33
thoroughfare vessels 44
threshold potential 28
thrills 69, 113
thrombi 80, 99, 114
thrombin 23
thrombinase 23
thrombocytopenia 23
thrombocytosis 23
thrombolysis 97
thrombolytics 97, 98–9, *98*
thrombomodulin 23
thrombosis *22*, 23, 98–9, *98*
thromboxane A2 23, 35, 51, 52, 99
tight junctions 44
tirofiban 99
tissue factor 23
tissue factor pathway inhibitor 23
tissue plasminogen activator 23, 97, 99
tocainide 111
torasemide 103
torsade de pointes 104, 109
training 65
trandolapril 77
transferrin 21
transient inward current 105
transient receptor potential channel 51
transmural pressure 41
transoesophageal echocardiography 71
transposition of great arteries 116, 117
transverse tubular system 13
Treppe effect 31
triamterene 103
tricuspid valve 37
triglycerides 78
tropomyosin 31
troponin 31
troponins 31, 90, 96
tunica adventitia 17
tunica intima 17
tunica media 17

umbilical arteries 57
umbilical vein 57
unipolar leads 73
urokinase 23

v wave 37
vagus nerve 61
Valsalva manoeuvre 49, 113
valsartan 83
valvular heart disease 118–19, *119*, 124
varicose veins 47
vasa vasorum 17
vascular anatomy 14–15, *14*
vascular histology *16*, 17
vascular remodelling 85
vascular resistance 43
vascular smooth muscle, excitation-contraction coupling 34–5, *34*
vasoconstriction 35
vasodilatation 35, 50
vasodilating metabolites 51
vasopressin 35, 67, 101
vector quantity 73
veins *10*, 11, *14*, 15
  as capacitance vessels 49
  see also individual veins
venous arterial compliance 49
venous return 49
venous system 48–9, *48*
venous valves 49
ventilation/perfusion ratio 57
ventricle 11
ventricular fibrillation 108, 109
ventricular function curve 39
ventricular muscle action potential 28–9
ventricular remodelling 95
ventricular septal defect 116–17
ventricular systole 37
ventricular tachyarrhythmias 108–90, *108*
ventricular tachycardia 108
ventrolateral medulla 59
venules *10*, 11
verapamil 30, 77, 83, 89, 111
very low density lipoprotein 75, 78
vimentin 17
Virchow's triad 99
vitamin B_{12} 21
vitamin K 23
voltage-gated channels 27, 28
von Willebrand disease 23
von Willebrand factor 23

warfarin 23, 99
water filtration/absorption 47
Wenckebach block 33
Wenckebach tract 33
white blood cells 11, 19
white coat syndrome 69
Windkessel function *42*, 43
Wolff-Parkinson-White syndrome 105, 107

x descent 37
X-rays 71

y descent 37

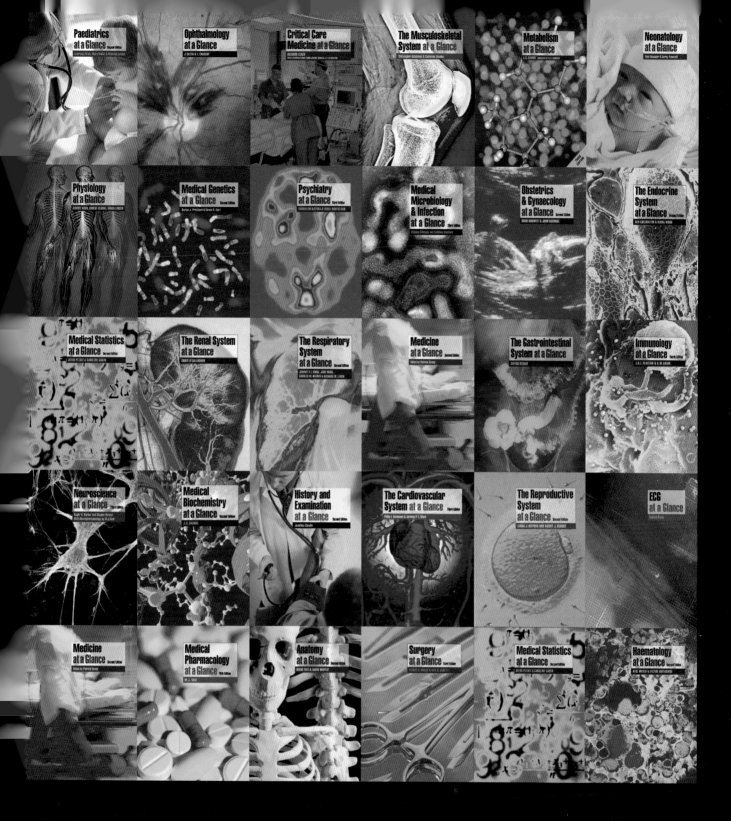

The at a Glance series

Popular double-page spread format • Coverage of core knowledge
Full-colour throughout • Self-assessment to test your knowledge • Expert authors

LECTURE NOTES

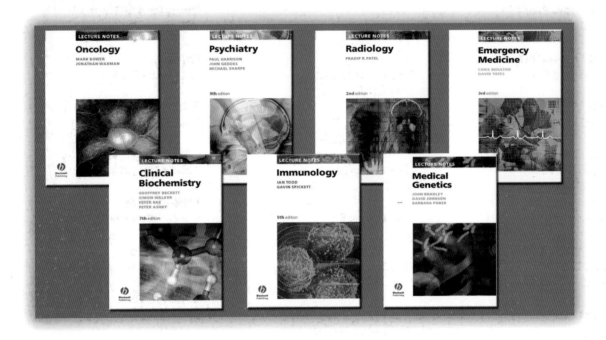

- Concise learning guides for all your subjects
- Focused on what you need to know
- Tried and Trusted

Titles in the LECTURE NOTES series

- Cardiology
- Clinical Anaesthesia
- Clinical Biochemistry
- Clinical Medicine
- Clinical Pharmacology and Therapeutics
- Clinical Skills
- Dermatology
- Diseases of the Ear, Nose and Throat
- Emergency Medicine

- Epidemiology and Public Health Medicine
- General Surgery
- Geriatric Medicine
- Haematology
- Human Physiology
- Immunology
- Infectious Diseases
- Medical Genetics
- Medical Law and Ethics
- Medical Microbiology

- Neurology
- Obstetrics and Gynaecology
- Oncology
- Ophthalmology
- Orthopaedics and Fractures
- Paediatrics
- Psychiatry
- Radiology
- Respiratory Medicine
- Tropical Medicine
- Urology

www.blackwellmedstudent.com

Blackwell Publishing